"*Hope's Edge* is not only a brilliant analysis of the global food and hunger challenge; it is also a philosophical work of the first order."

—Senator George McGovern, author of *The Third Freedom*,
Global Ambassador for Hunger, U.N. World Food Program

"With the help of her intrepid and observant daughter Anna, Frances Moore Lappé continues her paradigm challenging analysis of the plexus of food and freedom in this era of globalization . . . A thorough, often shocking discussion . . . The Lappés drive home their crucial theme: what's best for our bodies is best for our communities and for the earth itself."

—*Booklist*

"Absolutely one of the most important books as we move further into the twenty-first century."

—Jane Goodall

"In a bleak time, sick time, *Hope's Edge* is more than a palliative. It offers a way toward a cure."

—Studs Terkel, radio personality and bestselling author

"Some of the twentieth century's most vibrant activist thinkers have been American women—Margaret Mead, Jeannette Rankin, Barbara Ward, Dorothy Day—who took it upon themselves to pump life into basic truths. Frances Moore Lappé is among them."

—*The Washington Post*

". . . thought-provoking . . . passionately argued and deftly woven together . . ."

—*The Chicago Tribune*

". . . a powerful, beautiful, brave book—needed now more than ever. What is so fine is the mix, the shared experience of it, the raising of life and death issues, the inter-mingling of food—presented beguilingly."

—Howard Zinn, author of *A People's History of the United States*

HOPE'S

FRANCES MOORE LAPPÉ AND ANNA LAPPÉ

EDGE

THE

NEXT

DIET

FOR A

SMALL

PLANET

JEREMY P. TARCHER/PUTNAM

a member of Penguin Group (USA) Inc. *New York*

Excerpt from "Candles in Babylon" by Denise Levertov from Candles in Babylon, *copyright © 1982 by Denise Levertov. Reprinted by permission of New Directions Publishing Corp.*

Tomato Soup & Gingery Tomato Soup, Chinese Asparagus, and Parsnip Patties recipes reprinted with permission from The New Laurel's Kitchen *by Laurel Robertson, Carol Flinders, and Brian Ruppenthal. Copyright © 1976, 1986 by the Blue Mountain Center of Meditation, Ten Speed Press, Berkeley, California, www.tenspeed.com.*

Corn and Bulgur Salad with Cilantro and Lime and Butternut Squash Soup with Apple Confit from Fields of Greens *by Annie Somerville, copyright © 1993 by Annie Somerville. Used by permission of Bantam Books, a division of Random House, Inc.*

Most Tarcher/Putnam books are available at special quantity discounts for bulk purchase for sales promotions, premiums, fund-raising, and educational needs. Special books or book excerpts also can be created to fit specific needs. For details, write Putnam Special Markets, 375 Hudson Street, New York, NY 10014.

The recipes contained in this book are to be followed exactly as written. Neither the publisher nor the author is responsible for your specific health or allergy needs that may require medical supervision, or for any adverse reactions to the recipes contained in this book.

While the author has made every effort to provide accurate telephone numbers and Internet addresses at the time of publication, neither the publisher nor the author assumes any responsibility for errors, or for changes that occur after publication.

Jeremy P. Tarcher/Putnam
a member of
Penguin Group (USA) Inc.
375 Hudson Street
New York, NY 10014
www.penguin.com

First trade paperback edition 2003

The Library of Congress catalogued the hardcover edition as follows:

Lappé, Frances Moore.
Hope's edge : the next diet for a small planet / Frances Moore Lappé and Anna Lappé.
p.   cm.
Includes bibliographical references and index.
ISBN 1-58542-149-9
1. Environmental ethics.   2. Globalization—Social aspects.   3. Capitalism—Social aspects.
4. Vegetarian cookery.   I. Lappé, Anna, date.   II. Title.
GE42.L364   2002   2001048256
179'.1—dc21
ISBN 1-58542-237-1 (paperback edition)

Printed in the United States of America
10   9   8

BOOK DESIGN BY MAUNA EICHNER
ARTWORK BY ANNA LAPPÉ

For Grandpa John and Marjorie and Grandpa Paul and Helen
for helping to make it all possible.

And for Anna's grandmothers,
who taught us both how to listen to our own voices.

Hope cannot be said to exist, nor can it be said not to exist.
It is just like the roads across the earth.
For actually there were no roads to begin with,
but when many people pass one way a road is made.

LU HSUN, 1921

CONTENTS

THE BEGINNING

THE JOURNEY

THE HOMECOMING

TAKING OFF

COMING TO OUR SENSES

FOOD FOR THOUGHT

THE BEGINNING

AN OPENING NOTE

ope's Edge is about to go to press, and suddenly its meaning for us comes even more sharply into focus. It's September 11, 2001. Anna is on a plane from Paris to Nairobi; I'm traveling by train from Boston to New York. Both of us are turned back. In the next few days, as we watch the terrifying images on TV and frantically e-mail each other and those dear to us, we share shock, horror, and grief with millions, probably billions, of others across the planet.

We watch our own reactions, we listen to what the attack means to others. On the radio, I hear an attorney interviewed at random in New York City who says he's finding it hard to focus. His work doesn't have the same meaning, he tells listeners; it doesn't seem as important anymore. Millions ask: What can I do? They respond by giving blood or sending money, while acknowledging that these acts hardly feel commensurate with the enormity of the tragedy.

Such horrific shocks hold possibility. With our routines shattered, we can look at ourselves like that Manhattan attorney did and ask: Is what I am doing consonant with my own deep need to feel that my life counts, to know that I'm using each day toward ends that really matter and acting on the care for others that I feel?

Yes, to some extent a desire for retribution may be "natural." But surely just as natural is the desire to find redemption in our loss and pain. Like the grieving mother who found comfort in knowing that her son, a passenger on one of the hijacked planes, had prevented greater loss of life by helping to bring the plane down, might we each find comfort in recommitting ourselves even more fully to honor the preciousness of life?

Anna and I began to see that September 11, 2001, may be for millions, and could become for millions more, an instance of what the people in this book told us had transformed their lives. Suddenly, from one moment to the next—in what we came to call a moment of dissonance—their world just didn't fit together anymore. They asked themselves questions they'd long held at bay.

Unprecedented terrorism could trigger dissonance on a global scale. Our world cracks. In such moments, we have a clear choice: Do we continue burying our sense that something is profoundly wrong in the world we're creating, and therefore stay in denial of our truer selves; denial that produces fear so familiar we hardly recognize it? Or do we make another choice; do we choose to move into a cycle of hope?

Choosing hope means conscious risk; it means looking at the ideas that govern us. While it is easy to condemn terrorists who justify the destruction of themselves and others, a much greater challenge is to ask: Do we, too, hold ideas that end up placing other values before life? What belief systems allow people to tolerate day in and day out, for example, the devastation of nature and other species as well as the starvation and early deaths of millions of innocent people, and allow them even to benefit—in cheap food, fuel, and finery—from the poverty that so stunts and shortens those other lives?

Our book suggests that there is a profound disconnect between our inner lives—our deepest sensibilities and needs—and the world we're constructing from day to day. Instead of locking us more deeply into our fear, the monumental tragedy of September 11 could jar us into awareness of that disconnect. Awakened, we can ask: What might I reexamine in my own belief system that justifies what it should not? How can I align my actions with my deepest values?

Asking these questions pushes us to hope's edge. And that is where the people you'll meet in the book find themselves. By their willingness to seize the moments of dissonance in their own lives in order to break the cycle of fear, they push forward the edge of hope. We pray our book can help each of us to do the same.

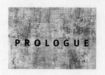

PUSHING THE EDGE OF HOPE

We're packed in on a flight from southern India to steaming New Delhi. The smell of curry fills the plane cabin. From her beaten-up backpack on the floor next to me, Anna pulls out a book to brush up on what we're about to see. Opening to a chapter on Indian food traditions, she starts reading aloud, but at the second sentence she stops. Puzzled, I peer over her shoulder and read, as she has, the Sanskrit word for food.

It is "anna."

We look at each other, stunned. Almost thirty years ago, at exactly the age Anna is now, I wrote *Diet for a Small Planet,* exploring the question: *Why hunger in a world of plenty?* It was a book that would set me on a lifelong path—one grounded, I only realize thirty years later, in the very name I had unwittingly given my daughter.

Anna turns the page, and we read on, learning that Annapoorna is the Indian goddess of food. We can't know what we'll find on the rest of our journey, but at that moment, we sense we'll need Annapoorna's spirit with us on our trip, one rich with discovery—and surprise.

Thirty years ago I wrote the original *Diet for a Small Planet* because I had to: What I was learning was too shocking. All around me experts were predicting famine, saying we'd reached the earth's limits to feed ourselves. *More chemicals! Bigger farms! More technology!* were the mantras of the day. Yet, in the basement university library where I had gone to pursue my curiosity as to how we might feed this small planet, I discovered that what I was hearing—the experts' call-to-arms—was, frankly, wrong. Not only was there enough to feed us all; there was more than enough. Worse than that, the strategies touted to bring us

5

plenty—the chemicals, the large-scale farms, the technology—might actually make the food crisis worse.

And, I learned that the very food I'd been raised on was part of the problem. Like every good Texan, I was brought up on meat and potatoes. Yet grain-fed beef, I suddenly discovered, is a symptom of an economic order actually diminishing the resources we need to feed ourselves. I discovered that we'd turned beef cattle into protein-factories-in-reverse, downing mountains of grain and massive quantities of water while returning a tiny fraction of the nutrients to us in meat.

Diet for a Small Planet became a from-the-heart story by a 26-year-old trusting her common sense. I remember photocopying the first version of *Diet* thinking I'd hand out the tiny booklet to friends and maybe plaster a few posters around Berkeley. Luckily, that little book got into the hands of Betty Ballantine, a founder of paperback publishing in America, who believed the message had to be heard. She published it and helped me reach what turned out to be millions of readers.

DARK BAR, TOUGH PITCH

This book was also an unplanned birth. It was a wintry day in the year before our Indian plane ride, and I'd come down from Vermont to New York City for the weekend to be with my children, Anthony and Anna. Outside it was drizzly and dreary, and after making our way through the narrow streets of the Lower East Side, we ducked into a neighborhood bar to dry out before heading home.

I wanted to talk about my future. My kids already knew that my dream—one combining family life with the launch of a new national news service, all on a spectacular piece of land in Vermont—was dead. So, huddled together, damp and chilled, we started talking about what I would do next. Out of nowhere, it seemed, an adventure began to take shape.

My children's clarity startled me. They knew *exactly* what I needed to do. I needed to return to *Diet for a Small Planet*.

Nearly thirty years ago, they reminded me, my book helped shatter the myth that hunger is caused by a scarcity in nature. It showed that the crisis is not a scarcity of food, but of democracy, as more and more people are denied a voice in shaping their own futures. But decades later, we admitted, the myth of scarcity is thriving.

"Thirty years ago," Anthony said, "you gave people a clear way to see the larger impact of their choices—even those as personal as what we choose to eat."

As we talked, sitting on stools in that dim barroom in Manhattan, I thought of the countless people who had reached out to me over the years, telling me how *Diet for a Small Planet* had changed them—how it had helped them see the insanity of an economic system feeding tons of grain to animals while people starve—and sharing with me the joy they derive from choosing the diet best for their bodies, knowing it is also best for the earth.

Over these thirty years, millions had turned to a plant-centered, whole-foods diet, yet I was aware that millions more around the world were devouring greater amounts of meat than ever. For the first time worldwide, roughly the same number of us—over a billion—are underfed as are overfed. And the fast-food/fat-food diet causing obesity to skyrocket in our country has taken off globally, and the overfed are eating more of the foods predisposing them to disease. So, worldwide, it's food—too little, too few nutrients, or too much—that's now the culprit in more than half of all disease-related lost years of healthy life.[1]

This sad paradox of the over- and underfed reflects, we agreed, a global economy that is creating never-before-seen wealth alongside deepening suffering. The pay of America's CEOs leapt 535 percent during the '90s, while most working people barely kept ahead of inflation. And those who now control as much wealth as half the world's people could fit into Anna's high school auditorium.[2]

I knew my kids were right—that their generation was frustrated and longed for help in making sense of it all. But I also knew that I didn't need to redo *Diet for a Small Planet*. It still stands. What was needed, we realized, was a book that takes off where the original stops. For over these three decades, despite accelerated environmental decline and worsening diets, I had been witnessing another story take shape. I wanted to tell that story—one of an emerging shift in our understanding of our place on the planet. That's what I wanted my children's generation to be able to see.

So on that gray day I became a seeker again, launched on a journey to places and to people who have taught me lessons among the greatest of my life. On five continents over the next year, I witnessed an emergence that is still invisible to most of us, but that, I'm now convinced, holds key to finding personal meaning and direction in our lives, as well as to healing our threatened, fragile, ever-smaller planet.

THE NEW BATTLE FOR OUR HEARTS

My children are acutely aware that the choices of human beings alive today are like none their forebears faced. Their choices—our choices—have ultimate consequences, not only for the thousands of species we're destroying each year but for us, the dominant species, as well. What a terrifying thought. What an extraordinary opportunity. But to perceive crisis as opportunity requires clear perception: We must grasp the nature of the crisis and what each of us can do to address it.

That's tough in any case, but it's especially hard to see opportunity when we're locked within a new ideological battle, one shaping our planet, one shaping our minds. The overt fight between capitalism and communism is over. But we're caught in a subtler yet even more profound struggle, one played out in small ways day by day, moment to moment. It is a battle over defining who we are as human beings, one staking the very edges of possibility for our species.

The new battle is not waged with tanks or measured in nuclear stockpiles; it's fought with ideas, the ideas that explain our world and determine what's possible in it, ideas repeated so often they become our own internal voice.

In the face of the unprecedented ecological and social crisis, our organs of mass media rarely do more than reinforce the notion that global corporate capitalism is our only hope. They feed us messages that the only way to feed the world is with huge agribusinesses relying on massive infusions of pesticides and chemical fertilizers, and on giant feedlots pumping cattle with tons of grain, hormones, and antibiotics. We seldom hear about the ways in which this highly concentrated factory-farming system is rapidly destroying the resources we need to ensure our long-term well-being. How often are we alerted to the fact that this system is a root cause of new threats to our health, ranging from heart disease to mad cow disease to the weakening of antibiotics' protection?

Headlines blast us with seemingly disconnected events—about genetically modified foods, the World Trade Organization, food trade wars—but our hunger to know what all this *really* means is rarely satisfied. Such concepts as globalization, even persistent world hunger, remain abstractions for most of us, and understanding how all of this determines the quality of our lives and what we can each *do* about it—that's even less clear.

If we do hear about people questioning the path we're on, they're often dismissed as hopeless Luddites or, as Pulitzer Prize–winning journalist Thomas Friedman called anti-globalization demonstrators, "flat-earth advocates." In the prestigious magazine *The Economist*, protestors against international financial and development institutions are reduced to mindless "rabble," and mocked as "warriors in the struggle between the forces of global capital and something-or-other."[3]

In other words, the key media shaping our view of the world cannot see what Anna and I saw on our journey. They cannot envision anything beyond today's world, in which multinational corporations, largely unaccountable private entities, wield more power than do elected governments. They cannot see what has been emerging in three decades: the innovations in creating communities that tap nature rather than squander it, and ensure community, not division.

To take off where *Diet for a Small Planet* stopped, I knew I had to describe this invisible unfolding. So this is the story of the something-or-other.

Most media cannot envision this emergence (and so give it less than a nod), partly because they have no language to describe it; they have no framing ideas to explain it. The media are as trapped as most of us are in the dominant ideas of our modern world, solidified in the last thirty years and reinforced daily by ever-more-concentrated media. These ideas have become "thought traps," making us believe our only path is the one we're on, blinding us to solutions already in bud and within the reach of each of us. The "thought traps" are literally life-stunting.

THE MAP WE TRAVELED

The three of us quickly realized I couldn't write such a book myself; it required the perspective of two generations. So with Anthony's unwavering support, Anna and I set out on this journey together, to learn from and to give voice to those who are freeing themselves from the thought traps. For clarity's sake, and because at times I reflect on my own life's evolution, we wrote the book largely in my voice, while Anna's accents each chapter. But it turned out to be truly our common work—each experience shared, each word mulled over by both of us.

Chapter 1: Maps of the Mind condenses the destructive thought traps to five, and suggests how they so stifle our imaginations that we end up creating the very polarization and destruction we so fear. Looked at this way, the crisis that my children perceive is actually a crisis of personal meaning—a profound disconnect between the direction our planet is headed and our own deepest sensibilities.

With *Chapter 2,* the journey begins. In a whirlwind that took us to five continents and nine countries, including the heartland of the United States, our travels became a snapshot of the planet. We take you from magical gardens in California to wind-battered shacks of formerly landless farmers in the Brazilian countryside. You join us in lush, remote Bangladesh villages and on rocky trails in the foothills of the Himalayas. You share with us the sweltering Punjabi heat as we talk with colorfully turbaned Sikhs, and you dance with us in a Kenyan village during one of the country's worst droughts. You meet renegade Wisconsin farmers struggling for survival, and you wind with us through the back roads of France's Brittany.

In all of these places, as different as they appear, we discovered people who are not accepting corporate global capitalism as it is, but are *evolving* it so that growing and eating good food—and economic life itself—is again embedded in life-affirming values and community. Across cultures and climates and cuisines, they—and millions more like them—are arriving at common insights about what human beings need to thrive. They are drawing a new mental map, one that is liberating rather than stifling.

Looking back to what people thought was possible when I wrote *Diet for a Small Planet,* I realize that if I had predicted any of their achievements, I would have been considered delusional!

In the book's closing chapter, we give shape to all we learned along the way, and share five liberating ideas we absorbed from the lives and work of those we met. We believe that these orienting ideas are as useful in our daily struggle to live meaningful lives as they are in sorting out the biggest global issues of our time.

Then, in *Taking Off,* we suggest entry points and offer resources that can help us to become co-creators of the world we want; entry points that flow directly from the lessons gathered on our journey.

Throughout the book, nestled between the chapters, you'll find vegetarian recipes to tempt your palate. And in the last section of the book, *Coming to Our Senses,* you'll discover dozens of recipes from chefs and cookbook authors—pioneers in whole-foods, organic, and vegetarian cuisine—recipes that are also a celebration of the distance vegetarian cuisine has traveled from the broccoli-stir-fry days of the early '70s. To awaken ourselves to new possibilities and sustain ourselves in the face of false messages of despair, we must engage *all* of our senses.

WALKING HOPE'S EDGE

To free ourselves from the thought traps—to bridge the painful disconnect between our inner and outer worlds—my hunch at age 26 was that food is a perfect starting place. Because food is our most primal need and our common bond to the earth and one another, it can ground us as we stretch ourselves to draw in all the interlaced threads—so we can weave a whole, meaningful picture for ourselves.

I still believe food has this unique power. With food as a starting point, we can choose to meet people and to encounter events so powerful that they jar us out of our ordinary way of seeing the world, and open us to new, uplifting, and empowering possibilities. They call us to travel "hope's edge."

By hope's edge we mean many things.

Yes, with global warming melting polar ice caps, with the obliteration of thousands of species each year, with the loss of almost one-third of our agricultural land over a single generation, our planet is nearing the point at which hope, honest hope, will no longer be possible. Yes, every day, we are pushing our little planet closer to hope's very edge.

But something else has been happening over these thirty years, too. The people we met on our journey are living this story. They are pushing forward the edge of hope with what they prove is possible. They are creating new space in which each of us can find hope.

We must warn you, though: This kind of hope isn't clean or tidy. Honest hope has an edge. It's messy. It requires that we let go of all pat answers, all preconceived formulas, all confidence that our sailing will be smooth. It's not a resting point. Honest hope is movement.

So you see, this one book is actually two. Yes, it is a *literal* journey of mother and daughter, exploring evidence of change afoot that's invisible to most of us. But it's another kind of journey, too. For to heal our planet and to find joy in this challenging time, each of us must also take an *interior* journey, one probing not only our unspoken fears but also our deepest beliefs about our nature as human beings.

Personal and social transformation can't be disaggregated. As we gain inner strength, we can perceive wider changes that before might have eluded us. As we gain confidence that the world can change, we can grow at the most personal level. So, Anna and I like to say that our book is not only about hope, but also about happiness. Through writing this book, we've become convinced that happiness is not a shallow, selfish goal; it's a virtue we cultivate by taking the leap—by refusing to be bystanders or victims of history. It is what we create by bringing all of ourselves consciously to the challenge of discovering our special place in that long walk, one pushing—and ever expanding—the edge of hope.

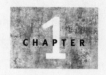

MAPS OF
THE MIND

Clear . . . your mind of old perspectives,
and new perceptions will rush in.
Yet, there is nothing we fear more.

DEE HOCK, *Birth of the Chaordic Age*

You can still buy tie-dyed T-shirts on Telegraph Avenue, and "Question Authority" bumper stickers may forever be in vogue here, but I discovered that something about my old Berkeley haunts had changed.

It's late afternoon before Anna and I can steal some time from our packed research trip to the San Francisco Bay Area to try to find the Giannini Foundation agricultural library, where I spent so many late nights sorting through facts and figures thirty years ago. For an hour we wander rolling green lawns and dimly lit hallways of the U.C. Berkeley campus trying to find the library.

"I guess they moved things," I finally conclude, disappointed that I can't show my daughter exactly where I'd sat. As we head toward the door, the headline of a single newspaper clipping pinned to a bulletin board catches Anna's eye.

"Look, Mom," she says, "'World Demand for Food Expected to Outstrip Production.'" For a second I think she's joking, ad-libbing a headline from the 1970s. Then I spot the dateline: *San Francisco Chronicle*, November 7, 1999.

Anna and I laugh in horror that even with all we know now, the same myths that spurred me on thirty years ago are being perpetuated. People are still being made to believe that hunger is simply the result of too little food. But that headline served a purpose. It felt like a lightning bolt sent from the heavens with one message: You have to write this book!

In that instant I was brought home again, home to the intuition that launched my adult life—that food is a powerful teacher, an unparalleled motivator. What's scarier, after all, than not knowing if what you feed your family is hurting them? And what's scarier than not knowing whether you can feed your family at all?

Nothing is more personal than food. Yet, in this increasingly globalized world, food is becoming frighteningly impersonal, further and further removed from something we feel we control. I think of the first big consumer scare with genetically modified foods, in the year 2000: the nationwide recall on taco shells with accidental traces of genetically modified Starlink corn not approved for human consumption. Just to pinpoint the error required private-detective-level sleuthing, tracking a chain of multinational companies across states and international borders!

Thirty years ago, my hunch was that food could be a great awakener—holding power like nothing else to open our eyes to what is amiss. But over three decades I'd also come to believe that food opens a path like no other to new possibilities, and I don't mean just new possibilities for feeding ourselves. I mean the whole enchilada—I mean that if we look at food, *really look,* our world can shift: We might just not only grasp for the first time the biggest ideas limiting our lives, but also discover for the first time whole new ways of seeing the world that release us from our march toward planetary destruction. That intuition sent me on this journey with Anna.

CREATING SCARCITY FROM PLENTY

I've said I wrote *Diet for a Small Planet* because I felt I had no choice. What I was learning was so shocking I had to share it.

It was 1969. I had dropped out of graduate school, opening the way for what became *Diet,* because I was scared. I was scared that I would arrive at the end of my life never knowing whether I had devoted my years on the planet to what mattered. Graduate school didn't appear to offer me the chance to find out. So, with my youthful passion in full bloom, I determined to dig to the roots of widespread suffering.

When I began, buried in books at that U.C. Berkeley agricultural library, I had one question: *Why hunger?* Since feeding oneself and one's offspring is the first concern of all living creatures—and since the headlines about hunger and starvation were blaring out to me that humans were failing at this primal task—I thought, What else matters? People have often asked me, "How did you get interested in hunger?" but I've never understood the question. To me all other concerns paled before this central one.

I was 26, and for the first time I became aware that fear served me well. The fear of never discovering whether my path made sense forced me out of a predictable graduate-school-to-career path. It forced me into thin air.

Mustering the strength and using my beginner's mind, my following-my-nose, question-after-question research, I unearthed a fact that changed my life forever: The world produces more than enough to feed us all, while millions go without the food their bodies need to survive. This shocking truth awakened me to other aspects of invisible waste. Most have only gotten worse since:

- For every human being on the planet, the world produces two pounds of grain per day—roughly 3,000 calories, and that's without even counting all the beans, potatoes, nuts, fruits, and vegetables we eat, too. This is clearly enough for all of us to thrive; yet nearly one in six of us still goes hungry.[1]

- Worldwide, we're feeding more and more of this grain, now almost *half*, to livestock, but animals return to us in meat only a tiny fraction of the nutrients we feed them.[2]

- To get just one calorie of food energy from a steak, we burn 54 irreplaceable fossil-fuel calories, so producing one pound of steak— providing less than 1,000 calories—uses up 45,000 fossil fuel calories.[3]

- To produce just one pound of beef takes thousands of gallons of water, as much as the average American uses for all purposes in several months—and this in a world in which two-thirds of all people are expected to face water shortage in less than a generation.[4]

Such measures of waste in the midst of hunger rocked me to my core. And soon my question changed. No longer "Why hunger?" but "Why hunger in a world of plenty?"

All around me, as I was researching *Diet*, authorities were worrying about impending food shortages, about frightening scarcity. And yet, I was learning, they were wrong. For a young woman still deferring to experts, it was a shocking revelation. The more I read, the more I discovered that in fact we are all part of a process that is itself generating scarcity, even destroying the very ground beneath ongoing food security.

Worldwide, topsoil is eroding as much as thirty times faster than it's being created.[5] It's gotten so bad that soil particles eroded from Kenya, for example, are blown as far west as Brazil and Florida.[6] So, in just the last forty years, erosion has made almost one-third of our farmable land unusable for growing food.[7] Water resources are being destroyed just as rapidly, not only through pollution of surface water but also, on every continent, by the rapid depletion of underground water by crop irrigation.

Since I wrote my first book, I've come to see the waste I had discovered in our food system replicated in every aspect of production and consumption. Just imagine: Here in the U.S., only one to six percent of all the stuff that goes into producing things turns up as products we can actually use—in other words, we waste more than 90 percent.[8] We can't blame nature. No, we humans are *creating* scarcity—exactly what we say we most fear. It was almost too unimaginable to believe.

With that realization came another big one, which hit me over the head again just recently.

I'm sitting quietly in a University of Montana forum entitled "Feeding the Hungry," listening to a professor of political science with a Harvard PhD tell his rapt audience about genetically modified organisms—GMOs. Almost three-quarters of all the GMOs planted worldwide are here in the U.S. Launched with our government's help but after virtually no public debate, genetically modified crops covered less than four million acres of U.S. cropland six years ago. Today, they're planted on 75 million acres, with more than half our soybeans and almost three-fourths of our cotton crops now GMO.[9] Walking down our grocery aisles, we can assume that more than half the products we see contain at least a trace of them.

I'd been increasingly concerned with this stunningly rapid agricultural revolution—one that has been largely invisible, especially for us Americans. So I am hoping I can learn something.

Apparently responding to anticipated criticism, the professor proclaims with Ivy League authority that, well, maybe we here in the rich countries can afford to be skittish about potential risks in the genetic engineering of seeds; after all, we have plenty to eat. But our skittishness jeopardizes the future of the poor abroad because they need genetically modified seeds to produce more food to stave off hunger. Then, for half an hour, the discussion hovers around only one question—the possible risks in using genetically engineered seeds.

I sit up straight with alarm, as I realize that even after all these years, no one is challenging the premise that scarcity causes hunger. I want to stand and shout out: We're still asking the wrong question! Not only is there already enough food in the world, but as long as we're only talking about food—how best to produce it—we'll never end hunger, nor create the communities and food safety we want. We must ask a different question:

How can we build communities in tune with nature's wisdom in which no one, anywhere, has to worry about putting food—safe, healthy food—on the table?

Asking this question takes us far beyond food and ultimately brings us back to food—as you will see in the lives of people we meet on our journey. It takes us to the heart of democracy itself: to whose voice gets heard in matters of land, seeds, credit, trade, food safety—all stuff that can sound dry and abstract. It can, that is, until it comes to life in real people risking their lives and claiming their voices—people like the Brazilians you'll meet who are facing down big landowners to create vibrant communities, the villagers in Kenya who are turning back the encroaching desert, and the Bangladeshi women who are taking huge risks to free their families from hunger.

Later that afternoon, sitting in the serenity of the Montana mountains after the professor's presentation, I suddenly see more. While little has changed, much has changed. Thirty years ago I couldn't have imagined the almost overnight, massive spread of genetically modified organisms (GMOs)—with incalculable risks of disrupting ecosystems; of creating new strains of super-resistant pests; of introducing new allergens, or something even more harmful, into our diet.

In one sense I see the genetic-engineering craze—absorbing hundreds of millions of dollars and untold time and energy both of promoters and doubters—as yet another catastrophic diversion from deeper questions about democracy itself. It keeps us from asking, *Why hunger?* It jumps over this question entirely, reinforcing the myth that inadequate production is to blame.

But I also see genetically modified seeds—just like the sudden emergence of grain-fed meat I wrote about thirty years ago—as a symptom. It is a symptom of our silencing. None of us called for genetic manipulation of seeds. Just as with the risks of feedlot beef, which now contributes to heart disease, groundwater depletion, antibiotic resistance, and more, no citizens were asked to weigh the risks of GMOs against possible gains.

So, might we come to see GMOs as a symptom of a deeper crisis?

Instead of distracting us from questions of democracy, genetic engineering could turn out to be our ultimate wake-up call. Where is democracy, we can ask, when just one company, Monsanto, controls 85 percent of all genetically engineered germplasm and has the power to saturate the commercial-seeds supply with genetically engineered varieties—with no input from the public, who must bear the consequences? Genetic engineering may be what *finally* shocks us into finding our voices to ask the questions we must if we are to heal our planet.

DEMOCRACY COMING TO LIFE

We go on swallowing the prevailing framing of the problem as scarcity, we go on bowing to "experts" promoting GMOs as the solution to hunger, such as the well-meaning professor in Montana—even when all evidence confounds their premises—in part, I believe, because we've lost confidence in the one thing each of us has: our common sense. Our capacity for basic problem solving—for putting two and two together and arriving at four.

We let paralyzing messages intrude—"They know better," "The market will decide," "I don't know enough," "These big questions are for somebody else." Even if we don't say these words, the feelings are often there. Despite the hype about our unparalleled democracy, our culture tells us something else: Democracy, well, it's risky, except maybe on Election Day. And in the 2000 presidential vote, Americans were reminded that, even here, it's not citizens' votes but ultimately the Electoral College, and sometimes even the Supreme Court, who choose our nation's leader.

Realizing how voiceless most people feel, I experienced an awful sinking feeling during the 1980s. Yes, I had gotten good at sounding the alarm. I prided myself on shaking up audiences with dramatic metaphor and precise numbers. "The death toll from hunger," I would tell them, "equals a Hiroshima bomb going off every three days." But, no matter how good I got, it dawned on me that I was making *no* difference—except maybe satisfying my own need for an ego thrill—if those moved by my words felt incapable of doing anything.

Without that, all my books, articles, speeches, and interviews were meaningless.

Yikes!

That's when I knew I had to push deeper, to cut beneath hunger, or any issue, to democracy itself: How do we discover our voices and use them to shape the larger world around us?

I realized that we humans can't do what we can't imagine and we can't imagine ourselves playing real, satisfying roles in creating life-serving communities—what I came to call "living democracy"—unless we see regular people like ourselves developing their power, their capacity to create. The problem is, the media doesn't show us such images.

That's why in 1990 I co-founded the Center for Living Democracy to shine the light on what is underway but still invisible; to show Americans that people just like themselves are stepping out in their communities, workplaces, schools—everywhere—finding their voices and becoming public problem-solvers. During this time I was nourished by living in a gorgeous old barn in Vermont, with the Center housed next-door in what had been an inn built in the 17th century. A sense of history emboldened me to believe that we can continue to create history.

In part responding to the breathtaking consolidation of our news sources since I wrote *Diet for a Small Planet*—now just six conglomerates control almost all of America's mass media, including publishing[10]—there in Brattle-boro, we had the audacity to think we could create the first independent news service in decades.

As founding editor of a news service about regular people engaged in their communities, I watched a world open up that I'd not seen before. My weekly headache turned out not to be the dearth of possible stories, but rather the flood of possibilities from which to choose. With every news story, my intuition about the capacities we each have to be contributors was confirmed.

And yet in some ways I became more perplexed, more acutely aware of a contradiction. Despite the islands of empowerment that our news service was highlighting, I knew most people's feelings of powerlessness were deep and growing.

So I was ready when Anthony, Anna, and I hit upon the idea for this book. I was ready with a new question I had to ask. The original question—Why hunger in a world of plenty?—had swollen into one even more puzzling: *Why have we, as societies, created that which as individuals we abhor?*

No one of us would choose to let a child die of hunger or preventable disease, let alone 32,000 children a day.[11]

No one would intentionally destroy so many species in just this century that it could take the planet 10 million years to recover.[12]

No one would seek to poke a hole the size of a continent in the ozone layer, causing cancer deaths to soar.

No one would decide to create a greenhouse effect disrupting life in ways we are only barely beginning to understand, or make our food production—our fossil-fuel-driven industrial model—into one of the biggest culprits, responsible for about one-fifth of human-caused greenhouse-gas emissions.[13]

No one would consciously design a world community in which a few hundred individuals control as much wealth as half the world's population; and where—as it is here at home—1 percent end up with more than do the bottom 95 percent combined.[14]

In other words, how could it be that we humans, the dominant species, are creating a world that at the deepest level we can't recognize as ours? A world of mega-cities with unbreathable air, of sterile strip malls, of beggars and billionaires? A world that we try to shut out because the pain of seeing it is too great?

My answer, in part, is that we don't experience ourselves as creating this world; we don't see ourselves as choosers at all. Our planet-in-decline is just happening. It feels as though it is happening to those of us who live amidst abundance as much as it does to the poorest person in the third world.

It feels as though it's just happening—and we're not choosing it—because, as I've said, we don't see ourselves as capable of being choosers in the public world. But at an even deeper level, it's that we don't perceive the assumptions, which, once in play, silently fuel this destruction of life. As long as we remain blind to these assumptions, other paths are invisible. And if we can't see other paths, we feel no choices are being made. No one is choosing: What we have is all there is.

THE POWER OF IDEAS

But how can this be? How could such a clever, heady species like ours be so nearsighted? What could be powerful enough to make us feel there are no other paths?

Clues came to me in the 1980s as I wrote *Rediscovering America's Values*, an odd book composed as an imaginary dialogue between a person holding the dominant worldview and myself. To write it I had to force myself to see the world through someone else's eyes.

That challenge made me realize just how much we humans live within frameworks of larger meaning, and it reminded me of the insights of social philosopher Erich Fromm. I loved reading Fromm in my college days—my generation would never forget his *The Art of Loving.* In my dog-eared copy of his later book, *The Anatomy of Human Destructiveness,* he confirmed what had long felt true to me—that we humans must have a "frame of orientation," some way of making sense of the world. Human beings cannot survive in a meaning void.

It is through these largely unconscious frames that we view reality; they determine what we allow ourselves to see, literally. I think this is what Albert Einstein was getting at when he said, ". . . it is theory which decides what we can observe."[15]

So, we're all like the Me'en people of Ethiopia: When given a photograph of themselves for the first time, they stared at it, crumbled it, nibbled at it. They literally *could not see* human beings on this tiny, shiny, two-dimensional surface.[16] It is hard for any of us to see what we do not expect to see; what our mental maps do not allow.

All this is well and good . . . maybe, *if* our theories, our maps of the world, aid us in problem solving, and if they align with our deepest sensibilities and needs.

But what if they don't and aren't?

Fromm argues that it's quite possible for there to be a mismatch; for our ideas to do us in. I had double-underlined a quote in *The Anatomy of Human Destructiveness* that I have pondered for years: "It is man's humanity that makes him so inhumane."[17] But inhumane means "not human." How can we do what's not human? The answer, for Fromm, is the power of our minds to invent ideas that snuff out our deepest sensibilities, even our common sense. We create a world that doesn't feel like ours because these big ideas can overpower our innate sense of connection to one another and cause us to suppress our need for power in the best sense of the word—power to express ourselves in the public world.

Over the years, it's become ironic to me that we view ourselves as thinkers. We think—that's what distinguishes human beings, right? We see ourselves stuck in Rodin's pose. But no, I've come to see that we're not only thinkers; we're also absorbers. We mold our perceptions of reality, and of ourselves, to conform to ideas we hold, ideas we often absorb *without* thinking. And we're adapters: We seek desperately to shape ourselves according to these ideas of who we are and what we believe others expect from us.

So there it is. We can only see that which fits into our "map"—what we expect to see—and mostly we can't even see the map. Yet we adapt ourselves daily to it. Quite a challenge! At the University of Montana gathering, I reflected on these ideas with students over a sumptuous organic lunch. I remember one whose eyes lit up, "Yes! It's like gazing through a screen; if you look long enough you don't see the screen at all."

We have gazed so long through the particular screen creating this world that we simply do not see it.

To begin to break free of life-destroying patterns, to create a world aligned with our truer selves in which no one goes hungry or is made sick from the food they eat, Anna and I believe we have to, and we can, gain new eyes. The challenge is enormous, but we can come to see the map shaping and limiting our vision.

So what are the big ideas of today's dominant mental map?

Anna and I have condensed them into the five that seem most potent to us—those that not only lock us into seeing scarcity in a world of plenty but that shape even our understanding of what it means to be human. They tell us where to look for solutions to the worsening global crises and ultimately influence what would seem to be the most individual choice of all: how we seek meaning in our lives.

Thought Trap One: The enemy is scarcity, production is our savior. In the original *Diet for a Small Planet,* I set out to explode the scarcity myth with mountains of evidence showing the abundance—and the waste—in our food system.

For me, discovering that here in the U.S. we feed sixteen pounds of grain and soy to cattle to get one pound back in meat was the first real wake-up call. Because so much of our harvested acreage goes to feed livestock, the waste is staggering. I calculated that the grain we annually feed to livestock could provide the equivalent of a bowl of food for every person on earth every day of the year! So, I thought, *anyone* who simply looked at the facts would be spurred to make big changes.

But I guess I didn't appreciate the strength of this thought trap's grip. Even now, thirty years later, the U.S. Department of Agriculture sees no problem at all. Its economists maintain that the grain-to-beef ratio is "only" seven to one—as if seven pounds fed to get only one pound back is some mark of efficiency. (To get their seven-to-one ratio, government analysts must credit grain and soy feeding with all the meat produced, although they know that more than half comes from grass, hay, and other things cattle eat.)

So, we've turned cattle into virtual protein disposals, and now we're doing the same with fish. During World War II, a government-issued poster read EAT FISH, THEY FEED THEMSELVES. But this is less and less true; we're now feeding fish to fish, shrinking overall supply. To get one pound of salmon, we use four pounds of what are deemed "junk" fish, including sardines, that are a vital pro-

FIVE THOUGHT TRAPS BLOCKING OUR PATH

The mental map that limits our imagination, helping to create the hunger, poverty, and environmental devastation all around us.

ONE: THE ENEMY IS SCARCITY, PRODUCTION IS OUR SAVIOR.

With the world's population potentially doubling in fifty years, there aren't enough food, jobs, land—or just about anything—to go around. We must keep single-mindedly focused on producing ever more, just to survive.

TWO: THANK OUR SELFISH GENES.

We are selfish by nature. To survive as a species, we had to be self-centered and competitive. While these traits aren't always pretty, they drive the entrepreneurial spirit and the creativity that have gotten us this far. Who can argue with survival of the fittest?

THREE: LET THE MARKET DECIDE, EXPERTS PRESIDE.

Since we humans are so self-seeking, thank goodness we can turn to the impersonal law of the market. What the market can't decide, we had best leave to the experts—the people who know what they're doing—because only our technological genius keeps us one step ahead of scarcity.

FOUR: SOLVE BY DISSECTION.

The world's problems are so huge that our only fighting chance to solve them is by dissection. We must break down our mammoth global challenges and tackle them piece by piece, one by one.

FIVE: WELCOME TO THE END OF HISTORY.

Communism, socialism, and fascism have failed. Human evolution has finally triumphed in the best system we can create: global corporate capitalism, in which everyone stands to benefit from the creativity and wealth it unleashes.

tein source for a billion poor people—exactly those who could never afford the higher-priced salmon.[18]

Neither do we register the literal waste created by our production drive— or that drive's environmental cost. Livestock waste in the U.S.—now *130 times* more than waste produced by humans—is polluting water and killing fish.[19] Waste from the growing livestock population now contributes 16 percent of global emissions of methane, a greenhouse gas 25 times more potent than carbon dioxide.[20]

A squinted-eye fixation on production blinds us to other ways in which we're destroying the very soil, water, and biotic life we must safeguard if we are to thrive. We are ruining topsoil many times faster than it is being created, as noted earlier. Fresh water consumption, much of it for agriculture, is almost two times that of its annual replacement. And 70 percent of the world's marine species are at risk of extinction.[21]

And then there's our health. Production myopia has spurred the shift to giant feedlots with thousands of head of cattle raised in cramped spaces. Cattle stressed by being shipped to big lots—then confined and fed a diet to which they aren't suited—commonly suffer lung disease. Acid indigestion, which can inflame stomach walls enough to slow nutrient uptake, as well as liver abscesses, bloating, and bovine polio, are also huge threats in these unnatural conditions. So cattlemen, pressed to produce, typically add antibiotics to feed—not just for the sick but for all cattle.[22] In fact, a recent study of antibiotics found that almost three quarters of antibiotics used in the U.S.— *for all purposes*—are now going to livestock.[23] Alarmed that this practice is transferring dangerous antibiotic resistance to us humans, even the American Medical Association has called on livestock producers to stop.[24]

Locked in the thought trap—the single-minded focus on ever greater production—we ironically cannot even see how we're reducing potential supply, destroying the basis of future security, and endangering our health.

Thought Trap Two: Thank our selfish genes. Linked to this fixation is the assumption that the only way to keep the machinery of production in highest gear is to rely on our innate selfishness. Not unlike our myopic focus on production, our vision of ourselves has become so narrow that all we can see is our basest survival drive.

A recent stroll through my local bookstore illustrated how widespread the view is that we humans are nothing but selfish egoists. The titles popped out at me: *Mean Genes, The Selfish Gene,* and even one entitled *How to Be Your*

Own Selfish Pig. Chart-topping shows like *Who Wants to Be a Millionaire?* reinforce the notion that our selfishness inevitably manifests as material greed, that we're all money-lusting. The dramatic conclusion of the hit TV show *Survivor* seemed to clinch the case: In this material world, it's the most manipulative and cutthroat among us who wins.

A few months ago the *New York Times* business section carried a story about a multimillionaire. Aware of the Internet billionaires barely out of braces, the guy asks: "What have I done wrong?" Now, this distraught multimillionaire isn't portrayed as pathetic and in need of immediate psychiatric help. No, the story tells us that here is a normal guy with a normal reaction. This is just who we are; we *always* want more.

The sad thing is, we've come to believe this caricature of ourselves, convinced that without these traits we'd lack the entrepreneurial heat that propelled us from cave to computer.

Sure, this view of ourselves is reinforced minute by minute through today's crass media messages, but we've also been absorbing it for a very long time. Seventeenth-century philosopher Thomas Hobbes put it quite bluntly: "Homo homini lupus"—we are to each other as wolves. Too bad Hobbes had no appreciation of the social nature of wolves; he meant that we are by nature at one another's throats. This view runs deep in American culture: Alexis de Tocqueville, revered for his penetrating insight into our national character, wrote in 1835 "Private interest . . . is the only immutable point in the human heart."[25]

Thought Trap Three: Let the market decide, experts preside. From this limited view of ourselves flows Big Idea Three: Since we humans are utterly ego-bound, genuine deliberation over our public choices—the ground of democracy itself—is suspect. The most selfish among us will only subvert it to their own ends. Best leave choices to the impersonal, neutral force of the market, which requires nothing of us except to be our selfish little selves.

While this thought trap has ensnared us for hundreds of years, in the last thirty it's acquired new vigor. "Market fundamentalism" is what financier George Soros calls it.

Seeing ourselves as narrowly self-centered, incapable of democratic self-governance, of course we distrust government. It's inept at best, corrupt at worst. With market fundamentalism in full bloom since the Reagan era, we've seen a rush to turn over to private companies essential functions long considered public responsibilities—from the incarceration of prisoners, to the schooling of children, to the control of the world's water. Already, sales of water worldwide total one-third again as much as pharmaceutical sales.[26]

We've also cut back government's role in regulating industries in the public interest. To cite just one example, in the '90s a new federal system for inspecting meat was developed with help from the meat industry itself. In it, federal inspection has been reduced to a sample of less than .01 percent of carcasses—even though the Centers for Disease Control estimate that almost a third of all turkey and six percent of all ground beef carries deadly salmonella.[27] And 76 million people each year suffer from food-borne illness; five thousand die.[28]

Bewitched by what Reagan called the "magic of the market," we end up weakening a powerful vehicle—accountable government—for coming together as citizens, from the local to the national to the international level, to resolve our deepening social and environmental crises.

This thought trap in which the only real threat is too-big government—since corporations are simply products of the all-good market—leads us in an ironic and scary direction. The biggest promoters of the market—private corporations—are killing it; they're destroying the diversity of players on which a free market rests. Since I wrote the first *Diet,* in every major sector of our economy a handful of corporations has come to dominate. Of course, it's hard to perceive this trend through the maze of ever-proliferating products, like Kraft cheese, Maxwell House coffee, Post Raisin Bran, and Altoids breath mints—all from a single company (in this case, Philip Morris).

It would be bad enough if such concentrated power only meant steeper prices from diluted competition. It would be bad enough if weakened competition only meant shoddier products and poorer service. But it's much worse. Once public elections are financed by private contributions; once private entities control more resources than do public ones, the stage is set for the massive disregard of public welfare.

Nowhere is this clearer or scarier than with regard to our food supply. The U.S. Department of Agriculture, for example, cooperated with corporations that were developing genetically modified organisms. So today, GMO products line most grocery shelves, yet Americans know virtually nothing about them or their risks. In fact, 70 percent of Americans still believe they have never eaten GMOs. Adding insult to injury, our government, yielding to industry pressure, refuses to mandate labeling GMOs so that the public might at least know what it's eating.

Would Americans be so ready to equate a "milk moustache" with good health if they knew that most milk is now laced with a dairy-cow-growth-stimulating hormone called rBGH—which the Food and Drug Administration approved on the basis of a 90-day test on 30 rats, when the standard cancer test for a human drug is two years and several hundred rats? Would they feel safe knowing that rBGH-maker Monsanto—the company responsible for cancer-causing PCBs and the chemical defoliator used in the Vietnam War— is so worried about what the public might find out that it threatened to sue dairies who label their milk rBGH-free and warned a subsidiary of Fox News of "dire consequences" if it aired a report on rBGH risks? (The station caved and even fired the reporters.)[29]

In the grip of this thought trap, we reduce more and more aspects of life to commodities for sale. Historically, funding for public schools has been worked out through public deliberation and carried by the public purse. Now, though, many Americans don't blink while companies, such as Coca-Cola, pay big bucks to schools for the right to exclude the sale of other beverage companies' products and gain access to our children, this despite the dramatic rise in childhood obesity and diabetes.

Previously, bushels and even shiploads of food could be owned, bought, and sold. Now, however, plant varieties and other forms of life are privately owned and turned into commodities on the market, a development the consequences of which we're only beginning to grasp. Just as we were finishing our book, two companies announced that they'd unlocked the genetic code of rice. Worried that this could lead to the patenting of the grain, an American professor responded: "How can a company own the most important food crop in the world? In Asia, rice is like a religion. To own a religion . . . can you do that? I don't think so."[30]

Mistrusting ourselves—our own capacities to bring wisdom and experience to problem solving—we defer to experts who we believe are, like the market, neutral and impartial arbiters. Such deference is dangerous even in the best circumstances, but what if the experts are themselves beholden to those whose interests are not ours? The American Dietetic Association, for example, is the voice of professional dieticians, isn't it? So, we can trust its impartiality. Or can we? Fifteen percent of its budget comes from food companies, and its Web site includes "Daily Nutrition Tips," many sponsored by the same companies that make the products.[31] On this site, for example, the dieticians in a "Nutrition Fact Sheet" assure us that biotech foods are safe for us and the environment. In small print we learn that Monsanto is helping to bring us these "facts." In part thanks to funding from Ajinomoto, we learn about the virtues of the flavor-enhancer MSG with no mention of the allergic reactions it triggers in some people. Or that Ajinomoto makes MSG.

And, within this thought trap's constricting hold, we don't think to ask: *Which* experts do we get to hear?

In one of the few early research studies on the effects of consuming GMO foods, Dr. Arpad Pusztai—who had considered himself an enthusiastic supporter of gene technology—was surprised when rats fed his genetically modified potatoes developed smaller livers, hearts, and brains, and when their immune-system organs such as the spleen and thymus were affected, too. And why haven't you heard about Dr. Pusztai's findings? He worked at the respected Rowett Research Institute in Aberdeen, Scotland, and in a television interview in 1998 he expressed concern about insufficient safety testing of GMOs. Immediately, the good doctor got canned. Not only did he lose his job, but the reputation of this author of 270 scientific papers was besmirched by the institute that had employed him for most of his thirty-six-year career. So that's one expert disappeared. Why? The authors of *Trust Us, We're Experts!* suggest that part of the motive might be that almost two-thirds of the funding for Rowett comes from the British government, which at the time was trying to lure biotech companies to Britain.[32]

Ironically, the core of this thought trap—the market, along with impartial experts, as the arbiter of happy outcomes—is supposed to free us. The market gives us all freedom of choice, yes? Yet Anna and I have come to see that this thought-trap increasingly robs us of real choice.

Thought Trap Four: Solve by dissection. Thought trap four springs from a view of our "world as machine," one that we can take apart, fix, and reassemble. This mechanical worldview emerged centuries ago—twenty-five centuries, in fact—as one of the many fruits of ancient Greek philosophy. Some Greek philosophers saw the world as composed of tiny and invisible bits of inert matter with everything easily divided up—down to the last atom, with atom meaning "indivisible." Rediscovered four centuries ago, atomism became a central piece of the Scientific Revolution.

Atomism also fed the self-seeking caricature of ourselves, because it encouraged us to see humans as walking, talking "atom equivalents." Philosophers presumed that, just as a physical atom pursues its own inertial trajectory in physical space, each of us—conceived as nothing more than a social atom—does the same. We doggedly chase after our own preferences in social space, all in splendid isolation from each other.

Unfortunately, this is no esoteric, academic matter! Our view of the world as a machine has had enormous consequences for the planet. Our belief that we could "solve by dissection," for example, led us to the Green Revolution, which bred seeds to produce higher yields—if, to be sure, the seeds are fed more chemicals and water. Still narrowly focused on the chemical fix, we go on blanketing the planet with agricultural pesticides—a billion pounds each year in the U.S. alone. But we fail to see the human and ecological ripples. Along with environmental devastation, worldwide these chemicals cause three million poisonings and over 200,000 deaths each year.[33]

Seeing only the pieces, not the pattern, we also ignore what we learned in Biology 101: Life evolves. Pest populations develop resistance to every new generation of poisons we throw at them. So, we're still losing as much or more to pests worldwide as we ever have, perhaps as much as *half* of all our crops.[34]

The real rub of this thought trap? Solving by dissection not only fails to fix the particular problem but blocks us from addressing the deeper question, one with multiple, interwoven threads: How can we have food for all while sustaining the earth?

Thought Trap Five: Welcome to the end of history. From these four thought traps flows the fifth: that the present system of global capitalism—no matter what its downsides—is the best we flawed humans can do. So Francis Fukuyama *was* right when he wrote *End of History and the Last Man* in the 1980s. Human history has finally culminated in a system that in a certain sense is the inevitable result of our nature. We've come to believe that any other system requires totalitarian coercion of people to act against their nature. If we want higher living standards, says *New York Times* foreign affairs analyst Thomas Friedman, there's nothing else from which to choose. Globalization—the worldwide spread of corporate capitalism—is it. All other ideologies have flopped in practice: ". . . there is no more mint chocolate chip, there is no more strawberry swirl, there is no more lemon-lime. Today there is only plain free-market and North Korea."[35] (And, of course, no one is about to choose North Korea!)

So, we've arrived. Whew. Now we can stop bothering even to imagine something different. Sure, we can soften capitalism around the edges—big-business volunteer days, pro bono corporate lawyering—but it's risky, even dangerous, to fundamentally change it.

Together, these thought traps pack quite a punch—they are the unspoken assumptions driving our planet. Within their confines, it's true, we have no choice but to continue to create a world so far out of touch with common sense, and with what our hearts desire, that we try to shield ourselves from it. These thought traps make it difficult, if not impossible, for us to express our true nature; to act on our need for effectiveness in the larger world and for connection with others beyond our immediate families.

Blocked from opportunities for effectiveness, creativity, and connection, most of us don't shrivel up. No, human beings are more resourceful than that! We turn to ersatz substitutes. And they're easy to find, with over $600 billion being spent each year on showing us the way to them. Advertising numbs us to deeper needs and keeps us grasping for *stuff*. Advertising tells us that if we can't have real connection, we can at least have status through our possessions; some standing with our peers. Accumulation becomes the substitute for effectiveness and community.

So the world we see today reflects not our true nature but in many ways a denial of ourselves. And that denial creates a world driven by fear—fear of expressing who we really are. For us, therefore, nothing is of greater urgency than reexamining the thought traps.

We must draw a new map to survive. It's that simple.

Now, some might ask, why not get rid of mental maps altogether? Well, we can't—however much we might like to. We human beings must have a way of understanding our world. We cannot just step into a "meaning void." So, it's difficult to let go of the dominant framing device, no matter how destructive it is, until we can see at least some inkling of a new one.

But, if we see only that which we expect to see—if we can't even perceive that which doesn't fit onto our mental map—how could it *ever* be possible to change? Aren't we frozen in self-destruct mode?

No, we don't think so. From my own life experiences and from the extraordinary people whom we meet on this journey, Anna and I have gleaned certain insights about breaking free, about doing the apparently impossible—perceiving the "screen" through which we now peer, seeing with new eyes, then moving forward with our fresh, improved vision.

One lesson is the value of a rude shock. Something must shake us up, rattle us out of our resignation or depression, or simply galvanize that vague sense that there must be more to life. Something must create internal dissonance.

In the lives of people you'll meet throughout our book, you'll see precisely those moments—moments when experience just doesn't line up with what they've been taught to believe. My own early moment of dissonance occurred as I sat in the ag library, astounded that the simple facts of abundance clashed with the news headlines warning of impending food shortages.

We can all expose ourselves to people, ideas, and events that create internal dissonance—that feeling that something just doesn't fit anymore. In such special moments, we can choose. Do we suppress the discomfort? Or do we listen to it, delve into the disconnect, and make the leap necessary to put the world together in a new way?

In making that leap, it helps to have an entry point: some hint of an immediate benefit to thinking differently—an incentive, if you will.

These precious moments of dissonance and entry points differ for each of us. What moves me may leave you cold. When I started the Center for Living Democracy, I thought democracy could motivate everyone—I thought democracy was, well, tantalizing! To me, democracy is an exciting, living practice, what we do every day. But to most, democracy still means something done "to us" or "for us"—it doesn't relate to our daily lives, and it sure isn't much fun. I now see that to engage in democracy, to jump into this living practice, we all need something tangible to act on. And on our journey, Anna and I saw just that—people discovering remarkably different entry points for meaningful action.

Despite their differences of focus, resources, climate, culture—almost everything—they share something striking. They are doing what the dominant worldview says can't be done. They are liberating themselves from all five thought traps. They are making the path as they walk.

EMBRACING FEAR

When we pay attention to those moments of dissonance, when we open ourselves to an entry point for the first time, something happens: We face fear. And, well . . . since fear doesn't feel good, it may be our struggle to avoid it that most traps us, and that most keeps us creating a society that violates our deepest selves.

To question ideas that have long given our lives coherence and meaning is just about the scariest thing any human can do. It's disorienting. It might even cause us to question the way we've lived. And questioning almost always means separating ourselves from at least some others, sometimes even others close to us.

We'll never forget the Wisconsin farmer telling us about the ridicule he faced when beginning to farm without chemical pesticides and fertilizers. His neighbor scowled and said, "Hey, what are you growing in that field—pineapples? I've never seen such lousy-looking corn!" Or the fear that the

Bangladeshi woman endured when her neighbors told her that if she borrowed money from the Grameen Bank, she would lose her husband and be denied an afterlife!

To make it worse, fear is hard even to talk about.

While it's socially permissible to acknowledge stress, anxiety, and burnout—in fact, admitting these feelings in some circles has become a badge of honor—acknowledging fear is verboten. It is a sign of weakness. So, if Anna and I are right that we must befriend fear to get at the root of the global predicament, we must drag fear out of the closet. That conviction was another kick that propelled me on this journey; I believed that the people we would meet could teach us a lot about fear.

It takes strong motivation to face fear, I know. And to find it, we must start with our own hearts. We must listen to ourselves. When we do, I believe that we begin to uncover our own unrequited yearnings; our unfulfilled need for genuine community and for effectiveness—our desire to be the problem-solvers we have all evolved to be.

I believe that, if we are to find courage, we must first let ourselves experience the pain of this unrequited yearning. The word "courage" comes from the French *cœur*, heart. Courage grows as we allow ourselves to experience our hearts' yearnings, no matter how painful, and allow them to spur us on.

We're then prepared to use our greatest vulnerability to our greatest advantage.

Here's what I mean: Letting others define us is part of what it means to be the social animals that we are. Yet this very quality is in some measure what has landed us in such a terrible predicament. Our need for acceptance, our need not to appear to be out of step with our tribe, means that we now go along with what is denying our deepest needs and destroying our planet. On the other hand, our desire for one another's approval, for acceptance—reflected in our taking cues from one another, mimicking one another—has its upside, if we use our noggins!

We change ourselves, helping to create communities that no longer deny but instead meet our deepest needs, by consciously choosing whom we bring into our lives. We can put ourselves in the company of those who are finding the courage to express their deeper selves and who, by their very being, remind us that the aberration is the world we see, not those who are out of step with it. We can seek them out. We can deliberately absorb them.

That's another way of explaining why we took this journey—to put ourselves and you in such company. Anna and I have learned that we can't rely on the media to tell us about the invisible emergence of the millions of people in every corner of the earth chipping away at the thought traps. From the delectable gardens in California to the tiniest villages in Kenya, we met people who are choosing what they want for their families, their communities, and their countries, and who are facing the fear of change.

The people we met are showing us that the thought traps are myths indeed. They're drawing the contours of a new mental map emerging, one that is liberating, not entrapping, and one I could never have imagined thirty years ago. Our journey allowed us, and now allows you, to rub elbows with such people—people who have changed us simply by letting us share in their experience.

They show us ways not to be better people but merely to become more fully ourselves.

THE JOURNEY

THE DELICIOUS REVOLUTION

Food is the one central thing about human experience
that can open up both our senses and our conscience
to our place in the world.   ALICE WATERS[1]

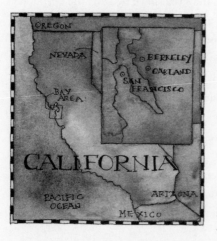

In 1971, nested in the U.C. Berkeley agricultural library—the one Anna and I searched for in vain thirty years later—I realized that, of course, food is about more than fueling our bodies. Embedded in family life and in cultural and religious ritual, food has always been our most direct, intimate tie to a nurturing earth as well as a primary means of bonding with each other. Food has helped us know *where* we are and *who* we are.

So, beyond the crisis of hunger itself, I was alarmed that this wider, richer dimension of food-as-relationship—with both the earth and one another—was eroding. What I didn't know was that, a few blocks away from where I sat, a woman named Alice, exactly my age, felt this loss with similar passion. She and I were products of the same Berkeley cauldron of we-can-change-the-world energy. I chose to invite people along a path by writing a book; Alice Waters chose to issue a similar invitation—to re-embed food in community—by opening a restaurant. Chez Panisse was born the very month, August 1971, in which my book first saw the light of day.

In the three decades since those intense times, Alice and Chez Panisse have proven it's possible to create haute cuisine using natural, locally grown food. Alice has helped bring us a world in which Portobello mushrooms go head-to-head with filet mignon; a world where granola is no longer a derogative synonym for "hippie," but a gourmet dish. She hasn't just changed the content of people's cupboards, though; she has also helped people to see the link between what we eat and our health, both our own and our community's. For many, she has come to symbolize the possibility of reclaiming our food cultures from the now-planetary trend of processed, uniform fast food—a trend that's gone into overdrive since Alice and I took our first steps in 1971.

Here, in one of the wealthiest countries in the world, we now face an epidemic of malnutrition. By malnutrition we don't only mean the plight of those Americans who aren't getting enough calories; we also mean that of the millions who are filling their bodies with foods that don't healthfully nourish them. Today *almost half the calories an American consumes come in the form of fat and sugar.*[2]

Fueling the epidemic are food companies that have become the corporate world's biggest spenders on advertising, primarily to sell us high-fat fast food. So, we're eating and drinking more processed, high-calorie-low-nutrition foods—from chips to sodas to burgers—than ever. One-fourth of all Americans now eat a meal from a fast-food joint at least once a day,[3] and if we choose a double whopper with cheese, we're downing in one meal 130 percent of the saturated fat we're supposed to eat in an entire day.[4] And, when we drink a Coke, we might as well be having a piece of chocolate cake—the sugar intake is the same.

Fast food has become a major U.S. export, with a new McDonald's opening somewhere in the world every five hours. Coca-Cola is now Africa's biggest employer, and Mexico just surpassed the U.S. in the race for the highest per-capita Coke consumption.[5]

America's grain-fed meat diet is also spreading faster than ever around the world.[6] U.S. beef exports have increased sixty-fold in the last three decades, while meat consumption in developing countries has doubled.[7] In countries like China or Thailand, the better-off are creating a demand for meat. This means that whereas almost no grain went to livestock in these countries thirty years ago, now more than one-quarter of their grain supplies are used to produce meat.[8]

While many Americans have chosen not to eat meat, some even foregoing all animal products, overall meat consumption per capita is up since 1971. Yes, we Americans are eating less pork and beef—though the typical sixty-eight pounds per person per year still reflects three to four burgers a week—but we're making up for it by eating almost twice as much poultry as we did back then. In fact, we're consuming so much animal food that the average American eats twice the protein that can be used by the body. (Nonetheless, think how frequently vegetarians are challenged: "But how can you get enough protein?")

Since poultry contains much less fat than red meat, Americans' fat intake would have fallen if it had not been for the striking increase in the consumption of cheese—pizza, anyone?—and salad and cooking oil. It's not simply that we're cooking with more oil, it's that fast food and processed foods are drenched in it. Think of Kentucky Fried Chicken or that almost half the calories in a Ritz cracker come from fat. Or consider that 17 percent of our vegetable consumption is from potato chips and french fries.[9]

THE EXPERIMENTAL DIET

This high-sugar, high-fat diet also bears no resemblance to the unprocessed, plant-centered diet of our evolving ancestors, in which meat, fat, and simple carbohydrates, like sugar, played minor roles.[10] The modern diet is the greatest experiment ever attempted on human beings, and we, the guinea pigs, aren't faring very well!

The health consequences are staggering. This experimental diet puts the weight on at unprecedented rates. Across the planet, more than one billion people are now overweight—that's one in every six of us. Here in the United States, 64 percent of adults and at least 15 percent of our children are overweight or obese[11]—higher today than at any time since records have been kept.[12]

Extra weight itself heightens the risk of a great many diseases, including hypertension, heart disease, and certain cancers, such as late-life breast cancer.[13] Therefore, obesity now ranks second only to smoking as a cause of mortality in America, resulting in 300,000 deaths each year.[14] Think about it: In America our diet claims ten times more lives each year than does gun violence.

Obesity is blamed in large measure, for example, for the skyrocketing rates of diabetes. Fifteen years ago, 30 million people worldwide were afflicted; today, 151 million suffer from the disease.[15] In the U.S. we spend close to one out of every twelve of our health-care dollars coping with the diabetes epidemic.[16] In total, one out of every nine health-care dollars goes to cover costs associated with excess weight.[17]

Eating meat itself brings with it higher risk of heart disease, hypertension, diabetes, and more, says the American Dietetic Association.[18] Male meat-eaters carry *twice* the risk of heart disease than do men who don't eat meat.[19] Eleven years after *Diet* was published, the National Research Council released the first major study implicating our diet in cancer.[20] By the year 2000, experts were estimating that our radical new way of eating—moving away from whole foods, grains, fruits, and vegetables—is linked to as many as four out of ten of all cancers.[21]

This giant experiment with the human diet has also triggered whole new diseases—eating disorders, for example. As a teen, I'd never even heard of bulimia and anorexia, but they've grown so fast that they now damage the lives of millions of Americans.[22]

Over the years, I've struggled to understand the meaning of this tragic and needless pattern of disease and death: Is the problem simply that because more of us can afford to eat too much, we do? Or do we humans perhaps just prefer foods that make us sick?

No, I'm coming to see that to find an explanation we must step back; we must perceive the ways in which more and more aspects of our lives—food only one of them—are being stripped of wider meaning, reduced to a mere commodity for sale. Alice believes we can reverse this trend, and we can start with food. We can begin to enrich our lives and regain our health by awakening our senses, which can then awaken our power to choose.

A CASCADE

"Simply saying 'I'm going to make a choice about the way I eat.' This is a giant step," Alice tells Anna and me in the dining room of Chez Panisse on a crisp spring morning. "This decision can send you down a beautiful path—a delicious revolution."

Alice's conviction is contagious, but we're unsettled, too . . . a delicious revolution?

Sitting amid the quiet elegance of Chez Panisse, with sunlight falling on white-clothed tables and a menu offering a $75 *prix fixe* dinner, we seem about as far away from anything revolutionary as we could imagine; as distant from the biggest questions about hunger and fairness as one can get.

Surfaces, though, can deceive.

"From the beginning, my strategy was seduction," Alice tells us with a slightly mischievous grin under her signature velveteen hat. "I didn't want people to come because it was good for them," she says of her restaurant's food. "I wanted them to come because it's delicious."

By choosing fresh, seasonal food grown near where we live by farmers who love the earth and therefore forego chemicals, Alice assures us, we begin to experience the world and ourselves in new ways. This one step, Alice says, can lead to a cascade of what can ultimately be new political and economic choices to heal our relationship with the earth and one another.

It's been this "cascade" possibility that has long excited me, too. I've always loved hearing from readers of the original *Diet* who've told me that making new choices about what they eat triggered a series of other new choices, even leading to new career paths—the physicist who became a community-health doctor or the sales manager who opened her own natural-foods restaurant. Alice's cascade has taken her far beyond cafés catering to the chic and powerful (Anna and I heard that the Clintons love Chez Panisse and that Alice had even been approached to open a restaurant at the Louvre). It's gotten her dirt-deep in a schoolyard's transformation down the street and even hooked her up with convicts planting gardens and trees across the bay in San Francisco. And for Alice and all those with whom she's working, the "thought traps" in the previous chapter are exploding right and left. Cascade indeed.

My Senses Dazzled

Entering Chez Panisse through the kitchen, we're bombarded with the smells of the early-morning preparations, the sights of golden onions, curly endives, and purple asparagus. It's easy to be seduced.

I'm reminded of my first "seduction" by food, my own sensory awakening. It was the late '60s, and, remember, the world was a different place back then. No housewife would dare call it dinner without meat—certainly not *my* mom. Bisquick, Jell-O, and pot roast were big in our family.

But once I began to awaken to the abundance beyond meat, I was dazzled by the world of plant food, whole food—food I barely knew existed, much less knew how to cook. I fell in love. I reveled in the amazing flavors. I discovered red and yellow lentils, azuki beans, millet and barley, bulgur and buckwheat. And seeds? Before, they'd only been bird feed to me. Now, roasted, they topped all my favorite dishes.

I read cookbooks as if they were novels, imagining the surprising taste combinations: barley, mushrooms, and dill? Overnight, meat and potatoes simply lost their appeal, so drab and lifeless were they in contrast. Then to discover that what was so tasty was *also* best for the earth and for my own health—what a happy convergence!

Over the decades, I continued to center my diet in the plant world, but along the way I lost some of the sensual wonder. My head seemed to take over. Unlike me, though, Alice stayed rooted in food and the senses. She believes now as much as she did thirty years ago in its power, not just for those who can afford her Chez Panisse entry ticket, but for everyone. And—funny thing— an offhand comment she made to a local newspaper reporter ended up offering her a way to reach . . . yes, potentially everyone.

THE GARDEN OF OUR IMAGINATIONS

Principal Neil Smith of Martin Luther King, Jr. Middle School, which is only blocks from Chez Panisse, was not pleased in 1993 when Alice made a disparaging remark about his school grounds' appearance and it showed up in a local newspaper. "So I wrote her a little note, and she called and asked me to lunch," he reflects when we talk with him just outside his office a few days after we spoke with Alice. "In our lunch, she raised the idea for the edible schoolyard."

It was a big idea: "The children create the garden, grow the food, prepare it, and serve each other," Alice explains to us. "Whether it's math or science or English, they incorporate what they're doing in the garden with their other lessons."

"Alice leapt way ahead," Neil says to us about his early conversations with her. "She was already at step ten; she wanted it all to happen at once. But," Neil goes on, shaking his head, "I told her we needed to start with step one, just creating a garden out of overgrown, infertile urban blight."

On this nippy early-spring day, we arrive just as King Middle School is letting out and run into a young boy. "What did you cook today?" asks Edible Schoolyard director Mildred Howard, with a broad smile that makes us feel her excitement about the wonders of her work with kids in the garden and in the kitchen classroom.

"Empanadas," he explains. "I folded the dough. Inside they've got carrots, potatoes, and onions." When we ask if they were good, he responds with a big grin and an emphatic nod.

Mildred walks us across a black asphalt playground, past a group of students playing basketball. We hear others shouting, a siren in the distance, and the school bell ringing. A blocky snack bar is selling kids that final bite before class.

And then . . . the garden. Entering, we move into what feels like a different time zone, a different latitude: It's cooler, shaded by overgrown flowering bushes and corn stalks. The air tastes different. In the garden's cocoon of bird songs, urban noises disappear.

No straight rows here. Beds of corn and amaranth, carrots and lettuce weave together. Arbors and curving fences made of branches and twigs laced with vines add a magical quality. With each step, I find it harder to believe that, just several years earlier, all this was merely an empty lot, a neighborhood eyesore.

Wooden, hand-painted signs tell us what is growing where. "Mashua," says one, and when I look bewildered, we're told it's an almost extinct ancient Incan tuber. Stopping at an artichoke plant as high as my chin, Mildred cuts three artichokes for dinner. "I'll make them tonight with Parmesan and butter," she tempts us, and I try to remember whether I've ever tasted a just-picked artichoke.

The abundance so early in spring speaks of the soil's fertility, so we're not surprised when Mildred tells us that the children regularly spread organic compost across the garden. They've added up to 200 tons over the five years since the garden was born.

Clearly, in all these years, Alice and King Middle School have gone well beyond "step one."

We hesitate to interrupt a man bent over in intense conversation, whose suntan and sunglasses make him look more like a lifeguard than the garden manager and teacher.

"I don't instruct a lot," David Hawkins explains, with a striking British accent, when we ask about his role. "I let the kids play. Experiment. They learn by watching. I don't teach them to use a hoe. I do it, then they try it until it works.

"We make every job a job a kid can do. We don't use lumber, just branches and vines—so every job is something they can succeed in." As we look around at intertwined branches forming arches and fences, it does seem impossible to build something ugly out of what nature has created.

Both David and Mildred make clear that the effect of the garden experience on the children may not be immediate; may not even be overtly measurable, but it's no less real.

"You never know," says David, who worked for years in London with children who'd been expelled from regular schools. "Last year, I was so frustrated with one kid. It felt like more trouble than it was worth just to get him to move a wheelbarrow across the yard. But this week, his mother came in and told me the garden had transformed her son.

"Of course, I didn't argue," David says with a laugh. "So she went on, 'He used to come home and play video games. Now when he comes home, he tells us stories about the garden, what you're planting, everything.'

"I never could have guessed," David stresses. "The garden is working *inside* kids; you can't test on it. It changes their way of being in the world. They know they've built this place. Where else can they have this kind of experience?"

As we linger, we start to see that, yes, this is a garden, but it's more, too. It's also a child's imaginary world. Behind us is a classroom created with jasmine twisting around branches, with hay bales for seats beneath. In front of us is a mound of hardened mud, with twigs protruding near the bottom. I'm stumped until we get the explanation later: It's a bird's nest the kids built big enough so that they could climb inside.

"Emotionally, many of these kids have shut down so much," David says. "Out here they can be themselves. They can make noise. You should hear one of the girls—she just perfected a haunting dove's call."

GROWN-UP PRECONCEPTIONS

Returning a few days later to see a cooking class, we're greeted by Ene Osterraas-Constable, the Edible Schoolyard jack-of-all-trades—part media liaison and photographer, part project manager, part cheerleader. In the kitchen, children are filling large bowls with tomatillos—small, green, and tomato-like—soon to be made into salsa.

I'm recalling that more than half of Americans' vegetable consumption consists of just three things—iceberg lettuce, potatoes, and canned tomatoes—when Ene tells us laughing that "The first food from the garden the kids prepared was braised kale. The teachers pulled us aside and whispered, 'We think this garden is a great idea, but couldn't we just skip the kale?'" Anna and I laugh, too, thinking kale was surely not the way to "seduce" children into the joys of garden-fresh food.

"We were all nervous, but the kids loved it," Ene says. "The kale was just picked, so it wasn't bitter. In fact, I saw one little boy hoarding five leaves under his napkin for later.

"Our most important accomplishment is demonstrating on a daily basis with diverse kids that this can be done, and done with beauty and joy. We're talking about food, and it can be really celebratory," Ene explains, beaming.

For Alice, as for Ene, the ritual of preparing, serving, and sharing food at a table covered, in this case, with red-and-white-checked tablecloths and terra-cotta plates, is just as much part of the learning as planting, weeding, and harvesting. As Alice had reminded us, "The table is where culture is passed from generation to generation. If it doesn't happen there, it may not happen. Most kids today rarely have a chance to eat a meal together with their families."

"Naturally, we're hoping the kids will use this time to talk about things that wouldn't come out in the busy-ness of the day," Ene says. "Once, I passed by a lunch table and heard a group of boys talking about someone's head being cut off and lots of blood. I was so disappointed. I assumed they were describing some horror movie. Later, passing by again, I realized they were talking about their class. They'd been studying Greek myths.

"This project has proven to me children are the leaders. The only thing holding them back is adult preconceptions about what they can and will do."

What began with one phone call and then one school garden, and grew through joint efforts with other groups, eventually triggered such responses from the community that by 1999 the local school board voted that all the city schools should have student-created gardens, serve organic foods, and buy from local farmers. And soon, the curriculum will embrace the entire ecology of food, from ground to gut.

Anna is amazed. Fewer than fifteen years ago, she attended a nearby public school, and she recalls that a good day was one when the french fries weren't too soggy.

Solving for Pattern

The Edible Schoolyard, we soon learned, is part of a resurgence of school gardens, which were the norm one hundred years ago. Already, a fifth of California schools use gardens for teaching, and thousands more school gardens have sprouted up across the country in recent years.[23]

The more Anna and I discover about the Edible Schoolyard, the more we return to one question: What blocks us from change? Why isn't a garden in every school deemed as essential as, say, physical education? At one time it, too, was considered beyond the educational pale.

"What's stopping us?" I ask, and Alice doesn't hesitate even a second.

"Fear of change," she says. "We've been educated to think there can be a kind of permanence about the world, about one's life. We even deny we're going to die. Other cultures bring children up with an acceptance of change as

IT'S TWELVE NOON—DO YOU KNOW WHAT YOUR KIDS ARE EATING?

When I was in junior high school, I usually ate whatever the cafeteria had that day: soggy french fries, doughnuts oozing with jelly centers, super cheesy quesadillas. My favorite, I must admit, were bigger-than-my-hand chocolate-chip cookies that got as soft as a wet paper towel when we heated them in the microwave. Imagine—even a kid like me, who came from a home where snack food usually meant crunchy peanut butter on rice cakes, was tempted by the draw of junk food at lunchtime.

More than a decade later, as I stand in the kitchen at the Edible Schoolyard with kids making fresh salsa and empanadas, my junior-high snack-bar days seem far, far away. I have the same shock when we learn about another local initiative, the Berkeley Food Systems Project, which is getting salad bars with locally grown produce installed in every cafeteria in the district. I try to imagine it, but it's a challenge. Remember, I'm part of the generation who grew up with President Reagan declaring ketchup a vegetable so that public schools' hot lunches could be called "balanced"—just add the condiment!

Still, the Bay Area is David against the Goliath force of fast-food companies making inroads into school cafeterias. School kids, after all, are a vast market, and corporate deals have been flying faster than a delivery of Domino's Pizza. Hundreds of public schools now have contracts with fast-food companies, and here in California, more than half of schools recently say they serve up food from Taco Bell, Subway, Domino's, or Pizza Hut.[24]

part of their lives," Alice continues. "They know they're going to go through this time of big change when they're teenagers. They're going to change at different periods in their lives. This is life. It's never constant. If you try to hold on, you're going to be shocked and disappointed. You have to let go."

As she talks, I imagine the children down the street witnessing change in the daily and seasonal life and death, the death and life in their own garden. And I see that part of my own fear—even as I have pushed myself to change over and over again—has come from this myth of permanence that I, too,

Beverage companies have also been getting in on the act, signing contracts with school districts for exclusive "pouring rights," paying pretty prizes of cash in exchange for a district's promise to sell only their company's soft drinks. (This, despite findings by scientists that just one more can of soda a day gave the kids they studied an almost 60-percent-greater chance of becoming obese.[25])

A look at what kids are eating these days is evidence of these inroads: A 1997 survey of high school students found that three-fourths of them are eating less than the advised five daily servings of fruits and vegetables,[26] with one-fourth of their servings of vegetables coming in the form of french fries.[27] Kids' health is showing it, too. Here in California last year, one in three children between the ages of nine and twelve is overweight or at risk of becoming so.[28]

But adults—and kids, too—have been rising up. In Berkeley, we learn Kentucky Fried Chicken had proposed building a facility at the high school, but a group of concerned teachers, parents, and students blocked the deal. In Madison, we'll learn later about citizens successfully blocking Coca-Cola from getting pouring rights in their district. And in Los Angeles, the entire school district voted to ban carbonated soft drinks and cut back on junk food in all its schools.

Maybe the new resistance is paying off. Today's newspaper says that Coca-Cola is backing away from its aggressive pursuit of school contracts and explains that the company is reacting to concerns about commercialism in schools.[29] It may just be this resistance that gets kids eating more salad-bar salads and less of those soggy french fries of my youth.   —Anna

have absorbed. It kept part of me assuming that if I *really* figured out life, I would be stable, and that meant *not* changing. But the question isn't, as Alice reminds us, to get beyond change. It's to develop the confidence that we can meet change full-face—embrace it, even.

Sounds great, but embracing change is challenging, especially when all we see are the gigantic problems facing our planet, from global warming to global hunger. It can feel overwhelming—just too much. So where do we find the motivation even to start?

Understandably, we're tempted to solve by dissection; to chop up our problems into bite-size, manageable pieces and solve them one by one. In Chapter 1, we dubbed this temptation "the solve-by-dissection thought trap." But the dissection strategy fails us if we take apart problems and ignore all the connections that have created them in the first place.

Thirty years ago, this model of the world as a take-it-apart-and-put-it-together machine held our culture's imagination. It still does, but it's gradually giving way to new images of how the world works. When I wrote *Diet for a Small Planet*, "ecology" was an obscure scientific term. Today, it's everywhere, eroding our mechanical mindset and teaching us to think in terms of relationships; to see the interconnectedness of all life. New communications technology—preeminently the Internet—encourages us to think not in isolated parts but in networks, in connections. And those distinct parts? Well, they dissolve right before our eyes.

To hurry this shift toward an ecological view of the world, physicist and author Fritjof Capra co-created the Berkeley-based Center for Ecoliteracy, which funds the Edible Schoolyard and assists in integrating the garden into the curriculum. Zenobia Barlow, a Center cofounder and its executive director, explains how we might get ourselves out of the clutches of the dissection thought trap, and how we might start to see patterns instead of pieces.

"Take the crisis in the local Sebastopol apple industry," Zenobia tells us, striving to make the abstraction real for us. "Cheap imports from New Zealand and now China have driven down apple prices; apple farming just isn't good business anymore, and farmers are ripping up orchards and the vineyards are moving in. We know how devastating this loss has been for these families who own orchards.

"So we here in Berkeley started asking, 'Why should we import apples and other produce halfway around the world?' We chose instead to buy Sebastopol apples for our after-school program. Just by making a few decisions, we're now buying as much as ten thousand dollars a month in local organic produce.

"We like to use author-poet Wendell Berry's term 'solving for pattern' to describe our approach," Zenobia adds. To her, and to us, the phrase conveys the power of grasping the connections that create a pattern among seemingly disparate problems, and then solving the pattern, not the pieces.

To illustrate, Zenobia ticks off a list of seemingly disjointed problems: "Take the loss of urban-fringe family farms, like those in Sebastopol; take urban sprawl; take the epidemic of diabetes and childhood obesity; take the loss of our open space and our kids losing reverence for nature. Solve for pattern.

Link those problems together and they become a solution. By buying food locally, at a lower price, and by using the institutional buying power of the schools, we help solve all those problems at once."

Anna and I come to see how "solving for pattern" is creating ripples well beyond apple farmers and schools.

But Anna and I don't immediately make the link when Zenobia says that "one of the biggest funders of school gardens is the solid-waste industry." "Schools are a huge part of the solid-waste problem," she explains, "a lot of it is from kids throwing away food they don't eat. Each day, tons of uneaten school lunches go into landfill, so the industry wants recycling in the schools. But mostly, they want us to feed kids something they *want* to eat, so it doesn't end up in landfills.

"People come to feel powerless fighting decisions made by anonymous corporations far away," Zenobia continues. "But we can easily influence our children's schools, and what they eat when they're there. That's within the reach of all of us."

Alice Waters had ended our earlier conversation by asking us to "imagine the effect if all Berkeley's schools started buying locally and organic." Like the chain reaction of her own restaurant's buying decisions—with more than sixty local farmers now regularly supplying Chez Panisse—this purchase choice has huge implications. Looking at us with the same mischievous twinkle we'd spotted before, Alice had said "And if all the country's schools followed suit? Multiply that out!" Her face had lit up.

Now, Anna and I are beginning to sense the possibilities that Alice and Zenobia do.

PRISONERS PLANT

Leaving behind the pleasure of relaxed wandering in the Edible Schoolyard, we head across the San Francisco Bay. Circling loading docks and tourist traps in heavy San Francisco traffic, we finally stop near Pier 28 to ask loaders in rubber boots and aprons, "Can you help us find the Garden Project office? Cathrine Sneed?"

Alice had told us in our first conversation that meeting Cathrine was a must. Alice's Chez Panisse Foundation was an early supporter of her work. But I needed no convincing. I had heard Cathrine speak the year before, and I couldn't forget her. I knew she had another piece of the puzzle I'd been trying to put together for thirty years.

Cathrine had kept her audience spellbound with tales of her journey from a household of fourteen kids in a tough neighborhood to law school to work with women in prison and, finally, to gardens. In the early '80s, still in her twenties, Cathrine was hospitalized with a kidney disease. For two years she fought for her life in and out of the hospital.

Then, just after her doctor told her in so many words, "You're going to die," Cathrine's boss and mentor San Francisco Sheriff Michael Hennessey brought a former teacher of Cathrine's to her hospital bed.

"My teacher said, 'You were a punk in high school and didn't read much. So here, don't just feel sorry for yourself, read this.'"

He handed her *The Grapes of Wrath.*

It held all she needed. "I felt the message. If people connected with the land, they would have hope," she told us.

Defying doctor's orders, she marched out of the hospital. A determined woman, she immersed herself in learning about gardening and demanded that Hennessey allow her to use some of the 145 acres around the city's jail to create a garden in which prisoners could work. By 1985, Cathrine had established an organic farm and greenhouse at the county jail. Today, more than 10,000 inmates have had their fingers in that dirt.

A few years after the garden's launch, Hennessey ordered a study of the impact that working in the garden had on prisoners. Starting in 1991, the study tracked 300 inmates. Did those who gardened reenter prison at the same rate as those who didn't? After three years, the evidence was in: Inmates involved in gardening were less than half as likely to return to prison.

Now, inmates who have worked in the jail garden have the opportunity after release to get a decent-paying job on a half-acre garden plot Cathrine created in the Bayview–Hunter's Point district—right next to a brand new police station.

We want to see Cathrine's magic at work, so we leave the Pier 28 office and land mid-afternoon in the ex-convicts' garden—a long, lush strip bordered on one side by a rain-faded wooden fence and on the other by a whitewashed side of a building with a bright mural.

"They want to talk to *you,* not me," Cathrine says, sweeping up a welcome gift of fresh green garlic in her long arms and sitting us down with Garden Project employee Anthony Travis. Anthony, despite his former street life and time in prison, looks far shy of his thirty-five years.

As Anthony chats with us across the picnic table, it's clear he isn't surprised by the sheriff's study showing that the garden experience makes a difference. "It's hard to get out of jail and stay out," he says. "There's no one to help you get on your feet. They say jail is about setting you straight, but it's really about breaking you down to keep you doing what you were doing.

"Jails are built for violent criminals," Anthony explains with a solid, earnest expression. "But a lot of people in there are just trying to make it from day to day; most aren't violent." And he's right: Two-thirds of the prisoners in our jails today are there for nonviolent crimes, a proportion that's been increasing over the past thirty years and that jumped way up in the '80s with the billion-dollar "war on drugs."[30]

Anthony echoes Cathrine's view that most people who end up in jail have been driven to crime by deprivation and hunger—in this neighborhood, mainly driven to dealing drugs, taking them, or stealing to get them. (As you weigh Anthony's and Cathrine's words about the impact of hunger, remember that, at any given moment, more than 20 million Americans are wondering where they're going to get their next meal.[31])

GIVE TO LIVE

How does gardening transform prisoners' and ex-convicts' sense of themselves, giving them power, both mental and material, to lead healthy lives? The healing power of nature may be considered the arena of poets, but Anthony offers an explanatory line that conveys perfectly the potency of this place.

"We always say, 'We don't just grow flowers and vegetables, we grow people,'" he tells us with total conviction. "This is a program built to help one another. If we can help one another, we can cut down on crime."

Some might overlook the "helping other people" aspect of why the garden works, but not Cathrine. "People need to feel useful," she tells us later around a kitchen table in a friend's house near the garden. "They need to feel their lives have meaning."

Seeing beautiful, nutritious food spring from a seed we ourselves plant certainly can make us mortals feel like miracle makers, but in this society we often think of *usefulness* purely in economic terms. Before arriving, Anna and I imagined the garden as more of a bootstrap-economics deal. We'd heard that it sold portions of its produce grown outside the jail to local restaurants, including Chez Panisse. But now we get it. The giving and sharing at the heart of what goes on here have nothing directly to do with economics.

"We no longer sell to restaurants," Cathrine tells us. "We now donate all of what we grow to people in the community, simply because the need—even in San Francisco—is so great.

"When I go to the bare basics of what we're doing," Cathrine says, "it's trying to replicate a family." She herself had thirteen siblings—"a Brady Bunch without the resources," as she puts it. She also raised eleven children; nine were those of close relatives.

"In a family, of course, whatever you have you spread however thin you need to. You spread it, and everyone gets some." Referring back to her own family size, she says "If you have a piece of bread, you cut it fourteen times."

Sharing and giving—including, during one six-month period, 20,000 pounds of broccoli, potatoes, zucchini, cabbage, and kale—are key to the project's transformative power. In a statement that is a far cry from the presumed human need for self-gain embodied in the prevailing mental map, Cathrine sums it up, "we have to give to live."

TOUGH COP

Later in the afternoon, we're standing in the police station with Captain Ron Roth and Cathrine. She says, teasing him, "Show them the picture, Ron!" Demurring at first, he finally pulls out a black-and-white eight-by-ten-inch photo. In full riot gear is a beefy cop with a scowl on his face, pulling the long hair of a young street protester.

"That's a picture of me from the early eighties—printed, page two, *San Francisco Chronicle*," Ron says, as if he can hardly believe it himself.

Anna and I are shocked, too. The friendly, fit man facing us in this airy office graced with inspirational posters and perky irises is unrecognizable as the man in the photo.

"After twenty-three years in the police force, I was transferred to this neighborhood. At first I didn't want to come here to Bayview–Hunter's Point," Ron says. I assume he means he'd just as soon have avoided a notoriously high-crime area. "I'd never heard of Cathrine's project."

So when he'd only been in his new job a few months and a dozen black men—with Cathrine in the middle—filed into his police-organized community meeting, Ron tells us, he was nervous.

"I didn't know if they were going to cause trouble," he says. "They seemed like they'd been in jail—they had that look about them."

Ron says that, despite his nervousness, he was touched as the men described the Garden Project, telling him that it offered them hope, and that they were staying out of jail, off drugs, and enjoying productive lives.

"The next day, Cathrine sent these guys over with desserts for my station.

She was trying to get on our good side, and it worked," Ron admits. One of Cathrine's secret food-to-heart weapons is a longtime relationship with the bakery Just Desserts, a Bay Area sweet-tooths' favorite that donated the original half-acre for the garden and has, over the years, hired graduates of the Garden Project.

"She made a connection," Ron tells us.

How sneaky this Cathrine woman is, I think to myself. With one speaking-from-the-heart session and a few tasty morsels, she'd accomplished step one in breaking the barrier of human stereotyping. Step two happened soon thereafter.

"I saw the guys working in the garden," Ron tells us, "and jokingly I said, 'Sure would be nice if you extended your project around my police station.' We laughed, and I walked away." But soon the ex-convicts were landscaping the station grounds gratis. They were sharing their skills, giving gifts of themselves, and the relationship with the police in this area of Bayview–Hunter's Point has never been the same.

Last year, Cathrine enlisted police officers in handing out 10,000 pumpkins at Halloween. "Seeing the mountains of pumpkins, the little kids were so excited, they were shrieking and grabbing the legs of the policemen," Cathrine exclaims. "These kids were hugging people in uniform they'd learned their whole lives to fear. And, once police officers have gotten that close to those kids, I believe it's difficult for them to see the black people in this community as the enemy."

If Alice's intuition is that food is the pathway to our senses, in every meaning of the word, then Cathrine's intuition is that food is the way through all our preconceptions. Via food—giving and sharing—we recognize each other as human beings. No longer a mere commodity, food returns to its bonding role in human culture.

And as the sharing of food has broken down barriers between the community and the police, Ron's job has gotten easier. "People are reporting more crimes," Ron tells us. "Now when there's a shooting, I might get a call right in my office telling me who the shooter is. Crime here in the last few years has gone down twice as fast as in the rest of the city."

PRISON PARADOX

As we talk with Cathrine, Anthony, and Ron, the cold contradictions of our society's approach to crime-fighting sink in. We see another way in which the dominant mental map leads us to create what we fear, and to generate scarcity.

We put more people behind bars per capita than any other country in the world, and then claim we can't afford better public education, job training, or other resources that help people stay off drugs or out of crime in the first place. Then, released convicts, many having been brutalized in prison and with no job on the outside, often become *re*-convicts: In California, a state with one of the largest prison populations, two of every ten prisoners released in the mid-'80s could be expected to return. Today, nearly *seven out of ten coming out of jail will return there.*[32] Trying to save money, we end up spending ever more in hard cash and even more in lost lives.

Anthony grins as he tells us that he's now earning more than twice the minimum wage as a manager in the Garden Project offshoot Tree Corps, which since 1994 has employed ex-convicts to plant and care for almost 10,000 trees throughout San Francisco. "My hands have been in all those trees," Anthony says, beaming.

Seeing the garden, Anthony's pride, and how relatively little it takes to create this opportunity and, ultimately, reduce costs to society, we're witness to another instance of how we as a society generate exactly what we say we loathe—in this case, heavy government spending and more crime.

Ron, the police captain, explained what it's usually like to put someone like Anthony back on the street after jail with no support. "Statistically," Ron tells us, "he's got a high chance of committing more crime. Think of one drug addict coming out of jail who steals cars to pay for his fix. Over the course of a year it can add up—in damage and in losses to the general public and to insurance companies—to *half a million dollars.* Compare that with paying someone less than thirty thousand dollars in the Garden Project. There's no comparison."

But while the logic holds, Cathrine battles for her shoestring budget, and the U.S. continues to prioritize prison funding over education and rehabilitation—spending roughly $40 billion a year on operation and construction of new prisons.[33]

But *why?*

"Prisons are big business," is Cathrine's four-word response. "We've created an economic imperative driving the status quo. The private prison industry is booming." And, we later learn, the California prison guards' union—with a huge stake in keeping that boom alive—was the biggest contributor to the 1990 campaign of Governor Pete Wilson.[34]

Sure, if we're trapped in the idea that we must leave outcomes to the market, we don't question the profit imperative that's driving what is certainly a public concern.

We haven't made a leap of perception. Media images reinforce the false-hood that it's violent criminals we're spending so much money locking up. "But most of the young men and young women in our jails are there," Cather-ine says, "because they're addicts and because they're poor, *not* because they're violent." We're made to feel they couldn't possibly have motivations and needs similar to our own. At the same time, many people see the beefy, hardened stereotype that Ron Roth once embodied as all that cops are and all that they can ever be.

But Cathrine is showing through the medium of food—growing it and sharing it—that it's possible to replace stereotypes with recognition of our common humanity.

Anna and I will never forget the contrast between Ron, the cop we saw in the newspaper photo, and Ron, the fellow who grins as he says, "If Cathrine and the guys don't call me by Monday afternoon, I call them. I'm away all weekend and I miss them. It's the best thing."

TRUSTING OUR SENSES

"Since I've come to Bayview–Hunter's Point, I'm probably the healthiest I've ever been," Ron admits. "I get disgusted when I think of what I was a few years ago. Now, I try to stay away from fast foods.

"When they're really rolling in the garden, we get deliveries every week. It's some of the best produce I've ever had. When I got home late from a com-munity meeting, I used to pull out something frozen for the microwave. Now I take the Garden's greens out of my car trunk and make a salad."

Ron tells us about the heartache he feels when he goes on a police call into a home and sees nothing healthy to eat in the refrigerator—and often nothing much at all. Remember, an estimated one in every five kids in our country lives in a home where not having food on the table is a constant threat.[35]

"I know there's a connection between healthy bodies and healthy minds," Ron says.

And we believe Ron is right, but the truth is that more and more people—both those with money and those without—are becoming caught in the corporate fast-food/fat-food snare we described in the grim health statistics that opened this chapter.

"Over the years, I've asked thousands of prisoners about their diets, and they all tell me the same thing," Cathrine says. "When they were growing up, there was little food in the house, no real meals, they grabbed what they could.

So, the first thing the guys do with their paycheck is to go to McDonald's. They're somebody then."

Cathrine is trying to break the spell of advertising that links fast food and the good life. It's not an easy task, when Burger King, McDonald's, and other fast-food companies have become ever more aggressive in capturing inner-city markets like Cathrine's. One out of every four hamburgers that McDonald's now sells is to an inner-city consumer and, disproportionately, to young black men.[36] It's also not so easy when the advertising clout of McDonald's is $800 million a year and, well . . . when was the last time you were seduced by a broccoli ad on TV?

"You don't know how to cook collard greens, girl?" Cathrine says, imitating herself talking to young black women in the neighborhood who grew up on fast food and never learned the healthy aspects of their traditional African-American cuisine.

As Cathrine talks about people awakening to the joy of fresh food, often including plants—like leafy greens—from their own culture's past, I recall my own thrill thirty years ago sitting in that stark basement library across the Bay: I discovered that, historically, every people in the world has created a diet by putting foods together in ways that heighten their nutritional value.

Combining legumes—including beans, peas, lentils, and peanuts—with grains creates protein that is more effectively used by the body than it is when the same foods are eaten separately. Corn and beans in Latin America, rice and lentils in India, pasta and beans in southern Europe, peanuts and millet in Africa: All these traditional combinations are ingenious ways of getting the most from plant protein.

I remember thinking, "Ah, what fun, we can be chemists in the kitchen." We can create more usable protein simply by doing what our forebears did intuitively. Pretty neat, and it's cheap, too.

What seems so obvious, though, was heresy when I wrote my first book. In fact, the National Cattlemen's Association felt so threatened by my questioning of meat-centered diets that it set up a panel of cooks to prove that my non-meat meals were inedible! They failed, and, as the recipes from leading chefs who contributed to this book celebrate (see *Coming to Our Senses*, page 331), an entire cuisine has evolved since then, centered in the plant world and in whole foods.

Before being dazzled by the world of plant foods, I myself was an obsessive eater. (When I told this to Anna recently, her mouth dropped.) No one guessed. I wasn't fat. I didn't talk about it, but secretly I compulsively counted calories and fantasized about the next meal as soon as I'd finished one. It wasn't fun; I felt trapped. But as I began to eat whole grains and beans, nuts and seeds, and unprocessed fruits and vegetables, my preoccupation and cravings stopped. My weight adjusted to exactly what felt comfortable for my frame and has stayed there ever since.

Thirty years later, scientists now have an explanation for my experience. Nutritionists can measure the rates at which we metabolize food. Processed food—refined sugars and other refined carbohydrates—are quickly metabolized; we therefore get hungry sooner and want more. A recent study of overweight teenagers found that those who ate a meal of whole foods—which metabolize more slowly than do processed foods—voluntarily chose fewer calories at their next meal than those who ate a meal of typical fast food.[37]

When I shifted to a whole-foods diet, my body's appetite came into balance with what it truly needed. And doctors are discovering my experience is hardly unique.[38] In effect, I learned that I could trust my senses to lead me to what made me healthy. My joy in then discovering that what's best for me—a whole-foods, plant-based diet—is also best for the earth has continued to propel me ever since. It's been a relief to shed my food obsession so that eating could become a source of pleasure and an opportunity for guilt-free camaraderie with family and friends—what eating had always been for human beings until this great, recent aberration.

And so, I find myself pondering again the question—why do we, as societies, create what as individuals we abhor . . . and now, why have we created a national diet that is so patently bad for us?

I've come to see the answer from two angles.

In the dominant mental map, we learn that we must leave outcomes to the "market," and in today's world, that means to an industry that disconnects the providing of food from what our bodies need to thrive. In fact, it means leaving our decisions about our diets to a very clever food industry that has hit on a glitch in our biology and exploited it big-time. The glitch is that we humans evolved what nutritionists call a "weak satiation mechanism" for fat and sugar—meaning that once we start eating them, it's hard to stop. Eons ago, when we were roaming hunter-gatherers and high-fat, high-sugar foods were scarce, the trait served us well.[39] When we made the kill or found the beehive, it was advantageous to binge, you might say. But when fat and sugary foods aren't scarce, the trait is mighty dangerous. Fortunately, I learned by my own little experiment on myself that if we eat more like our ancestors did, we don't have to fear our evolutionary programming.

Through another lens I see something more: Because so much about our culture denies our senses, we increasingly consume food that we take no time to enjoy and that is literally killing us. Once reduced to a commodity, food doesn't engage our senses. In fact, we are taught to mistrust them. We tolerate fast food not because we "lack good taste," but because we've lost touch with our natural sense of taste, with all its subtleties, and with the role food has always played in bonding us to the earth and to one another. Alice and Cathrine are determined to reverse this loss and help us reconnect with what our bodies want to tell us. In a sense, they allow us to see how we've been hurt by the thought traps and how we can free ourselves from them through our senses.

If Anna and I are right, awakening to our senses might well be a key to gaining the confidence we need to change the larger patterns that generate hunger and ill health out of plenty: The confidence Cathrine fosters in convicts and ex-convicts through her gardens every day and the confidence the children at the King School build as they come to be at home with the garden's earth, birds, worms, and plants may be the confidence each of us can gain as we reconnect to the earth.

COLD ABSTRACTIONS START TO BREATHE

In 1971, yes, I was pleased when many people who read my book stopped eating grain-fed meat or became vegetarians. I hoped they would experience the "cascade" of new choices that Alice and I so believe in. But I was also frustrated and yearned for a way to express more coherent guidance. For that, though, I had to live more, learn more.

Now, the Edible Schoolyard's innovation, Zenobia and Fritjof's initiative that is turning an ecological worldview into practical action, Alice's vision, Cathrine's success, Anthony and Ron's transformations—together they show the web in which our choices are enmeshed; how solutions arise in solving for pattern, not in dissection. Cold abstractions are starting to breathe.

Walking and talking through these urban gardens, Anna and I see even more clearly the many ripples of our choices:

- what we eat

- where we shop

- what we think are appropriate school lessons and lunches for our kids

- where institutions like schools buy food

- whether we continue to stash human beings away in prisons or invest in reconnecting them with community and the earth

But how do such choices become our choices? How do they become enlivening affirmations from within us, rather than heavy "you shoulds" from some exterior notion about "what's right"? The answer might be to start with choices that we feel will enrich our lives right now. I know I'm hardly "sacrificing" when I shop at my pleasant, human-scale Harvest Co-op in Cambridge and forego the massive, mobbed supermarket.

I love the story Alice tells to bring to life the idea that ultimately these choices are celebrations, not sacrifices.

"One of the teachers in Berkeley," Alice says, "tells about a time when her students washed and trimmed and cut up ingredients and made a big salad. 'Now wait,' she said, 'before we start eating, let's stop and think about the people who tilled the ground, planted the seeds, and harvested the vegetables.' The kids stood up at their desks and gave the salad a standing ovation."[40]

Yes, our new choices can be a celebration of life, but that doesn't mean denying the reality of needless suffering that still fills our world. We know that from California we're headed for lands where most people struggle even to survive, and we'll carry Cathrine's challenge with us: to be strong enough to embrace both the celebration and the pain of this era.

We'll carry with us Alice's reminder, too, that every choice we make about food matters. As she says, "the right choice saves the world," and then quotes artist Paul Cezanne: "The day is coming when a single carrot, freshly observed, will set off a revolution."

In one sense Cezanne's quote might seem silly. What difference could a carrot make, no matter how long you stare at it? But Anna and I have come to see that if you really were to stop and take the time to look at a carrot, you would have to think about the soil that it grew in, the water that fed it, the people who labored to tend it, and those who will—or will not—be able to enjoy its nourishment.

Whether Cezanne meant it this way or not, a single carrot *can* take us to the toughest questions of our time—to the life-and-death challenges, even, of the landless in Brazil who are struggling to turn idle land into life; to turn landlessness into hope.

CALIFORNIA: AWAKENING OUR SENSES

Food First Spicy Garlic Eggplant

Serves 4

Early in our journey we visited the Food First offices in Oakland, California where the staff served us a delicious lunch, as they do for each other every day of the week. Food First dining has come a long way since 1975, when Joe Collins and I—its founders—would rush down from our tiny headquarters over an A&P grocery store to grab a sandwich. This Food First recipe is a quick, easy dish with a complexity of tastes that lingers on the tongue. For dessert, try fresh fruit—a favorite is freshly picked raspberries over yogurt and dabbled with honey.—Frances

4 cups hot cooked brown or
    long-grain rice

1 pound extra-firm tofu

2 tablespoons sesame oil

3 Japanese eggplants (about
    12 ounces)

2 tablespoons soy sauce

3 tablespoons garlic black bean sauce
    (available in ethnic area of supermarket)

3 tablespoons cornstarch

1 cup water

½ cup loosely packed fresh basil leaves

1½ tablespoons garlic chili paste (available
    in ethnic area of supermarket)

Put up a pot of long-grain or brown rice (enough to make 4 cups cooked rice if you want a cup of rice per serving) to cook while making recipe.

Cut tofu into ½-inch slices, then cube into ½-inch size. In a medium-size skillet heat 1 tablespoon sesame oil, add tofu, and sauté until brown on all sides. Cube eggplants into ¾-inch size. In a larger skillet, heat 1 tablespoon sesame oil and add eggplant, sautéing over high heat for a couple of minutes until brown on all sides. Cover, and simmer on low heat until well-cooked (about 10 minutes). Add tofu and keep warm over low heat.

In a small bowl, mix soy sauce, black bean sauce, cornstarch, and water. Add sauce to the eggplant and tofu. Cook over medium heat a few minutes until thickened, stirring often. If the mixture becomes too thick, add more water a little at a time.

Wash, dry, and chop basil. Just before serving, add basil and chili paste to tofu mixture and cook over medium heat for two minutes, stirring, to get nice and hot.

Serve over rice. Pass a bottle of soy sauce in case people want extra. Serve as soon as possible, as this dish gets saltier as it sits. If you are reheating leftovers, add up to ½ cup water as needed to thin sauce.

The Edible Schoolyard Empanada

ESTHER COOK, EDIBLE SCHOOLYARD CHEF

This empanada recipe was first tried by a seventh grade Spanish class studying South America. This recipe is perfect for young people because it requires lots of chopping, grating, and rolling of dough, providing many jobs for everyone. Keeping with our efforts to recycle and reuse, we used plastic tops from yogurt containers as guides in cutting out the pastry rounds. These empanadas were a hands-down favorite with one and all.—Esther

PASTRY

1⅔ cups flour, plus extra for handling the dough

7 tablespoons melted butter

½ teaspoon salt

2 to 2½ tablespoons water, more as needed

Sift the flour and salt into a large bowl, stir in the butter and add enough water to form a soft but firm dough. Knead dough briefly, wrap in plastic wrap, and leave to rest for 30 minutes at room temperature.

FILLING

2 large waxy (Yukon Gold, red) potatoes, peeled and cut into ¼-inch dice (¾ pounds)

6 scallions, white and light green parts only, washed and sliced into thin rings

2 green chilies (about 2 tablespoons), chopped fine

1 cup (4 ounces) jack cheese, grated

½ teaspoon paprika

½ teaspoon salt

¼ teaspoon freshly ground black pepper

Cook diced potatoes in simmering water for 3 to 4 minutes. Drain well and let cool. Combine remaining filling ingredients in a mixing bowl, stir in the potatoes, and season with salt and pepper.

To Make Empanadas

Roll out dough on flour-dusted surface to ⅛ inch thick. Using a 5-inch saucer as a guide, cut out rounds. Knead and reroll any trimmings. Place one tablespoon of filling on each round, a little off center. Dampen the edges of the pastry with a little water and fold in half, over the filling. Seal the edges by pressing them with the tines of a fork. Place empanadas on a sheet pan and bake at 425° F for 10 to 15 minutes or until golden brown. You can also brush them with melted butter just before baking. Serve hot.

CHAPTER 3

THE BATTLE FOR HUMAN NATURE

What kind of Brazil do we want?

BANNER IN LANDLESS WORKERS'

SEMINAR ROOM

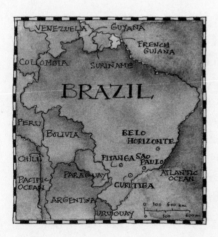

It's four in the morning, and the bus has just dropped us in Pitanga, a small town smack in the sparsely settled middle of the southern Brazilian state of Paraná. Waiting for our hosts, Anna and I watch as men in ponchos and cowboy hats greet the bus and then, in cars and trucks and on horseback, take weary travelers home. A woman with a baby bundled in blankets sits on the bench facing us.

We are in the coldest part of the country, at the coldest time of the year, during the coldest winter in history, and it's cold, even without the wind gusting through the open doors. We laugh, picturing the bathing suits crushed in the suitcases we diligently packed. (Obviously we'd seen too many posters of Rio beaches to believe it when we were told it was winter here.)

After a few minutes of huddled waiting, our guides arrive, their noses red. With hands like ice packs, they greet us, smiling, exuding unexpected energy that makes us momentarily forget the temperature. These two early risers are part of the Landless Workers' Movement, called the MST from its name in Portuguese, *Movimento dos Trabalhadores Rurais Sem Terra,* the largest social movement attacking the roots of hunger in Latin America and one of the largest in the world.

Amid the niceties, I find myself wondering: Do they have death threats against them? Have any of their family members been killed?

You see, in the process of settling a quarter of a million families on formerly idle land in the last sixteen years, thousands of MST members have been injured and more than 1,000 have been killed.[1]

But we don't take time to talk—it's 4:30 in the morning, after all—so my mind just races on its own as Anna, our interpreter Leo, and I stumble silently to the tiny hotel across the street. We fall onto plank-like beds, hoping to get some sleep before our first day in Brazil's countryside. (It's so cold that I beg Anna to push the narrow beds together so at least we can sleep under all four blankets!)

LARGER THAN LIFE

When I wrote *Diet for a Small Planet,* I'd never been to Brazil, but it held tremendous emotional power for me as I struggled to grasp why some eat and others do not. Brazil was modern skyscrapers next to frightening *favelas* (urban slums), huge *latifúndio* (estates) against starving peasants, natural abundance versus the plundering of the Amazon.

Hundreds of years of building walls of fear between people: That's what Brazil was for me. I knew that one percent of landowners had come to control almost half the country's arable land,[2] while almost five million rural people have no land at all.[3] The world's fifth-largest country with the eighth-largest Gross National Product, Brazil has become one of the world's leading agricultural exporters—while tens of thousands of its children die from hunger each year.

If there were ever a place in which hunger cannot be blamed on scarcity, it is Brazil. The country has among the world's most extreme inequalities of income and of wealth. (Only Sierra Leone is worse.) And because of such inequality, babies die in Brazil at twice the rate at which they do in much poorer countries, such as Armenia and Uruguay.

I also knew that owners of Brazil's vast *latifúndio* have gained and kept their land not only by controlling the political system, but even more effectively with guns. Every attempt by the poor in the countryside to claim land had been drowned in peasant blood.

In fact, I'd learned that it was partly the threat of land reform by a democratically elected Socialist president that triggered the 1964 U.S.-condoned military coup, which abolished democracy here for twenty-one years.[4] Under the military government, export agribusiness took off with a vengeance, and the distribution of land to the landless was hardly a priority.

In a country bigger than the continental United States, Brazil's problems—these obstacles to democratic change—had always seemed oversized to me, too. So when Anna and I set out to write this book, I was astonished to discover that, while I wasn't looking, something I'd least expected in this land of extremes had begun to take shape.

A growing movement was actually bucking everything I assumed to be "Brazil." It was wrestling land from large landowners to benefit the landless, challenging the large agribusiness model with small and medium-sized farms (many of them organic and cooperatively managed), and questioning the democracy of Brazil's relatively new constitutional government. This movement is the MST. With half a million members, it takes credit for settling a quarter of a million landless families dotted across the country on 15 million acres in 2,600 settlements and in almost every Brazilian state.[5]

Of course it caught our interest. Why does the MST seem to be succeeding, we wanted to know, when for hundreds of years all such striving for fairer access to land had been defeated? And what lessons does such a powerful social movement hold about how all of us—any of us—can break free from the dominant thought traps and effectively act from our own heart's yearning?

"It's Not Just About Land"

LAND REFORM FOR A BRAZIL WITHOUT *LATIFÚNDIO!* says the banner hanging across the front of the MST meeting room. (I can understand that much in Portuguese without our interpreter, I realize with a bit of satisfaction.)

As Anna and I walk to the front of the room to introduce ourselves, we leave a trail in the thin layer of sawdust on the floor and feel all seventy pairs of eyes on us. We don't talk for long, not wanting to interrupt this, the final day of a three-day seminar for MST representatives from across the region. It only happens twice a year, and they have a lot to discuss.

I feel immediately at home here. The sawdust casts the smell of a small-town hardware store, and the friendly robin's-egg-blue walls set off the bold red MST flags, caps, and T-shirts.

On the floor in front of us is a pile of dirt shaped like Brazil, its southern border roughed up by scuffling feet at the front row. Dotting the mini-Brazil are boxes the size of bread loaves and the shape of the hotels in a Monopoly game. Each box is carefully wrapped in black plastic. I whisper to Anna about what seems an odd choice. (It won't be until we visit our first MST encampment that I'll understand.)

Scattered among the little black boxes are paper tags with words in bold capital letters: HAPPINESS, TRANSPORTATION, HOUSING, LEISURE, PRODUCTION, SCHOOLS-PAULO FREIRE. In a glass half filled with dirt is stuck a single MST flag, and resting behind it in large letters is a sign that asks WHAT KIND OF SETTLEMENT DO YOU WANT?

Once we've eased into our red metal folding chairs, our interpreter between us, I look out at all the faces, of many colors, mostly men, some women, and even several young children, all enraptured by the presentation of Izabel Grein.

Izabel wears tweed trousers, a lilac jacket, and a white scarf, and her bearing is strong and clear as she discusses the upcoming Fifth National MST Congress. They're expecting more than 10,000 MST members to gather in Brasilia to confer about everything from the future of the Movement to farm economics. Something about Izabel's confident, kind carriage makes me guess that she's a nun.

After an hour or so, Izabel closes the discussion, erases the chalkboard, and writes one word: GENDER. For the next half hour, she and the group discuss what gender means and why women's equality is important to the Movement. She mentions an immediate goal: "We'd like half the people at the national conference in Brasilia to be women."

At the end of her presentation, Izabel asks for comments or questions. A man with an MST cap shadowing his face stands. "I think the Movement would be stronger if more women were involved," he says. "Women learn faster because they aren't afraid to ask questions or to show they don't understand something, the way men are." Before taking his seat, he adds, laughing, "Ladies, if the men want to beat me up after, please come help me!" And the group laughs with him.

After Izabel finishes, we listen as other facilitators lead discussions about everything from price formation for their traditional *erva mate* tea to special events for kids in MST settlements. But this is no ordinary meeting. Anna and I notice no milling about to ease boredom, no nodding off. Of all those present, I seem to be the only one having a hard time staying awake—and, keep in mind, this is after three days of transcontinental travel.

So I'm thankful that we're periodically roused by the designated musician sitting next to Anna, a young guitar player with plump, rosy cheeks and a strong, clear voice. When he strikes the chords, everyone breaks into song. "Land reform for a better Brazil!" rings out over one of the stirring melodies.

At the end of the morning session, a farmer with bright gray hair, one arm gripping a crutch and his right foot wrapped in bandages, hops toward Izabel. He hands her two packages of *erva mate* produced by an MST co-op and thanks her for her love of and dedication to the Movement. The whole room rises in a thunderous ovation.

Our interpreter leans over to us: "That farmer is a survivor of the massacre," he says. We both nod, but it isn't until several days later that we learn what Leo means.

At lunch, women who've been cooking in the kitchen just off the meeting room serve rice, beans, and cabbage from giant metal pots. Standing in a line that weaves out the door into the bright sun, we have a chance to talk with Izabel. I find out that I'm partly right; she was a nun for many years. She is also one of the founders of the MST.

Izabel wastes no time. "When they introduced you," she says in an almost stern voice, "they said you had written about the roots of hunger. But, please, in whatever you write, make clear that it's impossible to look just at hunger. We started out working on land but soon realized that every aspect of life has to be included—health, gender, education, leadership, philosophy . . .

"And I don't mean just included in discussions," Izabel adds, "I mean people gaining their own voices in bringing all these changes into their lives."

I think to myself: If only the professor I heard in Montana could be here, listening to people talk about what they really need—not another techno-fix, but knowing that their voices count in a "living democracy."

THE EYE OF THE BEHOLDER

On the plane to São Paulo, Anna had nudged me awake and pointed to our guidebook and a section about the MST in bold type. The Movement has settled hundreds of thousands of landless, the book says, but it is also responsible for much of the Amazon's recent destruction.[6] I am puzzled.

Then, after waking up on our first morning in São Paulo, we buy the day's papers, eager to know what the media is saying about a group that seems to defy Brazilian history. We're hit with a barrage: THE MST WILL BE CLOSED DOWN, declares the headline in the first local newspaper we pick up. It's a story about a lawsuit brought by a shopkeeper who charges MST members with invading his shop after he refused to give them liquor for a party. In another, we read that the MST leader whom we'd soon interview, João Pedro Stédile, is a dangerous revolutionary Marxist who is using children to create a paramilitary organization. Another reports the MST regularly strong-arms its members, even its poorest, into paying dues to the organization. We are told the MST is only able to carry on with its radical activities thanks to the fabulous amount of money it receives from abroad.

On top of all that, we read the MST doesn't even exist! It has no legal standing, and its legal arm is being sued not just for ransacking a small shop but also for siphoning off government money that should have gone to the poor.

I try to reconcile what we've read and heard about the MST with what we'd seen and heard at the MST seminar—deliberations about democracy in Brazil, kids running between people's legs, song and laughter in the next room, men and women serving each other steaming plates of food.

We turn to our interpreter to help us make sense of it all. He's a middle-class Brazilian, who—coincidentally—has recently been an interpreter for executives of Monsanto, the multinational corporation that is building a new facility here.

He explains that such press hostility toward the MST is relatively new. As recently as the mid-'90s, the MST enjoyed enthusiastic support. Public sympathy grew with the widely publicized police attack on thousands of unarmed landless during a demonstration in April 1996, our interpreter explains. Nineteen demonstrators were killed and forty more injured in a scene captured on film by a local journalist and broadcast across Brazil.[7] Two more have since died. Despite public outcry, no police have been convicted of the murders.[8]

Even a popular *telenovela* (soap opera), *O Reido Gado,* warmed Brazilians to the MST. Part indictment of the country's land distribution, *O Reido Gado* (Portuguese for "The King of the Cattle") aired every night for six months and became one of the most successful *telenovelas* in history. It also didn't hurt the MST that the sexy leading actor played a Movement member.[9]

As we can now see, though, the MST appears in the press as radical and dangerous. Good grief, we think, why this reversal of sympathy? What are we walking into? Are we about to meet a macho, cult-of-personality organization that is less about liberating people than about shepherding desperate peasants?

While these questions spin in our heads, our interpreter urges us to be wary of the Brazilian media. Most Brazilians, he says, don't trust the newspapers, knowing the media is controlled by some of the wealthiest people in

Brazil and operate in their interest, not in the interest of democracy. The founder of Brazil's near media-monopoly, Globo, even said not so long ago, "Rightly or not, I always had a certain enthusiasm for the military governments."[10]

Nonetheless, the news stories serve as a wake-up call for healthy skepticism. On that first day, we reaffirm a promise we make on our other trips. We take a few gulps and pledge to take it all in—whatever it is.

ENOUGH ALREADY

Despite all the controversy, one thing is indisputable: The MST's growth and impact arise from a long history involving millions of Brazilians, not just the landless themselves.

For centuries, only a few Brazilians owned most of the land—originally apportioned by the Crown to just fourteen Portuguese families. Over the centuries, land was more and more commonly sliced up illegally through what is colloquially called *grilagem*—for *grilo,* or "cricket." It became standard practice to create fake land deeds, making them look worn, old, and authentic by sticking them into drawers teaming with crickets who would chomp and stomp until the deeds looked like they'd been around long enough to be the real thing.

When we learn that most of Brazil's arable land is in the hands of a few large landholders who leave much of their land idle—in fact, the largest forty-six of them actually use only 17 percent of their land[11]—it becomes easier to understand how even the Brazilian city dwellers could have finally gotten so fed up that they said: Enough already.

From one of the MST's leaders—remember the scary "revolutionary Marxist" in the papers?—we learn more about how the Movement has channeled this widespread frustration.

When João Pedro Stédile walks through the door at MST's São Paulo headquarters—a converted upper-class home—we're greeted by a man with the build of a farmer and the intensity of a philosopher. João Pedro sits down, folds his arms, and—without dancing around with small talk—waits for questions.

Like millions of Brazilians, João Pedro comes from an immigrant farming family, so his personal story is the perfect place to begin to understand the national frustration with the concentration of land.

"My grandparents were immigrants from Austria," João Pedro begins. "They and my parents worked the land in southern Brazil for more than a century but ended up with nothing to show for it. I was one of the few to have a chance to study, and I was influenced by Catholic religious teachings. The church taught us that it was wrong to conform to inequity."

I like his directness and his clarity. I quickly see why his peers have chosen him to be their movement's chief articulator.

"When I was still in the university," João Pedro continues, "I started to work with the grape and apple unions. I was trying to teach them about 'price formation.' When I graduated in economics, I went back to work with the poor. Remember, this was during military rule, and no gathering *of any size* was tolerated. But we gathered ten thousand people and managed to raise the price of grapes.

"I was influenced by [U.S. farmworker leader] César Chávez," João Pedro adds, reaffirming my own sense that we open doors for each other through our examples. Here is evidence that it can happen across borders, even across continents—someone else's experience can become real enough that we believe ourselves to be capable.

At the same time that grassroots MST organizers like João Pedro and church groups were laying the groundwork for a national movement of the landless, Brazilians were experiencing the end of more than two decades of military dictatorship. In 1984, Brazil began the heady process of building a new democracy and, four years later, created a new constitution.

Imagine being alive for the writing of your country's constitution. If we Americans could start from scratch, what would we include? In 1988, while we were choosing between Dukakis and Bush, Brazilians were going back to the drawing board.

They chose to create a constitution much more detailed than ours, including specific land-reform provisions—thanks largely to continued pressure from church groups, unions, and the nascent MST. In the end, the constitution included articles that shock all Americans we've told about them: provisions requiring the government to take unused land and redistribute it to people with none. The constitution reads in part:

> It is incumbent upon the Republic to expropriate for social interest, for purposes of agrarian reform, rural property, which is not performing its social function . . . (Article 184)

But even with an elected government and a constitution with specific provisions for land reform, many felt land redistribution was proceeding too slowly, according to João Pedro. So, the MST, along with other groups working with the landless, decided to speed up the process. They chose a path we in the U.S. would call "civil disobedience"—saying, in effect, that the MST has the moral right to push the government to fulfill its constitutional duty to move land into the hands of the landless—even if that means the MST must break other laws, such as by trespassing, in the process.

Its strategy? Analyze which idle lands offer the most productive promise, bring landless people together, and—under cover of night—occupy the land. Using the old possession-is-nine-tenths-of-the-law thinking, MST members build temporary shelters and start working the land. At the same time, the MST presses the government to transfer title of the formerly idle land to the formerly landless occupiers.

The strategy seems to be working. João Pedro tells us that the government settled almost 400,000 families between 1995 and 1999, nearly twice as many as all of the families who acquired land in the entire *thirty years* since the first land-reform law, the 1964 Land Statute. In one sense, by organizing the landless into communities and evaluating which land is eligible for transfer under the constitution, the MST is doing the government's job for it.

Not long after we returned home, I would hear the head of Brazil's land-reform agency speak in a room down the hall from my MIT office. Given the Brazilian government's increasing hostility toward the MST, I was surprised when this man's chief assistant responded to a question about the MST by acknowledging that, of course, there would be no land reform without social pressure for it. Clearly not wanting to be heard as approving of the MST, he rushed on to accuse the Movement of "kidnapping," referring to an MST tactic of occupying government offices in protest and preventing officials' exit.

But here in Brazil, we hear João Pedro talk about such tactics in a wholly different light. What the government calls "kidnapping" or even criminal trespassing is, to MST members, acting in allegiance to a higher law—in this case, honoring the constitution's call to turn over idle land to those who most need it.

Aware of the obstacles the Movement faces—from government hostility to bad press to violent attack—it occurs to me to ask the most basic question: What made João Pedro think the MST could ever succeed?

His response is immediate and terse: "Being successful was never the motivation. We simply didn't have other options."

João Pedro talks as if it were the most natural thing in the world to proceed with no real hope of success, but he moves quickly from outcomes that they could not predict to what they are certain of: "There are no individual so-lutions in this world," he says emphatically, explaining that, within the MST, everything is done as a group. "We've seen what can happen with a movement that only has one strong leader. When we ask for an audience with the presi-dent of Brazil, he expects the president of the MST. One person. But instead he has to talk with the whole National Board, all twenty-one of us."

As we talk, the conversation turns back to the influence of early church teachings: how João Pedro learned that to be true to his faith he could not tol-erate inequity.

"The conservative church always used to say, 'Get used to being poor. God will give you what you want in heaven.' But my Franciscan mentors offered me a different version of the Gospel: 'God will help those who organize.'"

A Brazilian Manifesto

A few weeks after the national meeting in Brasilia that we heard Izabel and others planning, we receive a copy of the statement that the MST released at the culmination of the congress. It's called "Manifesto for the People of Brazil." When I hear "manifesto," I expect explosive protests of the violence against MST members, which has been severe; I expect complaints about the pace of government land reform, which has been slow. Instead, I read about Brazil's foreign debt.

At first, I'm surprised. The manifesto reminds Brazilians that last year the country's external debt was equal to one-third of Brazil's entire Gross National Product. It reminds people how many schools, hospitals, and new farms on idle land the $232 billion of debt could build. And it calls on inter-national political leaders to support debt relief.

Then I think back to the ice-cold seminar room and conversations with MST members. We heard it repeated everywhere: The vision of a better Brazil is for all Brazilians, not just the landless. I recall João Pedro's emphasis on joint effort and realize that, to the MST, "joint" reaches beyond its own members. After all, what could affect more Brazilians than millions drained from its nation's coffers each year?   —Anna

Laughing, I respond, "Hmm, an interesting twist on 'God will help those who help themselves.'"

João Pedro shakes his head, obviously frustrated that I don't get it.

"No," he explains, "one is a message to the individual to get up in the morning and struggle alone. The other, 'God will help those who organize,' is a message that justice will not be reached without joint effort."

FROM COLD MEALS TO CITIZENS

A few days later, we get to see the fruits of the MST's labors. Dressed in five layers against the cold, we head to our first "encampment"—an MST community living on occupied land, of which there are now more than 500 across Brazil. Today, roughly 70,000 families are waiting for official title while planning their new lives.

Driving out of Pitanga, with the morning sun glistening on the frost and our pint-size white Toyota raising a tail of red dust, we speed through the almost-fluorescent green landscape. Outlined against the sky are the strangest pines I've ever seen. With their largest branches on top, they look like giant green umbrellas.

"Most of the people you'll meet were called 'cold meals' before they joined the Movement," explains our driver, Adelir, a young man with chiseled features and curly brown hair peeking out from under his red MST cap. (Later, we learn he has been part of the MST since he was nine years old.)

"Cold meals?" I exclaim from the back seat, thinking I'd misheard our interpreter.

"Yes, because when you're landless, you have to work on somebody else's land, and you have to bring your lunch, and you work so hard you never have time to make a fire and cook hot food. By the time you get home you're so tired, you eat cold food, too. So landless workers are called 'cold meals.'"

Later, when we talk with Adelir's mother, Irene, about life before the Movement, she will say to us, "You see, before, we weren't just landless, we were everythingless."

Pulling into the encampment, we pass a wooden shack and three men lounging in the grass nearby. One sits up on an elbow, waves, and smiles. Another, leaning against the knocked-together wooden structure, gives a sort of cheery salute. An MST flag flaps vigorously in the wind.

"That's the guardhouse," Adelir explains as we drive by. "Most encampments have them." When the ninety families arrived four years ago, the landowner, like many, hired gunmen to get them off the land. Across Brazil, landowners have even publicly stated that they will "assassinate workers if they threaten their property."[12] Yet few have been prosecuted for violence against the MST. In fact, Adelir explains, local police, often siding with landowners, have been known to attack the MST as well.

"What would the guards do when the gunmen or police came?" Anna asks.

"The guards let off fireworks to alert people in the encampment. Everybody comes." As I imagine people rushing to the guardhouse to face down the threat, I remember João Pedro's words: "MST's strength is not weapons, it's people."

After a year of intermittent attacks, the landlord finally gave up, Adelir explains. Now, three years later, families here still have a tense wait while the government assesses the land's value and finalizes the transfer.

Minutes later, we sit outside an MST standard-issue. Every family here lives in a small shack of black plastic sheets. From a distance I assume the plastic is just waterproofing over walls of some sort. As we get closer I see that no, the plastic *is* the wall, wrapped around bamboo poles. Pulling out my notebook, it dawns on me that those black-plastic-covered boxes on the floor of the seminar room made perfect sense—this is what "home" looks like to much of the MST.

Baby chicks peep at our feet as we talk with a family who has been here since those early attacks—Luis and Selga Barch, their five children and baby grandson. Their blue eyes, blond hair, and weathered faces, like Dust Bowl portraits in a Dorothea Lange photograph, belie any uninformed notion of "Latin" America. Their stock is Polish and German. Adelir, our guide, has German roots as well.

Despite the midday sun, it's still so cold out that my fingers stiffen as I try to take notes. (How can they all be wearing flip-flops? I wonder.) Enjoying the faint farmyard smell and the sound of the plastic crinkling in the breeze, I'm immediately at ease with the Barches. I notice how affectionate they are with each other—passing a bubbly baby among family members, putting a hand on a knee or a shoulder, and leaning side by side during our conversation.

"We heard about the MST on the local radio," Luis tells us when we ask how they found out about the Movement. "They were calling for people interested in joining an occupation." We learn that the MST operates more than thirty of these community radio stations—all part of its attempt to counteract the mega-media monopoly here.

"Yes, we were afraid," Luis adds. "But we had no options; our land was too rocky, too small."

As I listen, I try to imagine living through four years of waiting for official approval, protected from the elements by nothing more than a sheet of black plastic. When I ask them about the earlier landowner attacks, they look at each other.

"Yes, that was a hard time," Selga says. "We would all go to the guardhouse when we saw the fireworks. We didn't want to leave the children alone, so we'd take them with us."

We talk about their wait for the government machinery finally to declare their legal right to the land as guaranteed in the constitution. Until the land is officially transferred, they are in limbo.

"We can't build, we can't invest," says Luis, wearing a red shirt and pale-purple pants, his leather shoes split at the sides.

As we all talk, Anna and I think about the productive potential being lost while the government delays the official transfer. So we ask how they explain the government's slow pace.

Adelir, our young driver, jumps in. "It's because the government's idea of development is worlds apart from the MST. The government wants everyone to move to the cities. They want the countryside for large export plantations."

His words might have sounded extreme if I hadn't known Brazil's history. Since the mid-'60s, government policies favoring large export plantations—which provide fewer jobs than do small farms and displace small landholders—have fueled the migration of over 30 million rural people to Brazil's cities just since 1970. Crowded *favelas* without the resources to build healthy communities have triggered an upsurge in Brazil's crime rate, terrifying everyone. In a São Paulo weekend, eighty murders is not unusual.

Adelir continues, "The Brazilian government is privatizing everything—electric power, transportation, sanitation. This system has created the inequality we have now—and wealthy landowners sitting on idle land, unwilling to give it up."

We're curious as to whether the Barches, and Adelir, too, believe they can reach wealthy people with their message; whether the landowners might change and willingly give up land, especially all those acres they're not using anyway.

"We don't know," Selga says, "Rich people are more interested in money, but we hope they'll do what's fair. It would make life easier, but we shouldn't wait for it."

I sense no hatred or demonization but a tough practicality in their stance.

Before Anna and I say goodbye, we want to understand better how they survive against all the challenges. Again, they look at one another.

"The poor don't have anything but their families," Selga says. "We don't have things; we don't have possessions. Everything that means something to us is in our families, and the family keeps us strong."

HOW CLOSE?

Months later, in my cramped Cambridge office, I'm distracted by an e-mail. It's a couple of lines long; a short report from a Brazilian news service. The title is simply: LANDLESS WORKERS KILLED IN CONFRONTATION WITH LANDOWNERS. This news is the latest reminder of the violence against the MST, a violence which has meant the deaths of more MST members fighting for land than all of the Brazilians "disappeared" during the country's twenty-one-year military dictatorship.

I read on. "Six gunmen attacked thirty landless families [in the encampment of] Lagoa do Serrote Fazenda, already in the process of official expropriation. One man, 28, shot and killed. Also shot, eight other landless workers including a 7-year-old girl and a pregnant woman."

I'm instantly transported from my centrally heated apartment, with its soothing music, to the Barches' shack. I'm there again: the bumpy wooden seat, the cold against our faces, the metal teapot hanging from a nail on the wall of their two-room lean-to. I hear the Barches telling us that even after official expropriation had begun—after the government land-reform agency had acknowledged their constitutional right to claim their land, but before official title transfer—they, too, had been attacked by the landowner's hired gunmen. How close, I wonder again, had they come to being killed?   —Anna

"CAPITALISM DOESN'T CARE ABOUT THE INDIVIDUAL"

After our visit to the encampments, we spend a few days in Curitiba, the capital of Paraná, before heading out into the countryside again. I'm intrigued by Curitiba, in part because, before leaving home, I'd seen a presentation at MIT about the city and its environmental-design breakthroughs. Today, I even forced Anna to photograph, of all things, city bus stops: gated platforms where you pay before the bus arrives, a small idea that saves fuel and time.

I find myself thinking about family again over dinner with two brothers, Dirceu and Vilmar Boufleuer, twenty-eight and twenty-two, and our interpreter in an all-you-can-eat pizzeria. Every few minutes with clocklike regularity, another waiter brings by platters of thin slices, each time with different toppings. In the packed restaurant, the dozen people at the next table talk heatedly about politics over their nth bottle of beer.

We've just met Dirceu and Vilmar at the MST's Curitiba headquarters this afternoon. We invited them to dinner so we could find out more about why they got involved with the MST. The pizza place was their idea.

"I was a seminarian," says Dirceu, whose cropped blond hair and flushed face make him look more like a surfer, "but felt I wasn't doing enough. I decided my faith called me to actually do something more practical." MST became that something.

"Christianity and MST are similar," Vilmar adds. "They both value people and oppose social discrimination. They are against the accumulation of capital by the few."

At this, most of the Christians I know would cringe. At home, most Americans assume that opposing capitalism is tantamount to endorsing communism—and communism, well . . . didn't Marx call religion the opiate of the people? But here, Vilmar is saying that it's impossible for him to be true to his Christian faith and, at the same time, to accept the suffering capitalism brings about in his country.

While Vilmar bites into an oozing slice of garlic pizza, Dirceu finishes his thought: "Capitalism cares only about production; it doesn't care about the individual."

It strikes me as we sit here with these two earnest young men, thousands of miles from our home in capitalist America, that what they're saying contradicts all we're taught about the value of capitalism: We're told it is the victory of the individual over the state. Here, Dirceu and Vilmar are saying that capitalism means the subordination of the individual to those who control production, and to the state backing them. Since we arrived, we've been hearing about MST creating businesses to function within the market, so it's clear that it's not the market *itself* that these young men find violates their faith. Rather it's the elevation of the market above all other values, including people's dignity and health.

FACING FEAR

We learned earlier in the day that Dirceu, this mild-mannered ex-seminarian, is being sued, personally, on MST-related charges. Now he tells us at dinner that he is facing thirty suits, and my mind boggles at the number. When we ask about the consequences if he's found guilty in any of them, our translator answers: "Lots of jail time."

Dirceu adds, quietly, "I've also had several death threats."

As the pizza and beer keep coming, we learn that Dirceu is hardly alone. A barrage of lawsuits is one strategy landowners and the government are using to thwart the MST. Dirceu's charges are typical of the ones faced by many others, including Izabel, the former nun whom we met at the seminar. Common charges include *formação de quadrilha,* literally "gang formation," which means associating with five or more people with clear intention of breaking the law. Since trespassing is breaking the law, it dawns on me that any meeting of the landless to plan an occupation of idle land could be considered "gang formation." Another is *porte illegal de armas,* which means carrying "illegal" weapons, including sickles, knives, and machetes—in other words, the farm tools typically carried by the landless during demonstrations.

Besides learning about the way the law is being used against the MST, we learn about another strategy—violence—as Dirceu fills us in on what we'd heard called a "massacre" at the Pitanga seminar.

In early May of 2000, fifty busloads of MST members heading to Curitiba for a demonstration calling for speedier land transfer were blocked by military police. (Estimates of how many police vary depending on who's making them—from dozens to a thousand.[13]) The MST reports that the police opened fire on the buses with a cocktail of rubber bullets, tear gas and live ammunition. An estimated 200 MST members were wounded, and two were killed.[14]

The police claim the MST was blocking the highway and that, while the police were removing the peasants, they attacked. To this day, the military police say they acted in self-defense.

This is the military police of governor Jaime Lerner—the same man whom I had heard so much about at the MIT presentation on Curitiba and later in Bill McKibben's book, *Hope, Human and Wild,* in which Lerner is the visionary genius of urban planning and transportation design.[15] But now, we hear nothing of Lerner's environmental consciousness, only that the violence against the MST is the worst in his state—and portends a national escalation of violence.

Sitting at the end of the table at the pizzeria, I see my reflection distorted by the cracked mirror-squares that make up the wall facing me. As I try to imagine the person I see in the mirror walking the path of these two brothers, I wonder what enables them to face their fear. Over slices of pizza improbably topped with corn and pineapple, the conversation moves away from violence, and something in what they say next begins to provide the answers I'm searching for.

FROM "YES SIR!" TO "I THINK THAT . . ."

As in so many conversations with people at every level in the MST, our talk soon turns to education. In its settlements, the MST works with more than 1,000 schools, reaching roughly 50,000 children. We're impressed by the scale. We're impressed that they're even thinking about education at all, given their survival challenges.

In describing the MST's curriculum, Vilmar says, "MST teaches philosophy to children in the lowest grades."

At this I am puzzled. My idea of philosophy is Plato or Kant, not exactly the domain of eight-year-olds. But then I brace myself: Maybe this is it. Maybe by "philosophy" they mean the kind of Marxist indoctrination the newspapers had warned about.

"We teach children to look around them and not to accept what they see as given," Vilmar explains. "By philosophy, we mean encouraging them to ask questions, to ask how things should be, and how they want them to be."

His words remind me of the picturebook that João Pedro had given us on the first day: a book of drawings by children in their settlements the MST publishes each year. This year, the children drew their images of the Brazil of their dreams. They were asked, *"What kind of Brazil do you want?"*

As Vilmar talks, I recall one most clearly. Above a Crayola-brown Brazil shaded in with green was a sun with words extending from each of its rays: *Justiçia, Igualdade, Paz, Amor, Fraternidade, Dignidade.* Justice, Equality, Peace, Love, Fraternity, Dignity. And I think of the model settlement on the tile floor of the seminar room in Pitanga, where these children's parents were being asked, *"What kind of settlement do you want?"*

The brothers explain that the MST curriculum is based on the insights of Paulo Freire—an internationally respected Brazilian educational innovator and writer. Freire's approach, spelled out in his *Pedagogy of the Oppressed*, liberates poor people's self-confidence through confronting unspoken assumptions that things can't change and encouraging students to value themselves and their direct experience—so devalued in most formal education.

I'm starting to grasp how these brothers might have found their strength to face the very real threats. First, we must believe that what exists now, what we see around us, is not inevitable.

The conversation brings to mind something João Pedro had told us when we talked with him about the earliest days of the MST. He explained the process of poor people gaining the courage to stand up for themselves—during a time, as he says, "when any mention of land reform could get you arrested, even though it was mandated by the constitution.

"The first step is losing naïve consciousness," João Pedro emphasized, "no longer accepting what you see as something that cannot be changed." (I'm amused by the irony that here in the U.S. it's the opposite. A person gets labeled naïve who believes that things *can* change.) "The second," João Pedro continued, "is reaching the awareness that you won't get anywhere unless you work together.

"This shift in consciousness, once you get it, is like riding a bike: no one can take it from you. So, you forget how to say 'yes, sir' and learn to say 'I think that . . .' This is when the citizen is born.

"This change of consciousness is hard to measure statistically," João Pedro reminded us. "You can't count it the way you can the number of families we settle or the number of hectares the MST makes productive. But it is equally, if not more, important."

João Pedro wants us to understand that the MST's biggest achievement may not be in land reform, exactly, nor in multiplying five-fold the incomes of the formerly landless, nor in helping people build dignified places to live, nor even in drastically reducing infant mortality in settlements.[16] It may be in its creation of citizens, people who believe they can create what does not yet exist.

WHOSE CHOICES? WHAT CHOICE?

João Pedro's thoughts and the voices of Vilmar and Dirceu sit with me—as do the countless slices of pizza. But the skeptic's voice nags.

If everything is done together, and at the same time, if critical awareness means knowing you can make choices and not just go along with the dominant voices, then within the MST, can you really opt for what *you* think is right for you, even if it doesn't fit the cooperative MST mold?

The MST says it's helping people make the internal shift from "Yes, sir" to "I think that . . ."—helping people free themselves from the fear of being out of step. But is it? Or is the MST just a different drumbeat with which one must align one's step?

Imagine being a landless worker, always doing the bidding of others, moving from job to job as a "cold meal"—through a lifetime of being told someone else makes the decisions, you do the work. Then you sign on to a land occupation out of utter desperation, and suddenly, almost overnight, you jump from cold-meal status to co-creator of a community. You are in charge.

Or are you? Is it even possible to become a decision-maker, given your limited and stunting life experience? Are you and other beneficiaries of land transfers necessarily at the mercy of the MST leaders' agenda, for good or bad?

We look for signs of real choice.

During the encampment stage, after you've occupied the unused land but still don't have legal status, you and the other families decide together how to organize your community. Or that's what MST official Geraldo Fontes explained to us on our first day at MST headquarters.

In my notebook, I have a neatly sketched replica of drawings Geraldo made to clarify his points. Geraldo is Mexican, and had once worked in radio in Denver, Colorado, but he came here because he so believes in what the MST is doing. I recall his delicate fingers holding each of the dozens of cigarettes he smoked with the same intensity with which he spoke. Over many hours, he filled pages of blank paper as he sketched this way through our conversation.

Geraldo drew three rectangles representing the way settlements organize themselves. Less than a third, we learn, choose to incorporate legally as a cooperative in which all work and profits are shared. Forty percent choose completely private plots. The rest opt for a large common area as well as private plots. Given the MST's commitment to cooperative values, I wonder how truly voluntary the choice is.

It isn't long before we will see these choices in action.

Only two days later, we're standing in the MST settlement *Perpetual Seguro* (Perpetual Security) near Pitanga—where the bus dropped us that first frigid morning. The settlement sits on a high bluff overlooking rolling green hills and, in the valley, a small pond. A dozen children giggle and point at us while they wait for the community bus to take them into town for school.

Our interpreter interrupts Nivaldo Fernando to introduce us. His sharp features and generous smile are marked by deep lines engraved by many days working in the sun, making him appear far older than his thirty-eight years. We learn that he has lived in this encampment, in black plastic, for four years, waiting. Waiting.

Now he stands, hammer in hand, building his own first home. When we ask how soon he'll be moving in, Nivaldo answers, "Helping each other, we can build a house in twenty-five days."

We'd been told that among the forty families here today, few were part of the original encampment, and we're curious as to why so many are newcomers.

"They have come because of our cooperative," Nivaldo says. "You can make more money with the co-op."

"Why?" we press further.

"Each individual can specialize," Nivaldo explains. "My specialty is building and also selling the quilts we make. In the beginning, everyone did everything. But this is better."

"Who decides on your specialty?"

"The group decides based on what people are good at and what's needed."

"And if there's a conflict?"

"We discuss it. But look, it was my choice to come here. It was my choice to be in the cooperative, so of course I'll want to do what the group decides."

"What if someone isn't doing their job?" Anna asks. "Couldn't they just slack off and still get their part of the profits?" I assume she's worrying about the "free-rider" problem economists obsess about—in this case, that without an owner in charge, lazy workers will shirk their responsibilities and take advantage of the hard-working ones.

"You record your hours, and you're paid based on how much you work. So people still see how they directly benefit from working hard." (Later we'll see a timesheet diligently filled in by women who make quilts.) "But in a cooperative, we also know that our hard work is going to help everybody else, too. It feels good knowing you're making a contribution. Plus, say I'm building houses and you're harvesting the corn and the weather is bad, we all share that loss. It's not fair to blame the farmer if it doesn't rain, is it?"

Of the forty families in this settlement, almost one-third work entirely cooperatively. Twenty-six work the land individually, but they share ownership of the machines—the tractors, harvester, and buses.

New Hope

It's late afternoon by the time we arrive at Nova Esperança (New Hope), but we still get the full tour of the settlement. We visit their school, meet the cows and pigs, and see the collectively bought gargantuan tractor that looks like something from *Aliens*. I'm still trying to fathom how the families built all this from scratch in just fifteen years when we meet the six women running the settlement's sewing cooperative.

The women decided to start the cooperative after they realized that MST members were buying their clothes from big companies outside the MST, when they could be making them themselves. So, the community paid for technical training, and the women opened this small shop that now sells its products to nearby settlements and encampments.

Silkscreens hang from the walls, and stacks of inventory are piled around us, ready to be moved out. As we talk, a newborn bundled in light-blue blankets is passed among the women.

When I ask how business is going, they laugh. "It's going well, but we just reopened." As a group of their children careens into the room, giggling and teasing each other, one woman explains: "We closed for a couple of months. One of us was sick and we wanted to help take care of her family and visit her in the hospital."

Talking with these women, I think back to my own attempt at cooperative living. It was a mediocre success, at best, and we had none of the real challenges these women face: We were just college students escaping dorm life and dining-hall food. I had wanted to believe we humans could share and cooperate, as this community does. But honestly, I didn't believe we could. These women, the calm baby, the giggling children, force me to rethink. Maybe we do have the capacity. Maybe this kind of cooperation is even happening all around us. But since our culture tells us it's not possible, we don't see it.

—Anna

"The cooperative seems to work well, so why aren't other families choosing to work this way?" we ask Nivaldo's wife, Doraci, a few minutes later in the quilt-making room down the hill.

"Most are still afraid," Doraci says. "Small farmers don't like to rely on others. They don't want to join; they're afraid they won't be as free. But we make the rules ourselves, for practical reasons. A lot of the original people didn't want to be part of the cooperative, so they went to other encampments. Now, many want to come back because the cooperative is working."

A lot of shifting and sorting out—that's what we're sensing here and elsewhere. People trying on new roles and seeing what works. Experimenting. They're experimenting not only with the organization of work but with the type of enterprise as well. Starting with nothing, the fourteen cooperative families have, in only a few years, created five "production units," Doraci explains—for grains, tea, milk, fish, and the quilts.

"We add ten-percent profit when we sell to others. Within the Movement, we sell at cost," she adds, to make clear another way that MST families benefit from these new productive activities.

From the quilt room, we walk farther down the hill to a sturdy brick building the size of a two-car garage that houses the donors of the fluffy stuff Doraci and her colleagues use to fill the quilts—dozens of healthy-looking lambs and sheep.

Furiously taking notes about everything we see, it's easy to let the real significance of it all pass us by: that landless, unschooled people, living under the most insecure, oppressive conditions, are able to come together, learn what they need to know—from fish culture to wool processing—to create new businesses and meaningful, dignified lives. And I thought putting together a small nonprofit in the U.S. was challenging!

To me, this creativity offers the most persuasive evidence that coercion in the Movement is low. In my experience, coercion and creativity don't mix.

WHO MAKES THE RULES?

From cold Pitanga we return to Curitiba, where it's so sunny we risk shedding a few layers. From there, we head more than forty miles south to a different-looking encampment. Here, the black plastic shacks dotting the earth make a striking contrast with what must at one time have been an elegant estate: a cluster of red-tiled stucco buildings perched on a hill with a view of rolling countryside.

We arrive at an encampment on the verge of becoming a legal settlement. The large manor house has already been converted, we soon discover, into an

MST training center. Modern track lighting shines down on what no doubt was the stately dining room of one of the wealthiest families around. Our hosts point out the window to former slave quarters.

We're happy that it's almost lunchtime, not only because our stomachs are growling, but also because we've been invited to dine inside a shack, where at least we'll be protected from the sharp wind.

Sitting inside on a wooden bench, we face a big iron cooking stove. Behind us is a blue-and-white sideboard with dishes and pots. Cradling a hot, hearty lunch of black beans, cabbage, thick noodles, and rice, we ask our hosts Antonio and Antonia Capitani, and several other MST members who've joined us, how life is organized in this soon-to-be-official MST settlement of 110 families.

They tell us that about half of the "family groups"—the basic unit of the Movement, usually ten families—have chosen to work the land cooperatively, half individually.

"The family groups might get together every three days or twice a day, depending on what's going on," Antonio tells us. "They deal with everything—work, health, education, marketing, finance."

Each family group elects a leader, and here Antonio is it. "But I'm not the boss," he jumps in quickly to clarify. "I don't have the right to decide for the family groups. My task is just organizing everybody."

Of course, I think to myself, with a quarter of a million families in several thousand settlements—like any community, they need rules. In the MST, settlement members come up with the regulations themselves.

"Drinking alcohol only inside your own house" is the first example Antonio offers. "Or theft—the rule here is that any stealing, no matter how small, means you get expelled. You also get expelled for hunting. It's not allowed anywhere in Brazil and not here, certainly. Each person has to sign the regulations to show their commitment," Antonio continues. "Here in this encampment, everyone has signed."

The black plastic around us ripples with the wind as we talk, creating a sound that's by now familiar, a constant reminder of the hardship these families endure.

"When we got married, we worked as sharecroppers," Antonio tells us, taking us back to the time when they were still landless. "We only got thirty percent of the crop we grew, and we couldn't make it on that.

"We heard about the MST from the farmers' union and the church, but at first it was hard to believe we would get a plot of land. It was too good to be true. We couldn't believe it because we knew the government was against it, too. But we had no alternatives.

"That was in the beginning, 1984, and there was still a lot of repression. When we first started, it was hard to talk about the problem of the landless. You couldn't wear MST caps or shirts. No one was allowed to gather in large groups.

"But then wasn't as scary as it is today," he adds, with no change in his serious but unagitated expression.

I'm surprised. "It's scarier now than under a military dictatorship?" I ask.

"We're aware of so much more now," Antonio explains. His friend sitting with us finishes his thought: "Before, we didn't realize how many poor people there were. The poverty is so much clearer now, and with any demonstration today we have police repression. Now that we're stronger, the repression is stronger."

"So do you think the MST will survive these attacks?" Anna asks.

Jacir Pagnussatti, a young man with light red hair and a worn-at-the-elbows jean jacket, answers with conviction: "The only way to end the MST is to end landlessness." Everyone nods.

DIFFERENT FAMILY VALUES

As in the pizza conversation with Vilmar and Dirceu, our discussion soon turns to what they are building, not what they fear. Jacir stresses that lack of education is one of the two major obstacles they are working to overcome. (The other is the media, not surprising after the portrayal of the MST we saw in the papers.)

Most people in the settlements have little education. "Generally, the child of a small farmer doesn't get to the fifth grade," Antonio tells us, helping us to understand why the MST schools are so important. As he talks, we can hear his four children playing just outside the black plastic.

"You learn more in one year here in our school than in eight years of typical school," says Jacir.

"So how is it different from the standard curriculum?" I ask.

"The first thing is effectiveness. Everything we teach is based in what the kids see all around them—agriculture. We teach math and science and biology through what the children see every day—growing corn, for example."

This Paulo Freire approach of starting with the known and building on the learner's direct experience has another benefit that MST members repeatedly stress to us. Implicitly, it communicates that a rural way of life has inherent value. This goes to the heart of what MSTers tell us their movement is all about—values.

And it's here—in the realm of values—that the MST differs, they emphasized, from the "neo-liberal model" that focuses narrowly on production unrelated to the well-being of the whole community. It's the neo-liberal model, they say, that's turned their country into one of the world's top three agricultural exporters and the number-one exporter of coffee, sugar, and orange juice. It's this production focus, with an eye on exports rather than on whether Brazilians eat, that has also pushed their country to second place among soybean exporters and third from the top in chicken and beef exports. It's also why two-thirds of Brazil's grain goes to feed not people but livestock.[17] All this production power, yet 23 million Brazilians go hungry—that's what's wrong with the neo-liberal model, we hear.

It's funny to our ears to hear unschooled farmers talk about the neo-liberal model, but that phrase has profound meaning for them—it is what the government is pushing and the opposite of what they see themselves working toward. The neo-liberal model, in their eyes, devalues rural life built around community and mutual aid.

"In it, people are used as means to an end," Vilmar tells us, "to produce for those who can afford to buy. In the MST, our goal is to treat everyone as a full human being, not as a means."

As we huddle on benches inside the shack, Jacir's wife, noticeably pregnant, joins us as if to underscore the importance of educating the next generation. Jacir continues to describe what is different about MST schools. "We teach children to think about the community, not just about the individual. We have to do this in schools, because TV teaches the opposite—only individualism."

"How can you teach kids to think of others?" we probe.

"Well, as an example, students help prepare meals for each other," Antonio replies, and Anna and I smile and tell our hosts about the Edible Schoolyard in California where students are doing just that. Later we learn that older children help out in the nurseries with the younger ones so their parents can work. "They start learning how to share," he adds.

As we talk, neighbors come in and out of our shack enjoying the ample lunch these families have cooked, not just for us but for them, too. And I'm grateful as Antonio adds a few more pieces of wood to the stove.

"For the older children, we help them understand what can happen to teenagers in the cities—the violence and high unemployment—so they don't get deceived by the glamour they see on TV," Antonio says. "We organize exchange programs with other settlements so our children get a bigger view of what the MST is creating. We also invite college students from the cities to work with us. A group of them made that map you saw on the office wall pinpointing all the MST settlements in Brazil."

Jacir returns to the theme we've heard from the beginning of our visit: developing the capacity to question *what is* and asking whether it matches one's own values.

"Children are learning to question their parents, too," he says. "That would have been impossible ten years ago. But kids are learning from their own experience that we all have the same rights. In some families, the parents don't like their children speaking out. They say, 'Okay, are you running this place?'" At this, everyone breaks out laughing, suggesting to me that some of these parents haven't always enjoyed it when their own children feel so entitled.

"My parents worked so hard day after day," Antonio says, trying to help us understand his motivation. "But at the end of the year they still had nothing—nothing at all. My father was filled with rage. When I was young, he would beat us with a whip."

Antonio squeezes his wife's hand and explains, "When our first child was born, we talked about what kind of parents we wanted to be. We didn't want our children to have the same life we did."

And we learn that this emphasis on values is connected to why, as a community, they decided to grow their crops organically, as part of creating "the Brazil they want." Nationally, the MST has been promoting organic and sustainable farming methods throughout its settlements. It's even funded some members to pursue higher degrees in non-chemical techniques. It was in fact the MST that created Brazil's first organic seed line, Bionatur.

"It took time," acknowledges Antonio, "for people to understand why we shouldn't use pesticides." He echoes what João Pedro lamented: It's tough to convince farmers to use an organic approach when chemicals give instant results.

At that point, Antonio's eight-year-old daughter, Franciele—her blond, shiny hair falling on a simple red dress—comes into the shack and leans against her father, as she has from time to time. Her cheeks are flushed after playing outside in the biting wind with her friends.

"I know what pesticides do," Antonio says. "I spent four days in the hospital with lung and kidney problems because of pesticides. The doctors who work for the landowners don't want to tell you that pesticides are the problem."

"So are the dangers of pesticides to you—the farmers—what is motivating the MST to try to shift members to organic farming?" I ask.

Jacir jumps in to answer, "It's not just that farming without using pesticides means less hazard and lower costs for us. Why would we go to all this trouble and risk to grow food that's just going to hurt people? We are concerned about the people in the cities, too."

My last image of the encampment is of Franciele and her buddies, healthy looking, with bright eyes and happy faces. In the late afternoon sun, they are laughing, teasing each other, and doing cartwheels in the tall golden grass near their families' shacks.

THE MARKET MIRAGE

So it's Franciele and her friends I think of when we return to São Paulo on our last day and learn from Geraldo that the MST is alarmed about a project designed in Washington.

Declaring that the present approach to land reform just isn't working—proven by continuing violence in the countryside and millions still waiting for land—the World Bank, with the Brazilian government's support, has come up with an alternative. It's been piloted in several Brazilian states and just received World Bank go-ahead.

The Bank calls its approach "market-based" land reform because it takes the government out of the process. In the present approach, it's the federal land-reform agency that determines which land is idle, determines its value in the courts, and expropriates the land for the landless—a process that can be excruciatingly slow. (Remember, the Barches had been waiting years for official title so they could move out of their plastic shacks.) So, says the Bank, remove the government, simply bring "willing sellers" and "willing buyers" to the table, and the result will be more efficient and effective.

But the MST disagrees. They, along with most groups working for land reform in Brazil, are worried about the World Bank plan. I think I understand, at least partly, why the MST is so worried.

The Bank's strategy, in a nutshell, is to encourage small groups of the landless independent of any organized movement to select land that they want and then negotiate a "fair market price" with landowners. The government then backs the landless with loans for buying the property and for initial investment to make it productive. It seems straightforward, but there's one big hitch. There is no such thing as a "fair market price" in Brazil's countryside. Most landowners didn't pay for their land in the first place. They either inherited it or received it in exchange for political favors . . . or, remember the *grilagem* (the cricket fraud)? During the 1960s and '70s, huge areas were essentially given away as the military government encouraged relocation into the country's interior. Also, the MST asks, how can a desperate, landless family with no social power hold out for a fair price from wealthy people who likely have no urgent need to sell? And why would the better-off sell anything other than the least-fertile pieces of their land?

That's why the MST sticks to its position: The *government* must remain responsible for determining which land is unproductive, assigning value to it, and transferring it fairly to landless people. And to keep the pressure on, the MST's land occupations are vital.

The World Bank perceives the market as working, but the MST says the market works only when the starting blocks are all set fairly and equally. Let the market reign free in a climate of extreme inequality like Brazil's, however, and you only reinforce historical, persistent injustices.

There's another perception gap, too. The MST sees the World Bank's approach as another sign that the Bank just doesn't get it. Escaping poverty involves the whole person, not just land, and, the MST is learning, that means building new communities—learning new skills and attitudes and creating new enterprises and schools. Any reform focused primarily on land exchange, argues the MST, cannot ignite this deeper process of human development.

THE BATTLE FOR HUMAN NATURE

Most people I know have become pretty suspicious of movements that claim great moral purpose. They get nervous. Given how self-centered most of us are, such movements become so frustrated with their raw material—we mere human beings—that they inevitably end up coercing, forcibly trying to get us to behave in ways that are not natural; they start using power for their own ends. That's the assumption, the fear.

So when we get a chance, we ask how the MST develops cooperative values among its members. One opportunity appears when we meet with José

Paulo dos Santos Pires, whom we had seen do his thing during the seminar: a mini-lecture on the economics of tea processing. Despite the late hour, he kept everyone with him. "He's the brains here," our interpreter had whispered to us as Paulo drew charts on the blackboard to make his points.

We're with him now at the MST tea-processing plant he manages, built with a Belgian charity's help. By marketing the tea as well as processing it, MST members capture greater profits from their labor, we learn. Clearly, the MST's critique of capitalism does not mean it opposes using the market.

Paulo, a serious but warm man in a red MST cap and sweatshirt, spends the afternoon patiently answering our questions. He's been with the MST virtually since its founding and acknowledges that the emphasis on values we've heard about from so many is "very recent." It's only been around in the last four or five years.

"You see, society as a whole cultivates individualism and competition," he says. "It rewards the people who have the most power. We in the MST have been brought up under this system. This creates problems in some of the older settlements where we didn't talk much about values.

"A lot of people thought that if they got land, that would be enough. But soon they find out that they are still facing so many problems; they are still il-literate, and they have no resources to make the land productive.

"They realize with time, not immediately but through debates and semi-nars, that land is not enough. They begin to understand that they have to get together to decide what to plant and how to get money to buy seeds. Their children have to go to school, but they have no school, so they have to build one. If they are sick and there's no one to help, they realize that land is not everything. They realize that if they want to make their lives better, they have to participate. They may have to join a demonstration, even occupy City Hall to get a school for their children. They acquire consciousness that they wouldn't be able to do any of this individually.

"The first ten years, we focused on land only, although the principles were born there. Creating our own schools helped us focus on values—what do we want our young people to learn?"

As we listen to Paulo in this cheery office, light pine walls and bookshelves reflecting the sun streaming in through the big windows, I see a man sure of his own values. But he is no zealot. "Practice is our middle name," he says, em-phasizing ongoing learning.

Always present in me is the skeptic's voice. Are these people trying to turn human beings inside-out? Or, could it be that Anna's and my hunch about human beings' need for connection with others and a purpose larger than ourselves is being born out by this extraordinary social experiment?

Here is one of the few places on earth where people are, in a sense, attempting a new society and one within an opposing dominant culture—global, corporate capitalism. It may be the only place on earth where people are attempting to meet this challenge on such a large scale, now directly affecting millions.

Many in the MST argue that it's not they who are trying to twist human nature into some unnatural contortion. That's what the dominant culture is doing to us every day. "The media and the whole culture are in a permanent campaign to project values," João Pedro told us as we sat sipping sweet dark coffee with him in São Paulo, "as if people are happy and important when they consume, and when they project their egoism and individualism. They tell us all we want is to consume. But these are fundamentally antisocial values."

I told João Pedro about an article Anna had shown me, which proclaimed that "the triumph of consumerism is the triumph of the popular will."[18] The media want us to believe that's true, João Pedro said, but he and the people in the MST think differently: "Human beings need something more to be happy."

On the way out the door to Logan Airport for our flight from Boston to São Paulo, I'd thrown a copy of Barry Schwartz's book, *The Battle for Human Nature,* into my backpack. I figured I might want to divert my mind at some point from harsh realities to more philosophic thoughts. It didn't dawn on me then that what I was about to witness in Brazil would be nothing less than that: the battle for human nature.

CHAPTER 4

BEAUTIFUL
HORIZON

*To search for solutions to hunger means to act
within the principle that the status of a citizen surpasses that of a mere consumer.*

CITY OF BELO HORIZONTE

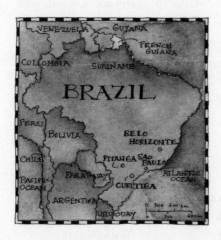

A long overnight bus ride north from São Paulo takes us to Belo Horizonte, Brazil's fourth largest city. We're in Belo Horizonte—"beautiful horizon"—for one reason: It's the only city we know of in the capitalist world that has decided to make food security a right of citizenship.

There are actually two Belos, we quickly realize, as on this morning we find ourselves at the crossroads between them.

On one side, a towering hill is dotted with palatial houses, their large windows glistening in the sun. On the other side, one of the city's worst *favelas* clings to a steep hill. In the crook between is a pond and a police station, with POLICIA in letters large enough to be read from either side. Just beside these towering letters we spot our destination—an airy, warehouse-sized market selling affordable, locally grown produce.

Walking inside, we are immediately dazzled by abundance: mounds of fresh carrots, peppers, eggplant, rutabaga, pumpkins, beets, watermelons, onions, you name it. Handwritten signs hanging above the wall-to-wall produce read 35 CENTS A KILO. We soon learn that the price is set by the city and is nearly half what nearby grocers charge. In exchange for keeping prices down, the city gives sellers like this one access to prime real-estate spots at cut-rate prices. With every item sold at the same low price, shoppers from both of the neighborhoods straddling the store eagerly fill their plastic bags.

Moments before, when we descended the narrow, steep streets of the nearby *favela,* giggling three- and four-year-olds waved goodbye to us from their nursery school's window. In a sparkling-clean lunchroom, we'd just watched them chow down on one of their four nutritious meals of the day, all provided by the city.

Earlier in the day, we'd talked with a local farmer selling fresh produce from a bright-green stall on city-owned land. In her cheerful green smock decorated with the words DIRECT FROM THE COUNTRYSIDE she grinned as she told us, "I'm able to support three children from my five acres now. Since I got this contract with the city, I've even been able to buy a truck."

Dotted around Belo are more than forty other farmers like her selling their organic produce thanks to a leg up from the city. Her success means even more to us when we learn that farmers' income in Brazil in the mid-'90s dropped by almost half.[1]

From the packed produce market, we head for lunch at the *Restaurante Popular*—the people's restaurant—another city-run operation, serving almost 4,000 hearty meals a day at less than half the market price.

EATING LIKE CITIZENS

In our country, we take the right to education for granted. And though we don't have national health care, we expect the government to pay for care for those with no resources. Of course, eating healthy food is a prerequisite both to learning and to staying healthy, yet for most people "eating" and "rights of citizenship" aren't chewable in the same mouthful.

Not true in Belo Horizonte.

The bustling produce market, the well-fed children, the local farmer's stall, the cut-rate lunch—all are examples of the dozens of striking innovations popping up since 1993 in this city. That's when the city started thinking differently about ending hunger, partly in response to the cruel fact that one-fifth of the city's youngest children were suffering from malnutrition and many in the city lived on the edge of poverty.

"We believe the status of citizen surpasses that of consumer," explains Adriana Aranha, the woman in charge of the many-faceted activities aimed at ensuring everyone in Belo has access not just to enough calories, but also to quality food.

Adriana, a tiny, vibrant woman with long, glistening black hair and a generous smile, is also our host here—tour guide to the city's innovations. In her bright office with a large ficus plant and a poster we quickly recognize as from the MST, she works patiently with our interpreter to help us understand what is behind this "new social mentality," as she calls it—what citizenship means when it comes to nourishment. "Everyone in our city benefits if all of us have access to good food, so—like health care or education—quality food for all is a public good," Adriana continues.

She explains that while food may be a commodity, "food security"—having enough food to feed yourself and your family—is a human right, a right by virtue of being a citizen. If the market is shutting out people too poor to be consumers, they are still *citizens*. It's the government's duty to step up to the plate and correct for this "market failure," as an economist might call it.

"The city decided we couldn't let people's nourishment be vulnerable to the market," Adriana says. This new attitude, she explains, "means letting go of any notion of charity. People having good food, even if they are poor, is not about charity. It's not about emergency feeding programs."

Once people started thinking this way—out of the charity trap—dozens of clever actions sprang up inside Adriana's city agency, many designed to improve the way that the market works, not supplant it.

The 35-cents-a-kilo produce store that we visited is an example. It's one of twenty-five similar sites around Belo. Adriana explains how they work: "City Hall arranges public bidding for entrepreneurs to create markets on city-owned spots around the city. For this advantage, the seller has to sell the fruits and vegetables at a price the city sets. Today's thirty-five cents was half the market price.

"For sellers with the best spots, there's another obligation attached to being able to use the city land. Every weekend they have to drive produce-laden trucks to the poor neighborhoods outside of the city center, so everyone can get good produce."

"So how do the sellers make money if they have to sell at lower prices?" Anna asks.

Adriana cites three ways: First, the city charges almost nothing for the spot. That helps, but the second part of the answer is sheer volume. And third, the seller's bottom line is boosted by the city in another way. Middlemen are cut out, so sellers are linked directly with local producers.

AGAINST THE TIDE

As we tour the city with Adriana and her colleagues, I admit to her that I'm baffled that a major Brazilian city could be successfully bucking the global ideology that says government is bad—stay out—and the market is everything.

Leaning toward me from the backseat of the van, she nods, not surprised by my surprise. "We're fighting the concept that the state is a terrible, incompetent administrator. In Brazil, it's true there's no tradition of state efficiency. But we are changing that. We're showing that the state doesn't have to provide everything; it can facilitate. It can create channels for people to find solutions themselves.

"We do things like helping to keep the market competitive."

As we bump along in the van on streets so steep that I think I'm back in San Francisco, she gives us an example: "At bus stops, over the radio, and in newspapers twice a week, we list the price of forty-five basic foods and household items at forty different supermarkets. So people know where the cheapest prices are. This makes the market function better."

We learn later that the city partners with local university researchers to keep the information current each week. Adriana continues, "We try to keep the market honest." How simple. Funny, I've never heard of a city government doing such a thing. Yet even an introductory economics course will tell you that accurate and complete information is essential to a functioning market.

I learn that what we're seeing is only a fraction of all the city's programs to make good food a fact of citizenship in Belo. Its Green Basket program links hospitals, restaurants, and other big buyers directly to roughly forty local, small, organic growers. In partnership with the city's environmental agency and a nonprofit organization, Adriana's department is also creating four "agro-ecological centers," not only to supply seeds and seedlings to its other projects, but to educate the public about eco-friendly farming techniques. The city also promotes dozens of community gardens as well as forty school gardens that are, like the Edible Schoolyard in Berkeley, "live labs," as they put it here, for teaching science and environmental studies.

"Many people in Belo came from the countryside," Adriana tells us. "They came here eating their traditional foods—dark-green leafy vegetables, fresh fruits, other vegetables. But they move to cities, see all this advertising, and start thinking it's cool to eat junk food, that soda is good for them. So part of our work is simply education—telling these people that what they ate all their lives is really healthy."

As Adriana talks, we pass through a congested neighborhood and, as if to drive home the point, the buildings and sidewalks that we see are crowded with ads promoting sodas, processed food, and fast-food restaurants.

FORTIFYING

Even in its more commonplace anti-hunger moves, Belo has figured out how to pack an uncommon punch.

In the cheery nursery we visited—with its brightly painted sidewalks and spotless interior—in one of Belo's worst slums, the city provides all four meals. And they're spiked with special flour, enriched with ground eggshells, manioc leaf powder, and other nutritious ingredients that would otherwise be thrown away. Most of the enriched flour—they give us a bag to sample—goes to 20,000 young children through the city's public health clinics. Three-quarters of the severely malnourished children receiving the flour are improving as a result.[2]

School lunches—not exactly what I usually associate with good nutrition—have had a different face, too, it seems, since the right to good food became part of citizenship here. Using the same meager thirteen cents per pupil per day that the federal government provides to all of Brazil's cities for school lunches, Belo has almost doubled the calories kids get.

But how? By using fewer processed foods and adding the eggshell-enriched flour, along with more fresh produce—bought from local producers and businesses, which cut transportation costs. Most obviously, the city increased the number of suppliers and simply let competition reduce prices.

As we hear about these commonsense strategies, I flash back to our visit to Berkeley, where the city council had just voted to serve organic, locally grown produce in its schools. Here on the other end of the globe, I wonder why more communities in between haven't hit on such sensible approaches.

NOT A SOUP KITCHEN

After a long, stimulating morning, I'm disappointed—but too embarrassed to admit it—that Adriana doesn't cut us into the long lunch line stretching out the door of the People's Restaurant. But I needn't have worried; the line moves fast, as it must to provide almost 4,000 meals a day. Within minutes, we're served large helpings of steaming beans, rice, salad, and mixed vegetables, and a banana. Others get chicken as well—and all this for about seventy cents. Despite rising prices for food, the city has held fast to this low price.

In the city's center, near the main bus station, this huge building with high ceilings feels airy, open, relaxed. We carry our trays to a long table which seems to offer the only empty seats in the house. I scan our hundreds of fellow diners and see grandparents and newborns, young couples, clusters of men, mothers with toddlers, and people eating alone. Some are in well-worn street-clothes, others are in uniform, and still others are in business suits.

No one has to prove they're poor to eat here.

"I've been coming here every day for five years and have gained six kilos,"

La Lanne Inspired

Later that night, in our Belo hotel room, I'm flipping through TV channels and stumble on the news. Stephen Sanger, Chairman and CEO of General Mills, is announcing the acquisition of Pillsbury—nearly doubling his company's size and making General Mills the fourth-largest food company in the world. Sanger proudly reports that Americans are now going to get more of what they *really* want: 80 percent of the company's products will now be "ready-to-eat" or will take less than fifteen minutes to make.

I think of the stores we just saw filled with mounds of inexpensive vegetables, and I flash to my New York City neighborhood and the offerings of my corner store. I didn't have a choice. It was ready-to-eat or it was wilted lettuce.

My head is still spinning with images of fresh carrots I can buy in one of the poorest *favelas* in Brazil—but not at home—when Larry King comes on. He's interviewing eighty-six-year-old 1950s fitness star Jack La Lanne, who is introduced as the only man who, at seventy years of age, has towed seventy boats carrying seventy people a mile and a half in the ocean, fighting strong currents, while handcuffed and with his ankles shackled. While I'm pondering beams one elderly, energetic man in a beige shirt and faded khakis. "It's a forty-kilometer trip," he adds.

"It's silly to pay more somewhere else for lower-quality food," an athletic-looking young man in a military-police uniform tells us. "I've been eating here every day for two years. It's a good way to save money to buy a house so I can get married," he says with a smile.

"I've also met a lot of people; I even organized some into football teams that play on weekends," he says, and adds, "I've been invited to barbecues—friendships grow out of eating here."

As we stand near the exit listening to this young man, we notice diners stopping on the way out to read clippings from today's papers pinned to the exit wall. "A lot of people who eat here can't afford a paper," explains Adriana.

the possibilities of that one, Mom reminisces about seeing La Lanne in stretch-suits on TV when she was a kid. He was the first Jane Fonda, she explains.

King starts firing away: "They say, oh, eat this, don't eat that. The average person out there, they're so confused. They don't know which way to go."

Jack replies, his sparkling eyes claiming the camera's focus: "If man made it, don't eat it!" I cheer him on.

Minutes later, King asks: "How come so many American children are obese?" Without missing a beat, Jack fires back: "Advertising!"

Mom and I do high-fives. Jack goes on. "You've got your great athletes. You've got all these guys selling their souls for millions of dollars. 'Drink this stuff.' 'Eat this stuff.' 'Have this candy bar.' 'Have this hamburger.' What do you think the kids are going to do? They worship these athletes. They're going to do what athletes want them to do.

"The body works for me. This body is Jack La Lanne's slave. That's why I treat it so good. You know, exercise is king, nutrition is queen. Put them together, you've got a kingdom."

With that, I'm down—I'm Jack La Lanne inspired—counting off my push-ups.

—Anna

Before we leave, we talk with the man who runs the operation. He knew Adriana in their university days. "I had my own fast-food restaurant before taking this on. Financially, that was much better," he says matter-of-factly.

"So why didn't you keep your own restaurant?" I ask.

"I like it very much here. It feels great that my work is helping people get access to food. Most people work for a goal—like getting a house—and when they've achieved it, they can work for deeper reasons; for personal satisfaction."

As we are leaving, I notice an elderly woman approach him, pat him on the back, and say softly, "It was delicious. Keep up the good work."

ONE PERCENT

As we leave the restaurant, our bellies full, and climb into the van for our next stop, I wonder aloud how other cities could ever be convinced to carry what must be the budget burden of all these initiatives.

"Actually, what the city spends amounts to less than one percent of its budget," Adriana explains.

I'm shocked at first, and then I realize that much of the city's role has been making things happen, not doing them itself. The first costs less.

"People are so fed up with government that they want to pass everything off to nonprofit groups or the private sector. But the government must keep its responsibilities and work *in partnership* with citizen groups," Adriana argues.

To make that partnership real, her department has created a twenty-member advisory council of citizen, labor, and church groups. We also learn that Belo, like many Brazilian cities, involves citizens in budget-making, a trend dating back to the '70s that became widespread in the '80s. Today, most major Brazilian cities now involve citizens in allocating city funds. Here in Belo, 600 people from all sectors of society gathered to vote on where city dollars should go, and the city's food initiatives, especially for children, got a lot of votes.

At the end of our visit, Anna and I sit down again with Adriana in her cheery office. We tell her how moved we've been by how much has developed in so little time, just since 1993. We also know that, a few months after we leave, Belo will vote for a new mayor. Can all that the city has done, all that we've seen, endure? The food-citizenship programs have already survived one shift in administration that put a different party in power. But can they last?

Adriana does not seem worried.

"I think we've shown this works," Adriana says. "We have popular support. At a time when record harvests in the country have not reduced the price of food, people know that here we've been helping make the market fairer."

I wonder if she appreciates how extraordinary her efforts are. Does she realize that her city may be the only one in the world taking this approach—food as a right of citizenship, of membership in the human family?

So I ask, "When you began, did you realize how important what you are doing was? How much difference it might make? How rare it is in the entire world?"

Listening to her long answer in Portuguese without understanding, I see her eyes moisten and try to guess why. Through our interpreter, I learn.

"I knew we had so much hunger in the world," she said. "But what is so upsetting, what I didn't know when I started this, is it's so easy. It's so easy to end it."

BRAZIL: AWAKENING OUR SENSES

Feijoada (Tangy Black Beans) Dinner

Serves 6   *This three-part recipe is one of our favorites from the first edition of* Diet for a Small Planet. *A Brazilian friend embellished it for the twentieth-anniversary edition, and we've added to it for this book—inspired by the delicious meals we ate from Belo Horizonte to Paraná. Serve the rice with sauce along with the beans and greens for a splendid three-course Brazilian dinner.—Frances*

oil for sautéing

1 large onion, chopped

2 cloves garlic, minced

2 green onions, chopped

1 green pepper, chopped

1 tomato, chopped

1 teaspoon cilantro (optional)

1 cup black beans

3 cups seasoned stock (or substitute wine
   for up to half the stock)

1 bay leaf

¼ teaspoon pepper

1 teaspoon vinegar (omit if using wine)

1 orange, washed but unpeeled, whole or
   halved

½ teaspoon salt

2 stalks celery, chopped

1 tomato, chopped

1 carrot, chopped (optional)

½ sweet potato, diced

Heat oil in a large heavy pot and sauté onion, garlic, green onions, green pepper, tomato, and cilantro until onion is translucent. Add beans, stock, bay leaf, pepper, and vinegar. Bring to a boil, reduce heat, and simmer for 2 minutes. Take off stove and let sit, covered, for 1 hour.

Add remaining ingredients and simmer, with lid ajar, for 2 to 3 hours more, until beans are tender. Remove a ladleful of beans, mash them, and return them to the pot to thicken the mixture.

I have done the whole thing in a pressure cooker, after first sautéing the onion and garlic. It is much quicker and still very good.

Rice with Green Chili Sauce

Rice

2 tablespoons olive oil

1 onion, chopped

3 cloves garlic, minced

2 tomatoes, peeled, seeded, and
coarsely chopped

about 4½ cups cooked brown rice (2 cups
uncooked)

Heat the oil and sauté onion and garlic until onion is translucent. Add tomatoes and simmer a few minutes. Stir in the cooked rice and keep warm over low heat.

Sauce

1 tomato, peeled and seeded

California green chilies, seeded to taste
(start with half a 2-ounce can)

1 teaspoon salt

2 cloves garlic

juice of 1 lemon

1 onion, cut into chunks

scallions and parsley to taste

¼ cup vinegar

In a blender, purée tomato, chilies, salt, and garlic until smooth. Add lemon juice, onions, scallions and parsley, and vinegar, and blend coarsely (do not purée). Just before serving, stir in a little liquid from the Feijoada pot.

Greens with Sesame Seed Topping and Orange Slices

1½ pounds greens (turnip or mustard
greens, collards, etc.), trimmed

olive oil for sautéing

1 clove garlic, minced

½ cup toasted sesame seeds or meal

1 orange, sliced (for garnish)

Steam the greens until barely wilted. Heat oil and briefly sauté greens with garlic. Sprinkle one heaping tablespoon of sesame seed meal on each serving and garnish with orange slices on top or around edges.

THE HYACINTH
PRINCIPLE

*I sincerely believe that banking establishments are
more dangerous than standing armies.*

THOMAS JEFFERSON, 1799

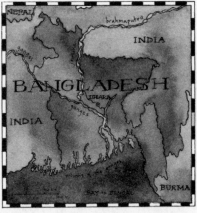

I'm already sticky hot at 8:30 in the
morning as I sit on a straw mat next to
Anna in a small, tin-roofed hut in the
village of Shauratoli, an hour north of
Dhaka, the capital of Bangladesh. Gazing directly into the faces of thirty
women, all swathed in vibrant-hued
saris of saffron, crimson, and turquoise,
I feel pale and plain in my simple black
skirt.

This moment, this country, these
faces, I've imagined many times. You
see, I've lived with Bangladesh for decades, although I'd never before set foot
in this lush land. Bangladesh is a place used by many people to make many
points in the development debate. Over the years, I'd used Bangladesh, too.

Henry Kissinger used Bangladesh in the 1970s to define "basket case," a
country so poor and hungry, so plagued by conflict and natural calamity that
one could only take pity. And since then, many have: Charitable agencies by
the hundreds have set up shop in Bangladesh.

Believers in American ecologist Garrett Hardin's "lifeboat ethics" used
Bangladesh in the same era to prove that some countries are just too poor and
overpopulated to have a fighting chance—and that, because there's only so

much food to go around, we'd better just let these sad nations sink—for the sake of the rest of us.[1] Others have used Bangladesh to make their case for intensive family-planning efforts. The list goes on.

I'd had my points to make, as well—mostly opposing ones. In books and articles, I'd argued that appearances deceive. Despite a population whose density is so great it is the equivalent to all the world's people squeezed into the U.S., Bangladesh has the physical means to feed all its people, and then some. Its ever-renewing alluvial soils and its unparalleled ponds, rivers, and canals give Bangladesh a Garden-of-Eden feel.

As our rusty white minivan speeds out of the capital, all those there-is-enough-for-us-all arguments I'd made in writing—based on other people's research—seem even more believable. Rice fields are everywhere; some harvested, others just turning golden, and others still a brilliant green. Mango, papaya, and jackfruit trees—with ripening fruit that look like pears on growth hormones—fill the sides of the roads. Here is a place where it would seem difficult to *prevent* food from growing, I think later, when a mango drops from a tree bursting with fruit and almost whacks Anna on the head!

I admit. I'd used Bangladesh to make my share of arguments about the causes of hunger. "You can't blame scarcity. Look at Bangladesh," I'd say.

And here I arrive in the country, finally, to make yet another point. Bangladesh is for many a mythical place of tragedy; I want Bangladesh to become my mythical place of hope.

THE DRAMA

You see, for years I'd been smitten by the drama of Bangladesh-born Grameen Bank, meaning "village bank" in Bengali. In less than two decades, Grameen has achieved what many thought impossible—built a lending institution for the poor that actually works, putting loans in the hands of over two million borrowers, almost all of them poor women. While the loans may seem tiny in Western terms—$160 on average—they make life-and-death differences here: often the difference between having a roof on one's house, or not; having food for one's children, or none.

Grameen's success has even generated a whole new buzzword—"microcredit"—and brought its charismatic founder, Professor Muhammad Yunus, international acclaim. The World Bank has tapped Yunus to advise on how to spread microcredit worldwide, and replications have popped up in more than fifty-eight countries. President Clinton even suggested that Yunus should receive the Nobel Peace Prize. Yunus himself claims microcredit is so potent it can "put poverty in the museum."

We wanted to go to Bangladesh to find out for ourselves what lies beneath the buzzwords. What lessons does Grameen hold about the potential of banks, one of the most basic institutions of capitalism, to serve society? And what does Grameen's experience teach about our potential as human beings, even the most oppressed among us?

After all, Grameen emerged in a uniquely challenging place: a country burdened by a legacy of colonialism, a costly war of independence, regular massive flooding, and poverty so deep that four-fifths of Bangladeshis survive on less than $2 a day and 700 children perish daily from malnutrition-related diseases.[2] Not to mention a coup shortly after independence that resulted in fifteen turbulent years of military rule and prolonged and entrenched corruption.

Grameen intrigues me, in part, because it has overcome such great odds, but also because, if truth be known, I was an early skeptic. In the '80s, in a public debate with microcredit true believers, I insisted that microcredit alone couldn't get at the root of poverty. It may give the poor a toehold into capitalism, but it does nothing to prevent the beneficiaries from replicating the injustice that they themselves had suffered, I had said.

Despite this skepticism, I was profoundly moved by Grameen's triumph. So I arrive with this push-pull in my heart—determined to remain open to whatever lessons are here—and knowing that to understand Grameen we must start with its own beginnings. We must start with Muhammad Yunus.

"I FELT COMPLETELY EMPTY."

On our second day, we wind our way through Dhaka's noisy streets to Yunus' office in Grameen's headquarters. Our guidebook tells us that 300,000 rickshaws—open-air, people-powered carts—are pedaled through these noisy streets every day, and I'm glad we aren't in one, as the lanes and stoplights seem optional here. This crush of traffic makes more sense once Anna and I learn that in the last thirty years this city's population has swollen from one million to eight million people.

After a hair-raising drive, we turn into Grameen's hotel-like circular entryway. Expecting something modest and nonprofit-looking, we find instead Grameen's twenty-some-story headquarters towering above its four-story neighbors. With more than 10,000 employees and 2.4 million borrowers, Grameen means business, and it looks like one.

A business born of suffering so extreme it's hard even to imagine.

While I was gazing out at the San Francisco Bay and writing *Diet for a Small Planet*, Bangladesh, then still part of Pakistan, was fighting a bloody war for independence. By the time the war ended, less than a year later, more than one million Bangladeshis were dead and ten million had fled. One-third of the nation's housing was destroyed. We were told that napalm, mass rapes, and targeted killing of intellectuals were all horrors of the struggle.

Now, sitting with Muhammad Yunus in Grameen's offices high above Dhaka, at first we seem far from that tragic time. He greets us warmly, his dark eyes framed by brown-rimmed glasses, and he talks with us as openly as if we're old friends. But with his first words, we're transported back to the painful events that triggered what would become Grameen Bank.

"Bangladesh was in terrible, terrible shape," he said as if living it again. "A lot of deaths. A lot of killings. During the war I was teaching at a university in Tennessee. But I decided I had to come back; I thought I should be useful in rebuilding Bangladesh. I came back and started doing the one thing I knew. I started teaching the same thing I had taught in the United States: economics.

"Instead of getting better, things were getting worse. Then in 1974 a terrible famine hit. People were dying in the streets. That's a rude shock," Muhammad says, as if the pain were still right there before his eyes.

"I lived in a beautiful bungalow on a hillside near the university and would walk by people who were dying. Then I'd come back to the classroom and give my big lecture, and I said: 'What is this?' I felt completely empty.

"I came to the conclusion that these theories were useless for these dying people," Yunus tells us. "I realized I could help people as a human being, not as an economist. So I decided to become a basic human being. I think that was a good decision for me because I no longer carried any preconceived notions."

Yunus's experience of dissonance reminds me of my own at the very same age. Everything I wrote in *Diet for a Small Planet* was sitting there for any nutritionist or economist to put together well before I did. But because I was untrained, I didn't wear the blinders created by being taught to perceive only within a set framework. Without those blinders, I could see that there is plenty of food for all; that we ourselves create the scarcity we fear.

For Yunus, as for me, an admission of "not knowing" was the beginning of real learning. But what Yunus did was much trickier. He had to *unlearn* what he knew, so that he could look at poverty anew.

Dropping his preconceptions and leaving his theories in the classroom, Yunus traveled into the villages near Chittagong University. He decided that to understand poverty and hunger, he had to listen to poor people themselves, in order to learn a new economics.

What Yunus observed in these villages seems, in one sense, utterly obvious. Those most hungry were those with no land. At the time, they made up at least half of the rural population. But instead of accepting what he saw, Yunus asked: *Why is it this way? Why can't it be different?*

He found that many of the landless struggle for income by making things to sell. But they must buy the raw materials, and to do that, they must borrow from a moneylender. By the time they repay the loan, plus interest (when Yunus began, interest could be as much as 10 percent, *per day*), what's left is never enough to live on.

Yunus's first "aha" moment was meeting Sufiya Begum, a twenty-one-year-old mother who fed her family by making bamboo stools. She bought the cane, her raw material, with loans from moneylenders who made her sell back to them at the end of each day. Her profit? *Two cents a day.*

Soon Yunus and his students had collected a list of forty-two people in straits similar to Sufiya's, and he provided each with a loan out of his own pocket. "My loan of only twenty-seven dollars spread among forty-two people was enough," he tells us. It was enough to liberate them all from bondage to the moneylender.

"YOU CAN'T EXPECT A MANGO FROM A JACKFRUIT TREE."

Where others looked and saw pathetic, hungry people who needed food, Yunus looked and saw resourceful people deprived of resources. To him, it was obvious that more than food handouts, they needed money to invest in tools of production. They needed a way to free themselves from dependency on the moneylender, to free themselves from vulnerability to hunger. Yunus saw credit as the liberator.

"But my loan was an individual response," Yunus says. "It stuck in my mind: *What about the bank?* This is what *they* should be doing. This is their job. So I went to the bank and talked to the manager. He was shocked and said, 'No it cannot be done, banks don't loan without collateral.' I told him, 'Look, I've shown that the poor are reliable, they've all repaid as promised. Will you lend to them?'"

"We won't believe you until you've tried it in more villages," the banker said.

"Not a problem," Yunus replied, and expanded his informal lending with success. He returned again to the bank. "Now will you lend to the poor?" he asked.

Each time, the manager demanded more evidence; each time, Yunus made more successful loans to the poor.

Ultimately, Yunus threw up his hands and decided that he himself had to create a new kind of bank.

"That bank manager did you a favor, didn't he?" we joke. "If he'd gone along with you, today there would be no Grameen Bank."

Yunus agrees, laughing, "Yes, I like to say the solution can be born in the womb of the problem."

And the problem?

Banks have rules, rules shutting out the vast majority of the world's people. Think about it: Only about 2 percent of us worldwide can get credit. Still, we've come to accept these rules, *as just the way things are.*

"But shouldn't the very fact that hunger and poverty exist make us question *all* our wisdom?" Yunus asks. The hunger and poverty he witnessed daily made him do just that, forced him to rethink bank rules—every one of them.

"People always ask, 'How did you get these ideas about lending to the poor?' I say: I knew I had to change the institutions themselves, and whenever I didn't know what to do I would look at the banks, and whatever they did, I did just the opposite. Every time I got into difficulty, I would just reverse the way banks do things, and that became the Grameen Bank," Yunus says, taking obvious pleasure in our looks of surprise.

"We have an expression in Bengali: 'You can't expect a mango from a jackfruit tree.' If you want a mango, plant a mango tree."

THE JACKFRUIT

Yunus believes he and his colleagues, through trial and error, have planted a new kind of bank bearing a new kind of fruit. Yunus really got us thinking. Just what *are* the assumptions that underlie our banks? Anna and I later teased out five that are so pervasive most people don't see them.

> *The Deciders.* Bankers decide who gets a loan and for what; only they have the expertise to tell a "good" risk from a "bad" one.

> *The Guarantee.* The bank's guarantee, if you don't repay, is its right to seize your property. So poor people can't get credit because they lack property; they have no collateral.

The Owners. A bank's shareholders are not the same people who are its borrowers. Otherwise, you'd end up with a mess of conflicting interests.

§ *The Secrets.* Banks can't do business in public or make their records public. That's private stuff.

The Motives. Banks are not in business to improve society but to make money for shareholders and to provide a service to those with money.

We all assume that somebody, somewhere, figured out that these rules had to be this way. In any case, they're working, aren't they? But to Yunus, the very fact of poverty is proof the way we are doing things is *not* working, so he took these five givens of banking and stood each one on its head.

GROWING THE MANGO TREE

Gazing into the women's faces that hot morning in Shauratoli at the first Grameen borrowers' meeting we visited, I imagined thousands of similar weekly meetings happening in nearly two-thirds of the country's almost 70,000 villages. Violating every single tenet of traditional banking, these women are . . .

the deciders. They, not bankers, choose who gets a loan and for how much.

the guarantors. Because Grameen has no power to seize property, its security is the bonds of trust among borrowers. Such trust-collateral begins with a group of five women, all poor and from different families, who come together and agree to back each other in good times or bad. They are co-responsible for the loans.

the owners. The Bank is owned almost entirely by its members, and borrowers elect directors from among themselves who head to Dhaka four times a year to directors' meetings where they make up nine of the thirteen board members.

As to the *secrets* and the *motives,* Grameen breaks the mold here, too:

the secrets. Discussions and decisions are public—as we see before our eyes at each of the meetings we attend in the small Grameen huts. As we sit watching, each group leader leans forward and passes the group's weekly payment to the bank worker, who records it in a notebook in full view of all the other women.

the motives. They are mixed and that's good, according to Yunus. The primary motive is eliminating poverty, and the goal of making a profit is consistent with that end, he believes.

All these features of Grameen create yet another difference. In Grameen, the bank goes into the community, seeking borrowers and encouraging them to participate. It doesn't wait for borrowers to knock on the door.

Now, while seeing the ways Yunus has "flipped banking on its head," I realize that most outsiders view Grameen as doing no more than bringing banking to the poor. (In fact the English-language version of Yunus's autobiography is titled *Banker to the Poor*.)[3] We tease Yunus about this (his relaxed and cheerful nature makes joking with him easy): "Isn't the popular view of your work 'Little loans for little people?' Grameen just miniaturizes capitalism so the system can work for anyone?"

Yunus laughs with us, but we don't admit aloud that we, too, had largely seen it this way before arriving. As we continue to talk with Yunus, we start to see Grameen as more than a miniaturization of capitalism—it's taking what works and challenging key premises that don't.

SIXTEEN DECISIONS

To begin to grasp the scope of Grameen, imagine this: You pass through the sliding glass doors of Fleet or Citibank and sit down at the customer-service desk to ask about a small business loan. "Sure," says the banker, "we can help you. But here are pledges you must take home and commit to memory. Come back when you can recite them, and then we'll proceed with your loan application."

You look down to discover that in order to get your loan you must pledge not to batter your spouse and to stand up against sweatshop labor abuses.

You are shocked—I would be—that a bank is getting "personal." How dare it get involved in strictly social questions!

Then I catch myself: U.S. banks *do* have social impact. Big time. Discrimination against minorities and banks' flight from poor communities go a long way to explain why many of our inner cities are troubled. So, I ask myself, as Yunus did: If banks have a social impact, why shouldn't they consciously acknowledge it and strive to have a positive one? Where is it fore-

ordained that an organization lending money can't also have the goal of improving society?

Fixed on the goal of ending poverty, Yunus and his colleagues soon learned
that progress involves more than moneylending. Today, every Grameen borrower memorizes and commits to a full sixteen pledges, called Sixteen Decisions, not too different from the imaginary ones we just posed.

Anna and I learn about them from one of Yunus's first students, Nurjahan
Begum, now manager of the Grameen's efforts to support microcredit programs worldwide.

We sit with her in the Dhaka headquarters, the whir of a fan and the din
of traffic far below mixing with our voices. As she talks, Nurjahan, a petite
woman with large-framed glasses and a voice made gruff from a cold, leans
toward us to make sure we get every word. With a directness that we both admire, she confesses her early frustrations.

"I told Dr. Yunus, 'Okay we're giving women in the villages microcredit,
but they have such large families. I don't think it will be possible for them to
improve their lives. So why don't you start family planning?'

"'Nurjahan,' he told me, 'you cannot sow two seeds at the same time.
This is not the right time. Later on we can do that.'"

For Yunus, microcredit was the entry point. It brought immediate relief
and more. It also built trust between Bank workers and village families. From
there, the Sixteen Decisions evolved, eventually touching on many of the interconnected problems that keep poverty entrenched.

"Now," Nurjahan explains, "we go beyond credit. But without credit—if
I couldn't loan women money—nobody would have listened to me."

The final Sixteen Decisions gelled in 1984 from long discussions with
Grameen borrowers. Among them is the pledge to keep the family small. Borrowers are, Grameen told us, 50 percent more likely to use family-planning
methods than the national average. Borrowers also pledge to grow vegetables
all year round, to educate their children, and even to build and use pit-latrines
(what we would call "out-houses").

Some critics look at the Sixteen Decisions and see paternalism at best,
brainwashing at worst. But, we remind ourselves, this effort to create new
norms emerged from the borrowers themselves. What's more, it's a lot easier to
criticize norms made explicit than even to *see* our own "Sixteen Decisions," expectations so embedded in our culture that they don't have to be explicit to
control us: norms like "Make as much money as you can; spend as much as
possible."

. . .

One of the Grameen Decisions is stunning in the magnitude of its implications: "We shall not inflict any injustice on anyone, neither shall we allow anyone to do so."

It's hard to imagine how such a profound and sweeping commitment would play itself out in real life. But we get a taste of it, unexpectedly, in a conversation with Dipal Chandra Barua, another of Yunus's first students, now Grameen Bank's general manager.

"Once when I was a local Grameen manager," he tells us, "a woman came into the borrowers' meeting crying. It took the others a long time to calm her down even enough to find out what had happened. It turned out the cow of a rich man had wandered onto her land and died. 'The rich man kept my cow as punishment,' she sobbed. After much discussion, the whole group marched to the rich man's house and confronted him for more than an hour. Finally, he agreed to pay for the cow. Individually, these women have little value or strength. Collectively, they became more powerful than a rich man."

It's impossible to know how common an occurrence this is, but as one Grameen trainer told us, "Just getting people to talk about what injustices they've experienced is an important first step. Many of them have never thought in this way before."

THE DOWRY SURPRISE

We soon learn more about another one of the Sixteen Decisions, which at first doesn't strike us as being nearly as revolutionary: "We shall not take any dowry into our sons' weddings, neither shall we give any dowry in our daughters' weddings. We shall keep the center [a Grameen group of thirty to forty borrowers] free from the curse of dowry."

Anna and I had both assumed the dowry—a payment to the groom by the bride's family—was a traditional practice waning in the face of modernization. On the way out of Dhaka to the first village we visit, we ask Fazley Rabbi, our patient Grameen guide and interpreter, about the dowry tradition. Actually, he tells us, as a significant practice the dowry is relatively new here, and it's becoming more common, not less.

The cost of "marrying off" a daughter is swelling, he explains, as advertising heightens appetites for consumer goods. Many men see the dowry as an easy way to quick cash, Rabbi explains. During the rest of our time in Bangladesh, we will read news accounts of women beaten by husbands demanding more dowry and even a case of a husband killing his wife who didn't produce the dowry he demanded.

Arriving in the village of Shauratoli with Rabbi's alarming words still with us, we're now ever more curious to find out whether borrowers really are following the dowry Decision as well as the others that require women to buck such powerful social norms.

As we sit with the thirty women at their weekly gathering, where loans are dispersed and paid under the thin tin roof of the Grameen hut, we ask: "Are you following the Sixteen Decisions?"

Here, as we will find in almost all the villages we visit, first we get smiles, then explanations. We imagine their expressions are saying, "We're trying, but we're not all the way there yet."

When we probe for details, the women gathered say: "Yes, we are digging pit-latrines, growing vegetables, sending our children to school. Yes, the younger women are having fewer children."

"And the dowry?" we ask.

One member near the front smiles with pride, "I have two married sons and didn't receive any money in their marriages."

Another acknowledges, smiling, too, perhaps with embarrassment, that she paid 20,000 *taka* (equivalent to about $400, or more than a year's income for the average Bangladeshi) at her daughter's wedding.

Others stir, seemingly uncomfortable, and repeat their disapproval of the dowry. The woman defends herself. "I had to pay a dowry, and one so high because my daughter's skin is dark." I groan inside, realizing that the Grameen Bank actually enabled this woman to reward sexism and prejudice by giving her the wherewithal to pay so much.

If the group disapproves of dowry, why did it approve her loan? How did that loan help her out of poverty? It doesn't add up. Then something cracks inside me, and the depth of repression against women here begins to sink in. As Yunus and Nurjahan realized, you can't just give credit; you must build new social norms—and that takes time.

TIN ROOFS TAKE ON A NEW MEANING

A few days later, after a second bumpy ride north of Dhaka, we arrive in the village of Azugara to sit in on another gathering of the basic cell of the Grameen Bank. We're here barely in time for the nine A.M. meeting.

"This is a mob," I hear Rabbi say jokingly, as the crowd following us from the van grows. Children jostle each other for a better view of these strange-looking Western women.

Stepping into the now-familiar tin-roofed hut, this time we're offered chairs at a table facing the group of forty women, many following *purdah*—from the Persian word *pardah*, meaning "veil"—by wearing the traditional Muslim dress that cloaks them in black cloth from head to toe. With sweat dripping down my back under my thin short-sleeved shirt, I try to imagine what being covered in yards of black fabric must be like.

We watch while the Grameen center manager conducts today's business and women from different groups request loans. When they're finished, we have time for questions. When we ask how they've been using their loans, the women respond with many of the examples we've heard at other meetings: "Yarn for weaving." "Feed for cow-fattening." "Small grocery items for selling in the stall." "A sewing machine."

"So, do the loans mean less hunger and better nutrition here?" I ask.

"Of course, we have more food to eat now," a slender woman in a periwinkle-blue sari responds. In her voice I think I hear impatience at such a stupid question; the answer is obvious. "Before, I was working on another man's land," she adds. "Now, I am taking rice from my own land."

Another explains: "Before, I was always paying a moneylender any money I made. Now, we have our own businesses. I can feed my family."

I'm glad that Rabbi then jumps in with his own question: "How many of you have housing loans?"

Hands shoot up—maybe a quarter of the room—and Rabbi smiles broadly. These are women who've built a credit history and secured a larger-sized Grameen loan to build their own homes. Walking back to the minivan, Rabbi points out for us the Grameen housing-loan huts, although their shiny new tin roofs are a dead giveaway.

Speeding past more green fields and water that extends to the edge of the horizon, I think back to my own heightened sense of security when I, on my own with two children, got my first loan for a home. I think I can relate to the women we've just met, but then Rabbi fills us in on the housing loans' significance, and I'm brought up short.

Over the clatter of the engine, Rabbi explains that until recently a husband in Bangladesh could divorce simply by saying *"talak, talak, talak"*—"I divorce you," three times. With these words, the wife would be out on the street—or, here, out on the dirt path.

"We decided to start offering loans for home construction, which costs a few hundred dollars, to women only," Rabbi says. "If the house title is in her name, it's the man who would be thrown out in divorce. Now, the husband has to think twice before divorcing."

Of course, a property title in a woman's name can only go so far in shifting deeply rooted injustice against her and in protecting her from an abusive husband—I had already learned that half the murders in Bangladesh involve women killed by their husbands. But Grameen's single-sex housing loans—all $186 million worth of them so far—undeniably give women one new source of power.

FREEDOM AND LIPSTICK

The first morning in Dhaka, I'm up at dawn, my internal clock thrown off by jet lag. Restless, I peer out my window and see through early morning mist a solemn march of women in bright-colored saris.

Later, in our first interview with Yunus, he tells us: "We have a thriving garment industry in Dhaka, and most workers are girls."

I think of the hundreds I'd seen that morning on their way to work.

"Most come from rural areas," he says, "where they'd worked day and night as domestics. In the garment factories they're paid cash—a small amount, but they're paid and they work regular hours. When they get their money they want some makeup. Now one million girls have started buying lipstick. Nobody ever thought Bangladesh had a market for lipstick!"

Despite his enthusiasm, I can't help but wonder: Are lipstick sales a barometer of progress? Just outside of Dhaka on our way to a village, we had driven by one of the new "export processing zones." I saw the barbed wire keeping people out, the hawkers and beggars nearby, and the long column of workers heading in.

So I don't automatically assume that girls working as day laborers are freer than when they worked in the villages. Of course not having to live day and night under the roof of your employer might bring more freedom, but I'm not sure working as a wage laborer here means you keep it.

You Can Always Get a New Wife

Back in Dhaka, I'm invited to give a talk at Naripokkho, an organization promoting women's rights in Bangladesh whose Bengali name means "pro-women." Again I find myself peering into the faces of Bangladeshi women sitting on straw mats in front of me. But everything else is different from the Grameen borrowers' meetings. Here are middle-class women in the capital, straight from jobs at hospitals and banks, universities and development agencies. As they enter the large meeting room, they are animated and energized,

> To me, these girls have taken their first step into a world of globalized work, where your wages are low, your rights weak, where your fate is determined by CEOs thousands of miles away. But they've also just taken the first step onto the brutal consumer treadmill—the more you buy, the more you see what you don't have, and the more you buy; the more TV you watch, the more you're shown what you should look like. I just read a Harvard public-health study on the effect of TV in Fiji: never-before-seen dieting, anorexia, and bulimia.
>
> Everyone we meet in Dhaka tells us about the country's latest epidemic: conspicuous consumption. *We used to be ashamed to show we had money,* one friend told us. *Now even those with very little flaunt it.* The occasional flashy car on Dhaka streets, the packed fast-food restaurants, and the gaudy jewelry all tell the same story. I worry that lipstick sales, in fact, may not be evidence of progress but of this disturbing trend.
>
> Grameen could be creating not only other economic options—businesses rooted in villages, with Bangladeshis themselves controlling conditions and earnings—but also an ethic of conscientious consumption, not conspicuous consumption. Their family of businesses grounded in Bangladesh are hopeful; but Yunus's enthusiasm for lipstick sales is unsettling. I don't say anything, though, not sure I feel so comfortable speaking up with my lipstick-coated lips.　　　　　　　　　　　　　—Anna

sharing warm words that I can't understand, but laughter that I can. I notice newspaper clippings tacked to the walls and a poster with a photograph of a disturbingly disfigured face, and I wish I could understand the Bengali words printed under it.

Sitting next to me in a cherry-red sari is Shireen Huq, a founder of the group, who interprets as I begin by explaining the meaning of Bangladesh to me.

I'll never be sure why, on this night, tears well up in me almost as soon as I begin to speak. To most Americans, Bangladesh is a sad place, I say, a country confronted by seemingly endless tragedy. I have worked for years to tell the world that Bangladesh has never been doomed to suffering. It has the capacity to meet its needs. I explain that I'm here now so I can continue this story—so I can show that what appears to be a tragic country holds powerful lessons of hope for the world.

Is this positive message of possibility what is bringing tears to my eyes? Or are the tears evidence that, as I begin to perceive the enormous gulf between men and women in Bangladesh, everything potentially positive becomes muddied? I do find my composure, and I speak, eager to share my experiences with these women.

But, for me, the most moving part of the evening comes during the questions and answers. As the lights—and fans—periodically go off, then on again, subtly shifting the mood from intense connection to subdued reflection, Shireen interprets a comment from her elderly mother sitting far in the back.

"What you are saying is true. There is enough food," she says. "Even in the worst famines, that has always been true. I remember in 1943, three million people starved while the warehouses overflowed with grain," she adds, speaking of the infamous Bengal famine when the country was still a British colony.

"I saw people crying out for rice, and I saw them become so weak that they couldn't even say the word 'rice.' I saw people dying on the street. If even one of the British had died, the colonial government would have called a national emergency, but they let millions of us starve."

Later that evening over dinner with Shireen and her family, we learn that in the famine her mother had almost died of hunger herself. She spent a year in a sanatorium, recovering. Shireen confides in us that at the time a friend of the family had asked her father: "Why don't you let her die? You can always get a new wife." Shireen's story reminds Anna and me that being within an educated circle is no guarantee that women will be valued as equals, or even as being fully human.

After dinner, Anna and I have a chance to ask Shireen about the images and articles on the walls.

The women and young girls pictured, she tells us, are survivors of acid burns. A recent phenomenon, the attacks are occurring mostly in rural areas. Primarily, young men are the perpetrators and claim the violence is justified "retribution" against girls who resisted their advances. Typically the men attack at night while the girl is sleeping and target the face, knowing that a disfigured face is a permanent, public punishment.

The preferred weapon is common car-battery acid, Shireen tells us. It's easy to find, cheap to buy, and melts the skin on contact. Most attackers have not been arrested, and those arrested are rarely sentenced. With little legal action against perpetrators, the incidents are increasing—doubling in Bangladesh in just four years. Shireen tells us last year almost 200 girls were burned.[4]

We remember the photographs on the wall. We understand now. We were seeing acid-attack victims—eyes and ears missing, skin frozen in melted screams, noses just sockets. I sense anew the terror women here must experience. I sense

THE BURGUNDY SARI

Driving through crowded Dhaka streets, the air thick, the sound of trucks and cars pounding, I search out, amidst the thousands of men in dark and graying white clothes, the rare flash of color. A woman. Their saris scream iridescent blues and golds, mustard yellows and lime greens, reds and bright oranges.

On our last day, I decide to buy a traditional Bangladeshi sari from Grameen's store. I choose a burgundy one with silver flowers embroidered delicately from head to toe.

Back at the hotel, I try on my new clothes, and as a finishing touch I take the long scarf and sweep it over my head and around my face, as I've seen the women in *purdah* do here. Only my eyes show. And I feel it as fast as turning off a light. I'm formless. I'm small. I'm suddenly invisible.

—Anna

it now on a visceral level. And I appreciate even more deeply the courage of Grameen women, both borrowers and staff.

Grameen's anti-dowry pledge, its policy of providing credit mainly to women, and even the women-only housing loans, all now hold new meaning for Anna and me. These are economic decisions, yes, but they're much more. They're also about changing norms, changing what is acceptable. They are about ensuring that women are equally included. They're about showing that women's rights are not just a question of justice for women. They are at the very heart of any movement for societal development. No society can become healthy as long as half the population is treated as less than fully human, sometimes as not even human at all. The loss is for the whole of society.

WOMEN CAN SPEAK

Despite Grameen's focus on women, after almost twenty years only six percent of the more than 10,000-person staff is female. And Yunus, looking pained, tells us that even this small percentage is getting smaller. When we ask why, he explains that many women are discouraged from working for Grameen, and that public disapproval of women traveling in the countryside alone means that the few women who are hired often leave before long. The pressures on women to stay home—and silent—are powerful.

I think of what Nurjahan told us when we raised questions about the Grameen salutes, chants, and exercises that are part of borrowers' meetings. To us, they felt authoritarian. They seemed to teach conformity, not independence.

"Well, the salutes are not really salutes," Nurjahan had said. "They are to recognize each other." Sweeping her beige sari scarf back into place, she continued, "When we started, most women came to us and bowed their heads in the way of tradition. So we wanted to find another greeting to express the dignity of each human being.

"A woman is given the idea that she should not speak, she should not laugh out loud. There is the common proverb girls learn: 'If you play a dumb role, there is no enemy.' This is what women are learning from childhood."

My own reaction reminds me again how quickly perception can change. The chants and salutes we had seen moments ago as signs of creepy conformity, now, like many of the Sixteen Decisions, appear as steps toward liberation.

Nurjahan continued, "We came up with the slogans for all women to say out loud, so they can take strength. Slowly, slowly she can come up with her own voice. You can see today, women can speak."

"Like a First Love"

When we ask Nurjahan how, in the early years with Yunus, she gained the strength to face her own fear of being out of step in her culture and confronted her family's disapproval, she takes us back to that time.

"Two or three years after I joined the Bank, I felt I just couldn't do this job. It was too hard to go against the culture. When I told Dr. Yunus, he told me that before I quit I should go and talk to some of the struggling women in the villages, find out how they live, what is their past and what is the future they want," Nurjahan explains, as she tosses her beige sari scarf over her head for the third time.

"I remember one woman telling me about the 1974 famine. Normally in our society, when anybody dies the body is covered with a new white cloth, but this woman said that when her eldest son died in the famine she was so poor she couldn't even afford a new white cloth. She was crying when she told me her story. You cannot explain this with words. I went back to Dr. Yunus and told him I would stay.

"It's being in touch with people's lives that is our biggest motivator," she states. "So we train our new staff by sending them into the villages to write members' case studies." (How quickly "case study" loses its stodgy, academic ring!)

"Going to the villages changes people's hearts," Nurjahan says. "It helps them to understand what kind of struggles these women are facing. It makes it hard to be indifferent. In Grameen we never recruit experienced people; when we recruit fresh people from university, they have energy to do something better."

Listening to Nurjahan, I think back to my life at the age she was when she helped launch Grameen. Three years before I wrote *Diet for a Small Planet* I worked as a community organizer in the ghettoes of Philadelphia. It was the early days of the Welfare Rights Organization, and my job was to go into the homes of welfare recipients, listen to their stories, and encourage them to join with other women to ensure that they were getting the benefits to which they were legally entitled.

Through my work there, one woman I came to love was Lillie. As I got to know her, I saw her suffer the stress of never knowing whether or not she could feed her children, or afford asthma medicine for her son, or keep coal in the furnace so her children would not freeze in the winter. Only months after we met, Lillie died of a heart attack. She was in her early forties, and I was convinced that poverty itself had killed her.

Looking back, I see, as Nurjahan does, that getting to know Lillie, working closely with so many other poor women, got beneath my conscious mind, beneath my fear of confronting authority.

Many of the senior managers we meet sound the same note. Umme Kulsum, who's known as Swapna by everyone here, was one of Muhammad Yunus's students and is now in a top leadership post in the Grameen Bank. "In the beginning I wasn't only criticized by men," she told us. "The other women wouldn't accept me as a bank worker, either. I wasn't following the culture's norms. So I carried a briefcase with the traditional dress for *purdah* inside. Whenever my role was questioned, I would pull it out of my bag to prove to the village women I was one of them." Swapna's yearning to connect with other women and be useful to them gave her courage to confront powerful norms and tap her ingenuity.

On a village visit with Mizanur Rahman, who was one of the "fresh" people and now is a tough-looking fellow in charge of Grameen's weaving spinoff, we ask what has been his favorite part of working with Grameen. He answers without skipping a beat: "It was when I was a branch manager. I was close to the people. I could see our work changing their lives. They could get loans. Their children started going to school. I could see the changes.

"It was like a first love. I'll never forget."

With his words, I think maybe my work in Philadelphia was my "first love," too, in which I first felt the enormous satisfaction of meaningful work.

THE FISH ARE FLYING

On our second trip out of Dhaka, we go farther, bobbing with the potholes as our driver speeds past packed buses, cars, and three-wheelers. Rabbi calls out to the driver many times a Bengali word we won't forget: *aste, aste*—go slow.

We fly by rice fields, coconut and banana and jackfruit trees. They are interrupted by clusters of small, rickety stalls selling packaged snacks, cloth, batteries, you name it. We begin to see how the equivalent of half the population of the U.S. can live in a space the size of Wisconsin—one cluster of human habitation simply follows the next.

Most striking is the water. There is no time during the two-hour drive during which we cannot see some form of water—there are ponds, marshy areas, and wide rivers. Water, combined with sun and heat, makes Bangladesh feel like an endless greenhouse.

In the village of Kali Kair, winding through ever-narrower dirt roads, we arrive midafternoon at the headquarters of Joysagar Farms, the pride of Grameen's fishery efforts. Flowering shrubs and trees hug the thick-walled, beige stone-and-plaster guest house.

Historically, ponds had always been a rich part of rural life and cuisine in Bangladesh. But as communal maintenance and use of the ponds gave way to private control during the colonial period, many ponds became silted up and useless. As Western aid agencies tackling the flood problem created dams and embankments and changed water flows, traditional fish populations were further decimated.

After the nation's birth in 1971, the government tried but failed to make the ponds productive again. It cried "uncle" in 1986 and, with a low-priced, long-term lease to Grameen, handed over management of 800 ponds. In other words, just three years after Grameen officially became a "bank" it had already gained enough credibility to be entrusted with this potentially rich resource. Grameen has since brought hundreds of ponds back to life. The Joysagar ponds alone cover more than 1,000 acres.

When we arrive at the fish farm, we're greeted by farm manager Akhter Hamid, a soft-spoken man dressed in a traditional white Muslim outfit and small white *tupi* hat.

Describing the Joysagar Farm, Akhter says, "At first it was hard persuading people to try the group fishing. But now, nationwide, there are over nine hundred fishing groups, and here in this area alone two thousand five hundred landless people are working in groups with thirty members—just like the Bank's centers.

"So far, we're reaching about half the poor people in this village," Akhter tells us. "But," he adds, repeating the Grameen mantra as if to remind us what this is really all about, "our goal is to eliminate poverty for everyone."

He urges us not to talk for long because he doesn't want us to miss the harvesting. "The husbands will be helping the members," Akhter explains as we're getting into the vans. He speaks English well, so I'm surprised when he says "husbands" but means "wives."

The sun is just beginning to set over the still water of a pond the size and shape of a football field. Roughly a dozen women, waist-deep at the pond's edge, grip the large, tightly woven fishing net. Their colorful saris darken and fan out in the water. A few yards out, an equal number of men, bare except for the traditional waist-cloths called *lungis,* grasp the net's outer edge. As a group, they steadily pull the net closer and closer to the shore, their focused bearing

PITFALLS OF NOT SOLVING FOR PATTERN #1

Bangladesh had always held an epic quality for me, too. I saw it as a land cursed by never-ending flooding. So when I heard that since the '70s development agencies have been trying to control floods by continuing the colonial British solution of creating embankments to prevent floodwater flow, I thought "That's exactly what Bangladesh needs: the Southeast Asian version of Dutch dikes."

What I didn't realize, and apparently many experts didn't either, is that floods weren't just a problem to eradicate, they were also a vital part of life here.

Over the centuries, native fish had evolved with the water flow, spawning and swimming and flourishing in the ever-moving streams and rivers, even in the rice paddies. And the villagers had evolved a fishing culture in sync with the flows; the native fish varieties, an estimated *260 to 500* of them, had become a diet mainstay, with the average Bangladeshi villager eating between *50 and 75 species a year*.[5]

But embankments designed to control water flow blocked fish flow, too.

contrasting with the wild energy of hundreds of trapped fish whizzing high in the air to escape their fate. Some do, but not many.

Watching this scene, I try to imagine how powerful the forces of colonialism and then Western-aid strategies had to have been for people to let go of such traditional fishing practices that now had to be regained . . . and how devastating for the people of this verdant land.

COMING OUT AT MIDNIGHT

Roughly a dozen men stand in the shade of a tall, leafy tree to weigh and send off to market today's catch. The women, dripping from the waist down, some holding babies on their hips, gather around to talk with us. I realize only now that Akhter did not misspeak when he told us the husbands were the helpers. This *is* a female fishing group.

Initially, Grameen fisheries assumed fish culture was not appropriate for

At the same time that villagers were losing native varieties, they were encouraged to introduce exotic species. Native fish—the tiny, bony ones—were "junk fish" in the eyes of experts, who preferred exotic varieties big enough to sell in Dhaka; big enough to bring "real" return. With the introduction of exotic species, native fish were hit with a whole new problem: not just blocked waterways but new fish diseases, too.

What the experts didn't see, in their "control-the-flood" focus, was that solutions to flooding could have been found without this chain reaction. Especially if those on the ground, villagers themselves, had been a bigger part in the process.

A friend told us a story about visiting a Bangladeshi village years ago. He met a young girl who was coming back from the river with a bucket full of the day's catch. When he asked what she had inside, she showed him and named, without a second's hesitation, all twelve species.

I think about this little girl as I stand on the edge of this pond, knowing that swimming in it are big, fat, exotic fish that the men will weigh and ship off to Dhaka, the tiny, native ones like those our friend found in the young girl's bucket long since gone.

—Anna

women, just as the Grameen Bank had made that assumption about microcredit only to discover women were more reliable and used their loans to better effect. Now, of the more than 600 Joysagar Fish Farm groups, forty are made up of women, and more female groups are planned. Nationwide, a little more than one-fifth of the fishing groups are female.

Standing in high green grass, I spot a leech heading straight for Anna's ankle—more proof that she's the world's best pest deterrent. In any crowd, the pests go for her alone. We both laugh, get out of the way, and then try to purge leeches from our minds so we can focus on the gathered fisherwomen.

"Before, we never ate three meals a day, only two," one woman, Anwara, wrapped in a forest-green sari, tells us. "Sometimes only one. We hardly survived.

"In the beginning, people laughed at us. They had a lot of superstitions. They tried to frighten us. But now they see. We have food, clothes. We eat three times a day. We are sending our children to school. My son is going to college."

"How much will you make this year working in the fisheries?" we ask.

"Eight thousand *taka*."

I do the rough division and come up with about $200, meaning these women are at least doubling their income with work taking up less than half their time.

"Other women told us, 'You are working like a man. If you join with Grameen, you are not part of our culture.' People said Grameen was using money that came from Christians and was trying to convert us. There were even rumors that Grameen would take us away to some island.

"Now these same women want to join us."

"We're more courageous now," another adds. "When we have to take our fish to market, we even dare to come out at midnight."

THE HYACINTH PRINCIPLE

Leaving the fish farms, we head back to Dhaka, where we meet Farida Akhter, another of Yunus's former students and a cofounder of Nayakrishi, a movement of 50,000 farmers here who are reviving traditional crops. For centuries, rural people have saved, stored, and shared seeds they carefully bred as the basis of their household's food security. But under colonialism, these practices eroded in favor of growing a limited number of crops for the market.

Now, tens of thousands of farmers, in movements like Nayakrishi here and throughout Asia, are reviving the traditional practice of seed-saving and -sharing, we learn. (In the next chapter you'll learn about another such movement.) They're rediscovering the wisdom of seed diversity and breeding for specific, varied local conditions. They're awakening to the vulnerability built into a world in which a handful of corporations control much of the global seed market, and where some companies even take farmers to court for saving seeds that the companies have patented.

Sitting in Farida's second-story offices, whose tall windows overlook a narrow Dhaka side street, we get a botany lesson.

"Our movement is growing because farmers are talking with farmers and sharing ideas, seeds, and knowledge," says Farida, a tiny woman with an exuberance that brings the dimly lit room to life. "We don't go out to villages from a head office and tell them what to do. We work like the water hyacinth." The water hyacinth seems like a particularly apt metaphor, I think, in a country whose rivers and ponds are filled with the plant, its dark green leaves dotting the water like lily pads.

"The hyacinth sends out shoots horizontally, and a new plant sprouts," she tells us. "It grows so fast. Each plant sends out shoots to a new one. That's how our movement is growing—farmers teaching farmers."

Driving back to our hotel through the darkening Dhaka streets, we talk about how many of the people we've met are hyacinths, all in their own ways. About the way the Landless Workers' Movement in Brazil is sharing ideas, even promoting exchange programs to help landless in one settlement learn from those in others, or how the Edible Schoolyard in Berkeley shares its experience with teachers, principals, and schools far and wide.

We see Grameen, too, as a hyacinth in action, sparking ideas and spreading not just inside Bangladesh, but also beyond its borders. Microcredit programs have already sprouted in dozens of countries. This year, 37 million people worldwide, each of whom lives on less than $2 a day, have access to microcredit. Expecting a speedy spread, the global microcredit consortium, on whose board Yunus sits, hopes to reach 100 million people by 2005.[6]

Here in Bangladesh, Grameen has already spun off roughly a dozen new enterprises, mainly in the last six years. Grameen's sister-shoots are companies involved in weaving, renewable energy, marketing, communications, software development—even a mobile-phone company that makes telephoning possible for the first time in many villages. Grameen has also created a kind of health insurance for its members, and it even offers educational scholarships. Many of these ideas are offshoots of others, building and growing as a hyacinth grows.

WE'RE ALL BONSAI TREES

One evening, over our third plate of mangoes in our stark hotel room, Anna and I reflect on the staff that has created Grameen and instigated these off-shoots. We scratch our heads: Just where did Yunus find such talented people, many of whom have been with him since their university days?

When we have time with Yunus the next day, we ask what to us is an obvious question: "When you chose the students to work with you, how did you identify potential leaders, students who would be honest enough to be trusted with collecting the deposits and sensitive enough to work well with people?"

"I was not selective; they just happened to be around," Yunus answers, and my mind flips to the many impressive people in key roles whom we've met here. They are people who "just happened to be around?" Wow.

Yunus continues, "I think all people are honest; circumstances make them dishonest. People get pleasure from being honest. But then opportunities come, temptations come, or things are done in such a sloppy way people feel that, 'Well, why don't I do it, what difference will it make?' So they *become* dishonest.

"I came to see that you could create an environment that would avoid those temptations, and people would be happy to be honest.

"Today, Grameen Bank has more than ten thousand staff, and they work in remote villages with families, collect money, and carry it back to the office. Each one carries cash; lots of cash, say thirty thousand *taka,* and in Bangladesh that's like carrying thirty thousand dollars. He could do anything . . ."

"Like get on the next airplane," Anna jokes.

"He doesn't even have to wait for the next airplane! Look, it's simple, you tear your shirt, put on some blood or something and say, 'Oh my god, I've been robbed!' You've got your thirty thousand *taka*. Because it's an isolated place, nobody saw it. 'I was attacked, look at me, look what happened, and I saved my life.' Everyone is relieved you're alive. In the meantime you're thirty thousand *taka* richer.

"Remember, Bangladesh is a corrupt country. Everywhere you turn is corruption, but in Grameen this has never happened, *not once.*

"I've had to recruit a lot of people. I often am asked: 'What qualities are you looking for?' I say 'nothing.' There are too many applicants. I'm just trying to weed some out. Every one of them would be as good. It's the job that creates them.

"If I reject him, he may find another job, like with the police. He'll become a policeman, a corrupt policeman. If I had recruited him, he would have become an honest Grameen Bank staff member, dedicated to poor people— the *same* person.

"Human beings are like bonsai trees. I'm a tall, tall tree, a giant tree, but unfortunately I'm planted in a small pot, so I become a tiny little thing. It's the fault of the pot. It's the society, global society as a whole. The pot is the important thing. I could grow tall, if there was a place to support me. We're all bonsai trees."

WE MEET THE PERDUE LADY

Seeing how Grameen borrowers use their loans, we better understand why Yunus sees credit as a key missing nutrient for all us bonsais. Grameen borrowers frequently invest in materials to develop small enterprises, as Sufiya, the earliest borrower, did in her stool-making business. A common investment is a cow, and in the villages we visit we see many of them mingling with the children and goats. Chickens are common, too. Until we reach the village of Borodol, though, we hadn't seen anything more than a few hens scratching out survival in the family compound.

That was before we met Dahlia, one of the few stocky women we see in our time in Bangladesh. Wrapped in a dark red-and-gray sari, Dahlia proudly shows us her Grameen-supported enterprise. Starting with a loan to buy seventy-two chickens seven years ago, Dahlia now has a booming poultry business. Standing in her open courtyard, she shows us her chickens—all 1,400 of them.

Rabbi explains that Dahlia is one of those whom Grameen dubs its "golden members," women who have proven so reliable and entrepreneurial that they are eligible for loans of 100,000 *taka*—roughly equivalent to $2,000 but effectively worth a lot more here.

"Ten or twelve others are following my experience and asking my advice," Dahlia tells us. "I even sell chicken feed to some of the women who've started their own businesses."

As she talks, I can't help but notice the chickens trapped in tiny mesh cages madly pecking at each other's throats, and the piles of feces beneath them, and I wonder, and worry, about Dahlia's village-wide impact.

Back in the van, Anna and I don't exactly whisper, but we're not sure we want Rabbi to hear us. Trying to guess what we might find if we came back in five years, we dub Dahlia the "Perdue Lady."

Like Dahlia, poultry tycoon Frank Perdue started small, but today Perdue Farms is a $2 billion business in an industry notorious for low wages, dangerous working conditions, harsh treatment of the chickens, and serious pollution. Certainly, Perdue is no model for liberating people or protecting the environment. So what would keep Dahlia from following in Frank's footsteps?

When we ask Yunus, his answer is intriguing.

Part of it, he believes, is that Grameen builds in peer pressure. "She still has to go to center meetings," the weekly member gatherings like those we visited, at which women make loan decisions face to face. "She is still part of a group," Yunus reminds us, "no matter how rich she is."

For Yunus, part of it is also simply the magic of microcredit. Credit availability itself is protection. "This person cannot exploit Grameen members, because what she has, they have, too: access to credit. So, if they think, 'I can do that,' they can borrow money and follow her as a role model, as a mentor."

But the idea that the availability of credit protects against exploitation assumes everyone can be an entrepreneur. As I look at my own country and my own experience in two nonprofit start-ups, I know how hard it is to make a business go. It is exhausting and totally demanding. Does everyone have even the physical stamina? Perhaps Yunus is right that virtually any of us could successfully manage our own at-home weaving operation or a small stall selling groceries, but as Bangladesh becomes a more complex economy, so will the generation of small businesses.

But more important, even if we all really are entrepreneurs trapped in wage-laborer bodies, does Bangladesh want several million Perdue Ladies? I think about the cruelty to animals and the harm to rivers and estuaries, and to air and earth that the waste of factory farming generates.

Yunus took his capacity to rethink institutions from the bottom up and applied it to banking. It's possible, we hope, that this questioning—*why does it have to be this way?*—can inspire rethinking of all the businesses Grameen spawns. Grameen can help the potential Perdues of Bangladesh, for instance, rethink the poultry business, as is already happening here in the U.S., in Europe, and elsewhere, too. In France, for example, we will later meet a farmer who proves that commercial chicken production is possible without confining the birds in tiny cages, pumping them with antibiotics, or polluting the environment with their waste.

"Don't We All Want to Live Happy?"

We're still stirring with these questions when we meet another Grameen-inspired entrepreneur. In a region near Dhaka known for its traditional weavers, we're here to see firsthand one of the many hyacinth-like spinoffs—Grameen Uddog, a company in the "Grameen Family" that is reviving Bangladeshi traditional weaving.

We arrive at the local Grameen offices well after noon and welcome the lunch we're invited to share. The rain hits with a high-speed drumbeat, and hundreds of Grameen loan notebooks, warped by the hot, moist air, line the walls behind us. Dish after dish—eight in all—are laid out on a long table. I love the fish most. They're tiny native varieties with lots of needle-thin bones that I carefully tease out. Well, almost. One lingers mid-throat, and I silently pray for something to wash it down.

"Traditionally, Bangladesh was known for our weaving," Mizanur Rahman, who is in charge of Grameen Uddog, explains. "But for years, Bangladesh had been importing Madras Check cloth from India, and our own weavers were dying out. We had to do something. So, about six years ago, we created Grameen Check and formed a company to bring in big orders from abroad and give weavers better return for their work.

"Before, there were seasons where weavers would have no work at all, so they would get in desperate situations. Now, they get a steady flow of work."

We're eager to talk to a weaver and thus delighted when Santahar, wearing a colorful Grameen Check button-up shirt, joins us. Launching right into his story, he tells us that six years ago he was making $1.50 a day weaving on another man's loom. Today he owns eight looms and employs eight men.

Distracted momentarily by the tiny fish bone still in my throat (ah, the joys of native fish over commercial varieties!) I wonder, as with the Perdue Lady, what prevents Santahar from paying his workers a pittance so he can line his own pockets? When we ask how much he pays, he says, "I pay my workers eight hundred to twelve hundred *taka* a week," which is two to four times more than what he had made as a day laborer.

Suddenly, the electricity fails, and the light and (much more importantly) the fan go off. A lantern is placed on the table along with a bunch of small, fat bananas. My prayer is answered. With my first bite, the last little fish bone slides down.

Continuing the conversation in the shadows of the lamplit room, we ask Santahar how he determines his workers' salaries. "Couldn't you pay them less?" I ask.

"I could—but don't we all want to live happy?" he responds as if it's the most obvious thing in the world. "My laborers would not be happy if I paid them less. Now I see my workers putting tin roofs on their houses, and I feel proud."

PUTTING POVERTY IN THE MUSEUM

Bangladesh pushes Anna and me to keep asking ourselves: What is poverty, anyway? Yunus loves to repeat his vision that one day "poverty will be seen only in a museum, and we'll have to explain that awful thing to our grandchildren." But what is it?

Poverty, we're convinced, has actually very little to do with "things"—with what we can buy or how much we own of what. Beyond, of course, our most basic needs, our "things" are really tickets, passes to inclusion.

When we ask Yunus about his own definition of poverty, he answers by saying, "When Grameen was still a small organization, a village woman said to me, 'You people don't think we belong to this country, do you?' What she was saying is that, in the eyes of people who are *not* poor, she—a poor person— was not even there."

"She was telling you she felt invisible?" I ask, making sure I understand his message.

"Yes, invisible." Poverty, Yunus reminds us, is being excluded from community. It is internal exile.

But if poverty is exclusion, then it's not enough just to help people get "things"; to bring people into the economic fold through microcredit, for instance. The mores, the norms must change so that it is no longer acceptable to exclude, to leave people out of what they need if they are to be members of the community.

And if we don't? Just look at our own country where, despite growing national wealth, our poverty and hunger—exclusion—are continually recreated. While the top 1 percent of our population saw its wealth grow by 40 percent between the early '80s and the late '90s, at the end of the millennium almost one in five American children still lived in poverty, and millions of Americans work full-time and *still* don't have enough money to put food on their tables or adequately house themselves and their families.[7]

So, I look back on Santahar with hope. With his words, Anna and I sense a shifting norm: Santahar is practicing an ethic of inclusion—and we hope Dahlia will, too. Santahar is saying, in effect, "I will not pay my workers so little that they remain invisible, exiled." But will Santahar's ethic infect his whole community? I wonder.

I think back to Brazil and the MST's new emphasis of using dialogue to develop social values, both in its settlements and in venues like the seminar Anna and I attended. But here in Bangladesh, face-to-face dialogue is still inhibited. The social distance between men and women limits it, and even the format of Grameen meetings hardly facilitates free discussion. In borrowers' meetings, women all face the front and look at the bank worker, who is usually male, and not at one another. Here, involving a whole community—men and women together—in discussing what kind of village they want, as the MST is attempting to do, is unthinkable.

Then again, I remind myself, twenty years ago the taboo against contact between men and women was so entrenched here that Yunus had to talk to Grameen's early borrowers through bamboo walls.

During our last visit with Yunus, we discuss the importance of insuring that the values of Grameen are embedded in all the norms it encourages and the new businesses it spawns—like Dahlia's and Santahar's. We gently suggest a Seventeenth Decision: "If I become an employer, I will pay a living wage—a wage that provides enough resources for a dignified life."

Yunus smiles graciously but notes that sixteen is already an awkwardly bulky number. Also, Yunus says, "Helping others, doing justice to others is already in the pledges members make: 'We should not do any wrong to others and we should not tolerate any wrongs to others.'"

We keep pushing, though, to understand how Yunus's institutions do what he says, get at the root of poverty—exclusion. "You've moved one-third of your borrowers out of poverty," I say, hoping I convey my appreciation for the enormity of the accomplishment. "But you're still lending them money, even though they aren't poor, by your definition, anymore. And, you're no longer focused on expanding the number of borrowers. Why do you still loan to Golden Members like Dahlia?"

"Dahlia is an owner of the bank," Yunus says. "She has improved her life, and that is a success story of the Bank. I'm only an employee of the Bank, so who am I to tell her 'You leave the Bank'? She is the owner, so she can decide for herself whether she would like to stay with us or leave.

"Besides," Yunus adds, "now there are many other microcredit programs in Bangladesh that can reach people Grameen isn't reaching; we can't do the whole job."

YUNUS'S WATCHDOG

I understand Yunus's explanation, but I'm worried, too. If Grameen moves in a straight line from here, it will be a bank for people like Dahlia, no longer a bank of the poor. But when we learn of what we come to call Yunus's watchdog, we start to see another way Yunus is creating new norms, planting a new tree.

"We have to go to the root of the creation of poverty," Yunus says, "and that's what institutions are. So I'm trying to create new institutions—ones by and for the poor. That's why we created the Grameen Securities and Management Company."

We had been hearing about this new company since we arrived, but we had never understood its significance. Now, talking with Yunus, we come to see it as potentially the most creative piece of the ever-expanding hyacinth.

"The Grameen Securities and Management Company is creating mutual funds that own shares in Grameen family companies," Yunus explains.

"So the management and the oversight of these companies are with this mutual fund. It's sort of a brain trust, a social trust, to make sure these companies do the right thing; they don't go doing fishy things and shift their weight somewhere else.

"Business can run in all directions. We want to persuade all Grameen businesses to go in the *social* direction.

"Like we now have GrameenPhone," Yunus says, "which is a mobile-phone company. The mutual fund is a minority shareholder, but we have influence because we have thirty-five percent of the shares, and we have helped them to create an additional dimension of that company—bringing phones to the poor women in the villages.

"And we're hoping to go beyond Grameen companies to bring the social objectives to companies who never thought about it before. Like a ceramic factory in Bangladesh, why can't we become an owner of this company and channel it to poor people? We can do that, too."

Yunus reminds us, "The world has always visualized capitalism by saying the driving force is greed, but Grameen is a capitalist institution. Make no mistake. We're maximizing profits. But you can't say greed is moving this bank. Our social objectives are. So the theory needs a big reinterpretation. Social consciousness can be just as powerful a driving force for capitalism as greed. We must put this social consciousness to work."

Yunus's fund reflects a global trend to widen the logic of capitalism, a movement we can now measure, for example, in the two-trillion-plus dollars selectively directed by U.S. investors into companies based on their social impact. Yunus's enthusiasm about his new mutual fund brings me back to the hide-and-seek game in my mind: Grameen as a miniaturization of capitalism as it is, on the one hand, and Grameen taking capitalism beyond our limiting assumptions, on the other.

In the unique structure of Grameen that defies the givens of banking, in Yunus's "watchdog" mutual fund, as well as in the Sixteen Decisions that are beginning to form new social norms—in all this, Anna and I see that Grameen *is* evolving capitalism. It is showing that we haven't arrived at the end of history, as promoters of corporate globalization tell us, but are walking an ever-evolving path.

THE HYACINTH CAUTION

The Sixteen Decisions, the unconventional structure of the Bank, the mutual fund, all illustrate that for Yunus and his colleagues credit was never an end point, only an early entry point. Still, many see Grameen and see only one thing: microcredit—a single financial intervention. Locked into the "solve by dissection" thought trap, some believe they've uncovered in microcredit a straightforward economic formula to end poverty. Others beg to differ.

During our travels, we meet an American nun who tells us about working with a church-sponsored microcredit program in San Francisco. Microcredit was surely no quick fix in her eyes. As she put it, it takes a lot more than a small loan to start a viable business in the U.S., where marketing has become a virtual science and filing business tax forms uses a small grove of trees. For her, in an American urban setting, microcredit did not get to the root of the poverty everywhere around her.

So we become a bit uneasy with our metaphor. The hyacinth principle suggests the way ideas can spark and spread from person to person, generating ever-expanding spinoffs. But what if the new hyacinth sprouts—the micro-credit start-ups that Grameen has ignited in roughly sixty countries—are replications of the Grameen model but not its guiding ideas?

When we voiced our concern, Yunus said, "Yes, people are sometimes impatient. They want a quick fix. People don't want to understand first. They say, 'Oh, I got it!' But because they don't go into the philosophy of it, they are just imitating the grammar of Grameen."

To us the "grammar" of Grameen is microcredit as a single intervention. Its philosophy—and its essence—is a process of continuing to listen to the people themselves and to innovate in response to specific circumstances; to push assumptions about even the most seemingly rigid structures, like a bank, beyond the known. Fortunately, many of the hundreds of people and organizations inspired by Grameen understand this. They are not cookie-cutter copies. They're listening to the needs and possibilities of their own situations, experimenting with what might work best for them.

When we leave Bangladesh, though, it's the possibility of the transference of the "grammar" that unsettles us and our metaphor. We want the hyacinth to be spreading not a rigid formula but a liberating philosophy.

We're sorting through all of these impressions when we come up against the water hyacinth—the real one. We've just left Dhaka and are on our way to visit villages in the southern Indian state of Kerala. As our boat glides through water shimmering like aluminum foil, we hear our Indian guide grumble, "Damn water hyacinth!"

Catching our puzzled looks, he asks, "You don't know about the hyacinth? It was brought here by some idiot. It's not native, and it's dominating our waterways. Boats can hardly pass through some rivers now."

Aha, we think, this hyacinth overgrowth is a perfect caution that, like the plant, no idea can be transferred wholesale from one place to another. To learn from one another, we must discover the essence of the other's experience—in Grameen's case, putting an ear to the ground and keeping it there. Grameen is a willingness, as Yunus says, always to come back to the question: *Is it working? Is it really getting at the root of the problem?* Slipping through the narrow Indian river, Anna and I look at each other: *This* is the full hyacinth principle, we realize.

DISTURBING HOPE

Reflecting on Grameen now, we see it not as a product, microcredit, but as a daring process—of listening, of continual renewal by commitment to one precept: *What is, is not what has to be.* Grameen means never being afraid to question a given, even a given you yourself have created. Yunus becomes for us a symbol of our innate capacity to see beneath the "givens," to listen to our deeper intuitions, to have the courage to create.

Yet the Bangladesh experience is also profoundly disturbing. So many questions haunt us: such clear progress for the millions of women borrowers of Grameen, yes, but at the same time violence against women is increasing and female representation on the Grameen staff is shrinking. Yunus's beautiful vision of putting poverty in the museum moves me, but credit doesn't necessarily prevent Grameen entrepreneurs from reproducing the exclusion at the root of poverty. Will new norms of inclusion continue to evolve, or will growing consumerism, fed by multinational advertising, overwhelm Grameen's best efforts to nourish them?

When I left home, I thought I could use Bangladesh to prove somehow that hope is justified even in one of the world's poorest societies. But instead, Bangladesh used me to teach a deeper truth.

It taught me that no one can "justify" hope by proving something good and positive. Hope is more verb than noun—an action, not a stance. It is movement. It is jumping into the messiness of it all. It is listening, learning, trying, stumbling; it is false starts and contradictory evidence.

Bangladesh taught me a kind of *disturbing hope*—hope I can't let go of but that leaves me restless. A hope that doesn't satisfy but gnaws at me to keep pushing.

BANGLADESH: AWAKENING OUR SENSES

Bengali Lentil Soup

Serves 6   *This recipe was inspired by recipes from Professor Muhammad Yunus and the women of Naripokkho in Bangladesh. The soup will take you less than a half hour to make, and it's extraordinarily tasty and healthy.*

1 cup red lentils
4 cups water
½ teaspoon turmeric
1 cup canned tomatoes
1½ teaspoons salt
2 tablespoons vegetable oil
½ teaspoon cumin seeds

½ teaspoons yellow or black mustard seeds
2 teaspoons jalapeno pepper (½ small), seeded
4 cups onions (2 large), finely sliced
5 teaspoons garlic (3 to 4 cloves), sliced
½ cup fresh cilantro leaves, chopped

Add lentils to water in a large saucepan. Add turmeric and stir. Bring to a boil and then simmer for 20 minutes until the lentils are soft. Add tomatoes and salt, and cook for a few minutes longer. Reduce heat.

Meanwhile, heat oil in a skillet. Add the cumin seeds and mustard seeds and sauté until fragrant, for just a few minutes. Cook at a low heat and be careful not to burn the seeds. Add jalapeño, onions, and garlic, and cook until golden brown (about 10 minutes).

Add onion mixture to lentils and cook for a few minutes longer, stirring occasionally.

Remove from heat. Add fresh cilantro leaves to the lentil soup and cover to steep for a minute. Serve while hot. For a final touch, scoop a dollop of fresh yogurt on top.

CHAPTER 6

SEEKING ANNAPOORNA

Ours is not a problem of scarcity,
It's a problem of plenty.

SHANTA KUMAR, MINISTER, CONSUMER
AFFAIRS & PUBLIC DISTRIBUTION
GOVERNMENT OF INDIA

Lifting off from the Kerala airport at the southern tip of India, all we see below are endless stretches of coconut palm. As we head north to Delhi, through the most spectacularly sculpted clouds I've ever seen, my thoughts drift back to the early 1970s.

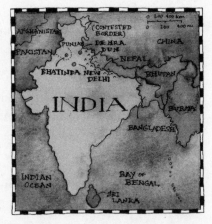

That's when I met Joe Collins, my co-conspirator in creating Food First and in writing the book of that name. At that time, the Green Revolution—the spread of hybrid seeds fed by chemical fertilizers and protected by pesticides—had just dramatically upped grain output in North America. One of the leading Green Revolution scientists, Norman Borlaug, had won the 1970 Nobel Peace Prize for his high-yielding wheat varieties. The Green Revolution was a proven success, it seemed.[1]

So, the logic went, why not transplant this neat package, plus farm machines, to the hungry third world as quickly as possible?

The unstated assumption: When it comes to relieving hunger in the world, the active players are Western philanthropic foundations, development agencies, scientists in elite research centers, and CEOs in big companies. The inert recipients are poor people abroad . . . waiting—hungry—for their answers.

Joe and I argued that more food by itself couldn't end hunger, and we said that people in the third world were not waiting passively—they had the savvy, hands-on experience, and indigenous knowledge on which to create their own food security, if obstacles like landlessness and antidemocratic authority structures were transformed.

But the Green Revolutionists scoffed at us.

Now Anna and I are on our way to see with our own eyes what truths thirty years have revealed. In India—home to one out of every four farmers in the world—the proving ground of the Green Revolution was to be the Punjab, the Indian version of our Midwest breadbasket. Soon we will actually be there.

DÉJÀ VU

From our stuffed backpacks, Anna and I pull out and divide up reading materials to prepare us to speak intelligently in Delhi, not just about the Green Revolution but about the latest promise of Western agriculturalists and agribusiness: the "Gene Revolution"—the new practice of combining traits across species in ways nature never could to engineer pest-resistant and higher-yielding crops.

As we read, the corporate arguments for bioengineering are eerily familiar.

"Worrying about starving future generations won't feed them. Food biotechnology will," claims Monsanto, whose seeds account for more than 90 percent of all acreage planted with genetically modified organisms (GMOs) worldwide. Monsanto and other companies getting into biotechnology also promise that GMOs will reduce pressure on the land, help us become less reliant on chemicals, and even protect the rainforest.[2]

Ironically, studies of Monsanto's genetically engineered soybeans in the U.S. have found their yields to be *lower* than those of other varieties, and that the amounts of herbicides used on them are *greater*—this according to work of a prominent former member of the National Academy of Sciences.[3]

In case you don't know Monsanto, it's a company that helped develop the atom bomb, produced cancer-causing PCBs, and brought us the dioxin-containing herbicides used in Agent Orange—notorious for its use by the U.S. in defoliating Vietnam. It's also the company that threatened to sue a potential publisher of Anna's father's book *Against the Grain,* a scientific evaluation of the company's genetically altered seeds.

We read about another "revolution" I could never have imagined when I wrote *Diet for a Small Planet.* In just the last few decades, national and international laws have changed, allowing companies to patent genes from living organisms. The result has been a further skewing of world resources. Today, corporations in the industrialized world—not third-world governments, research institutions, or companies—hold roughly 90 percent of all the world's technology and product patents, many of them derived from plants cultivated in the third world.[4]

In a few hours, we'll be stepping off the plane to meet leaders of an Indian movement that is questioning the wisdom of all this: the Green Revolution and its 21st-century redux, the Gene Revolution, as well as new international rules governing patents, including those on life forms such as seeds.

"AND OLD EXPERIENCE LABORED OUT ONCE MORE"

When Joe Collins and I wrote *Food First,* Anna was still a baby. (The first time he visited me in Hastings-on-Hudson, she fussed so much for her food that it was a challenge to get across just how much I wanted to work on the book.)

In *Food First,* Joe and I argued that what was missing was not Western technologies, not more pesticides or exotic crops or large-scale mechanization, but what I came decades later to call "living democracy"—people developing their capacities to work together to build on traditional wisdom to find solutions. Class, caste, and the legacy of colonialism, we argued, meant that new, purchased technologies would further separate poor people who couldn't afford them from the land and jobs they needed to feed themselves.

Joe and I predicted that the Green Revolution plunked down in the Punjab would ultimately impoverish many people and drive the least-advantaged among them off the land. To produce high yields, the hybrid seeds need costly pesticides, fertilizers, and often irrigation, too, so they require farmers to take on debt—loans that only those who are better off can carry.[5]

Though yields from the hybrid seeds are typically higher, they also involve greater risk, because the crops are more vulnerable to pests and to variations in weather. The Green Revolution also brought "monoculture"—the spread of only a few seed varieties at the expense of diverse crops and varieties—thus further heightening farmers' vulnerability to pests and weather. Again, it is the better-off, not the poorest, who can afford to risk losing a crop.

Also, hybrid seeds are often sterile. Those seeds that do reproduce often fail to pass on the high-yield traits, forcing farmers to purchase seeds each year. Farmers who relied for centuries on saving and sharing seeds no longer could.[6]

Our arguments seemed strong, but honestly, I had my secret fears. Were Joe and I being naïve? We couldn't deny that grain yields did jump dramatically with the importation of this technology.

Recently, in a Harvard debate, I heard the father of India's Green Revolution, Dr. M. S. Swaminathan, repeat what Joe and I heard so often: that the Green Revolution bought time—prevented starvation while population growth was slowed—allowing India to move from "begging bowl" to "bread-basket" almost overnight.[7]

Joe and I didn't question the increased production. We asked whether there were better ways both to grow food and to ensure that those who needed it had access to it. But were Joe and I just young idealists refusing to face tough trade-offs? Anna's and my journey to India brings us back to these questions. I want to know—were our instincts right?

Stepping off the plane, I'm slapped out of my reverie by the Delhi heat. Sticky and exhausted, Anna and I arrive at an ashram where our hosts had arranged for us to stay. Our room is stark and hot—very, very hot. This night we discover one of what turn out to be a dozen uses for our Grameen Check sheet, bought from village weavers in Bangladesh. As we lie under the ceiling fan, the blue-and-yellow-striped cloth, sprinkled with water, becomes our makeshift and oh-so-welcome air conditioner.

Finding it hard to sleep in the heat, Anna looks for some non-research reading. In a motel room at home, she'd no doubt have found at least a Bible, but here, on an almost barren shelf, she finds only the writings of the ashram's founder, Sri Aurobindo, a 20th-century spiritual leader for Indian independence. Opening one of his books to a page at random, Anna reads aloud. The first passage ends:

And all that was destroyed must be rebuilt;
and old experience labored out once more.

Sri Aurobindo's words lull me to sleep, and I drift off wondering what we will find here. Maybe it will turn out that Sri Aurobindo hit it right on the nose.

THE "FREE TREE"

The next morning, a beaten-up, British-style black taxi takes us to the offices of Dr. Vandana Shiva, founder of the research center and farmers' movement we hope will help us untangle our huge questions.

Vandana has been called everything from quack scientist to the new millennium's Gandhi. Sari-cloaked and heavyset, with a voice that booms across stadiums of thousands, the former nuclear physicist is unarguably one of the world's preeminent global environmental activists.

As our taxi dodges bicycles, motor scooters, and thick car traffic, Anna and I talk about Vandana's seeming omnipresence. In the past year, we've seen her rouse crowds ranging from pierced anarchists in Seattle to $3,000-Armani-suit-wearing executives in New York City, and we've read dozens of articles by her or about her in publications ranging from *The New York Times* to *The New Hindu*.

It's been five decades since India won its independence, and Vandana sees herself waging an equally important battle. This time, the fight is against the CEOs and trade commissioners whom she claims threaten Indian independence as much as the British imperialists did fifty years ago.

So, when we turn into a narrow residential street, we're surprised when the cab stops in front of a small house with a modest sign announcing Vandana's organization: The Foundation for Science, Technology and Ecology. We see now the value of the organization's clunky and self-important name, which fooled even us. It's a good reminder that you can't equate influence with resources.

We climb the porch steps past a generator with the look of a car engine and the sound of a tractor. Spotty electricity makes it an essential backup for computers whose Internet connection is this organization's lifeblood.

As soon as we enter, I can't help but notice a mural painted across the office's tall, light-green wall. With Grandma Moses charm, its colorful branches reach toward the ceiling, and intricately drawn animals perch here and there.

"That's the neem tree," says one of the several people milling around the homey office. We have no idea of the neem's immediate significance, but the staff is quickly abuzz, filling us in.

In 1994, a patent on a fungicide made from Indian neem-tree oil was granted to the U.S. Department of Agriculture and W. R. Grace, one of the world's mightiest chemical conglomerates.[8] (Remember the movie *A Civil Action*, with John Travolta? Based on a real-life lawsuit, the film also stars W. R.

Grace as one of the two companies whose factories allegedly contaminated the water in small-town Woburn, Massachusetts.)

Vandana's Foundation, along with several other international groups, filed suit, arguing that the USDA-Grace patent unfairly claimed "ownership" of knowledge developed over centuries by Indian farmers and healers. As many as 2,000 years ago, Indian texts allude to neem's numerous uses.

"As a kid, we used neem to clean our teeth, as a shampoo, for soap," Kusum Menon, a Vandana colleague, explains. "It's not something of the distant past; neem is part of everyday life."

Today, neem is used in all these ways and more—as an insect repellent, in cosmetics, even as a contraceptive.[9] It's also good against the Medfly, which we've been warding off back home with mandatory sprayings of malathion, even though serious health questions have been raised about its use.

In the fight against the neem patent, an Indian delegation that included representatives from Vandana's group delivered to the European Patent Office in Munich a petition signed by half a million Indians—farmers, children, housewives, and businessmen—demanding that the patent be withdrawn.

We're here just two weeks after the May 10th victory. And this morning the excitement is palpable. The Patent Office overturned the USDA-Grace patent, concluding that the "claims were not novel in view of prior use, which had taken place in India."[10] The decision builds on the 1997 U.S. Patent Trademark Office repeal of a turmeric patent because the company in question couldn't prove "novelty."

"You need to realize that winning this case is not just about the neem," clarifies Afsar Jafri, a scientist with the Foundation whose wispy frame and smooth skin make him look even younger than his twenty-nine years. "It's a precedent. It makes challenges to other patents more likely to succeed."

After our crash course on the neem, we sense more potently how a patent system developed in industrial society doesn't fit uniformly all around the world. For one thing, we in industrialized countries are used to thinking of inventors "tinkering" with objects, creating technical innovations. But what if the real value is what nature *itself* created, not what people devised? What if the people-contribution is mostly in discovering nature's genius?

We're told we need patents, that without them we'd never get innovation and individual inventors wouldn't get their due reward for cleverness. But what if much of the world's inspiration for innovation has been driven not by monetary rewards but by a sense of community self-interest? And what if the creativity that's sparked when knowledge spreads freely—without patents and legalese—has been the very thing that has brought us the innovation we so cherish?

So it seems with neem.

Patents like the ones on the neem bring big financial gain for those to whom they're granted, but the real "inventors," Indians who long ago discovered neem's many uses and shared their knowledge openly, get nothing.

The way our patent system—now going global—works, it doesn't matter if, for instance, Kusum shows her grandchildren how to use neem as a toothpaste, or for fevers, or headaches, or diarrhea. It's not an invention until the knowledge is translated into the language of Western science. Only then is the "inventor" acknowledged and rewarded with monopoly property rights. Our patent system just wasn't created to recognize and reward the fruits of community innovation.

But remember, this patent paradigm is brand new.

India has historically prohibited the patenting of any life forms, and so, too, did the U.S. Not until the early '70s did our laws change, allowing the patenting of sexually reproduced plants. And, in 1980, the Supreme Court effectively reversed laws preventing the patenting of living organisms. I recall no broad public debate, yet it's hard to imagine a decision with wider public impact than the patenting of life. This may be especially true to people in less-industrialized countries, home to two-thirds of the world's plant species.

And it's especially true for farmers here in India. Eighty-five percent of the seeds they use are not patented, purchased seeds but seeds that exist as a "commons," in effect, saved or exchanged among themselves. Now, because of new World Trade Organization requirements, patent laws around the world may soon look just like ours, opening the door for multinational seed patenters. Or, maybe not. The European Parliament has taken a strong stand against the patentability of life forms. And almost 200 citizen organizations and tribal bodies in both northern and southern countries are developing a proposal for an international Treaty to Share the Genetic Commons which would disallow the patenting of life.[11] Costa Rica has already banned all patenting of, and profiting from, the genes of native Costa Rican plant and animal species by foreign countries.

At the end of our conversation, Kusum leans in close and says, "You know what 'neem' means? The tree was actually named thousands of years ago in Persia. They called it *Azad-Darakth,* 'the free tree,'" she says with a smile and a wink. "Our ancestors knew."

But this ancient tree has still more battles in store to remain true to its name. In the early '90s, when the USDA-Grace patent was granted, there were only four other patents on the neem. Now, the "free tree" has ninety official patents on parts of its essence and forty more pending.[12]

THE NEW SPINNING WHEEL

We're still absorbing the neem news when Vandana arrives, greeting us with hugs and a friendly effervescence that shows the other side of her powerful, can-do public persona and her full frontal attack on the process of corporate globalization. She claims it is literally killing hundreds of Indian farmers and threatening the livelihoods of millions more.

Vandana has only a short time with us before she has to depart for a government meeting to weigh in against privatizing Delhi's water. Maya Jani, one of her colleagues and a friend since college, tells us that government agencies increasingly ask Vandana for advice on a range of issues, water being just one.

Sitting with us at a large wooden table with the neem mural behind her, Vandana launches right in.

"The turning point for me was 1987. I was at a conference called 'The Laws of Life,' which attracted a lot of biotech companies. A representative from the multinational Sandoz predicted, 'By the turn of the century there will be just five of us [big agrochemical companies], and we better have patents on seeds.'

"That one sentence triggered a whole redirection of my work," Vandana continues.

"When India was a British colony, the country, like most colonies, produced commodities that were extracted at a painful price for us and sold cheaply in the British Empire.

"For Gandhi, liberation, independence, would come in part from reclaiming national industries and Indian traditions. So the textile industry was critical to Gandhi's struggle, and the spinning wheel became his symbol.

"What's happening now is a new kind of colonization by the Novartises of the world [explained shortly], who are monopolizing control of our agricultural knowledge and traditions." She pauses and looks at us with resolution. "So I asked myself, what's our spinning wheel?

"My answer was the seed."

The seed, I think, may be an even more powerful symbol than the spinning wheel. The seed is life itself. In India, where agriculture has been practiced for thousands of years, local seed varieties are the living history of an entire people.

And about the Sandoz representative's predictions that triggered Vandana's early moment of dissonance? They were surprisingly on the mark.

Since his 1987 forecast, multinational mergers have quickened at a breathtaking pace. In 1997, Sandoz merged with Ciba Geigy to form Novartis. In turn, Novartis recently merged its agrochemical and seed divisions with AstraZeneca's to form Syngenta—now the largest agrochemical corporation and the third-largest seed company in the world, and Monsanto has become part of the giant Pharmacia. Thirty years ago, a multitude of seed companies sold seeds around the world; today just ten global seed corporations control approximately one-third of the world's commercial seed market, and many of these companies also dominate markets in the related fields of pharmaceuticals and argochemicals.[13]

With genetically modified seeds, the concentration is tighter still: Just five companies sell all transgenic seeds planted worldwide.[14] And two—Monsanto and Syngenta—have locked up patents on key techniques that scientists use to develop new biotech seeds.[15]

PANNA HEAVEN

After Vandana rushes out to her meeting, we realize it's unlikely we'll see much of her. In the morning, we head for the foothills of the Himalaya, where we don't know what's in store; we know only that we'll get to meet farmers in the Foundation's movement. Called Navdanya, meaning nine seeds, the movement was founded to help preserve India's agricultural diversity and promote food security.

Navdanya has an urban strategy, too. In part through its Delhi-based shop and festivals highlighting Indian food traditions, it's linking countryside and city. Maya prepares us for what we're about to see—and taste—at one such festival this afternoon before we head out, and up, to the villages.

Now that India's economy has opened to multinational business, Maya explains, the country has become a hot spot for new industries. "But despite growing wealth here—just look at all the billboards for high-tech jobs—food insecurity is worse," she says. "Violence against women is worse. Market forces are creating pockets of beneficiaries who are becoming more callous.

MODERN-DAY PIRATES

Between interviews, I browse the Foundation's dozens of books: *Cargill: The New East India Company, Seeds of Suicide,* even one called, *Rani and Felicity: The Story of Two Chickens,* a children's book about factory farms.

Sitting on a comfortable couch, I flip open *Biopiracy* and learn about another heated debate: RiceTec Inc.'s patent on Basmati rice lines and grain that small farmers throughout India and Pakistan had developed over centuries.[16] In 1998 Vandana's organization, other Indian groups, and the Indian government took it to court, claiming that its patent is derived from Indian varieties and is not "novel"—a criterion for any patent.

Likened to the pirates of centuries ago, RiceTec is allegedly stealing knowledge earned by the hard work and innovation of people here. (Reading a report by a Canadian group fighting the patent, I learn that RiceTec is wholly owned by Prince Hans Adam II of Liechtenstein; the pirate metaphor gains strength.) If RiceTec keeps its patent, Vandana's group, and the Indian government, too, fear for the two million small farmers who depend on the Basmati cachet for their livelihood.

After several years of legal battles, RiceTec is losing ground. They lost the right to use the name "Basmati," and all but three of their patents' claims. The courts agreed that "Basmati" is the name tied to the place where the rice was originally developed, and it's in India, not Alvin, Texas.[17]

But as I put the book down, all I can think about is that several months ago, craving Basmati, I bought the closest thing I could find. Now with a half-full jar of RiceTec Jasmati™ at home, I feel like a pirate's accomplice.

—Anna

Even the old charity mentality is going away." Maya's words seem to resonate with what we've just heard in Bangladesh.

In the fewer than ten years since Pepsi and Coca-Cola were allowed back into India, they and their local brands have flooded the market. Coca-Cola is now one of the largest foreign investors in India.[18] In my research for *Diet for a Small Planet,* I was horrified to learn that, as mentioned in *The Delicious*

Revolution, drinking a can of Coke or Pepsi is the sugar equivalent of eating a piece of chocolate cake, with no redeeming nutritional benefit.

Navdanya fears that Indians are being sucked into this radical, experimental diet—the one spreading from America to the rest of the world, bringing with it heart disease, cancer, and diabetes. They fear, too, that the meager health-care resources—in India, less than 1 percent per person of what the industrial countries spend—will be diverted even further from the health needs of the poor, who are still fighting infectious disease, and to the rich, who are getting sicker with diseases like diabetes, thanks to this high-fat, high-sugar diet.[19]

"Navdanya," Maya explains, "wants to retrieve indigenous food and drink from extinction through pleasure—and fast, before our taste buds are completely stolen by Pepsi and Coke. Our festivals are a way to help people regain confidence in their traditions."

It's late afternoon by the time we arrive at Navdanya's outpost in a Delhi open-air market. The heat has made us droopy and incredibly thirsty, so we both perk up when Maya tells us our arrival luckily coincides with Navdanya's *panna,* Hindi for "drink," a festival celebrating traditional cooling beverages.

"We want you to sample them. You'll love them," Kusum tells us, but we need no convincing.

On the edge of a busy boulevard, the market's stalls overflow with saris and trinkets, and a mixture of tourists and locals meanders past dozens of vendors. Among nondescript stalls, Navdanya Foods' elaborately decorated store stands out. Providing a selling point for indigenous crops threatened with extinction, this Delhi shop is Navdanya's bridge between ecological farmers and urban consumers.

Handmade paper lanterns and dried seeds hang from the ceiling, and bordering the store are painted white swirls dotted with bright marigolds. "We put these out today in honor of your visit," Kusum tells us.

As we chat at a stone table with Navdanya staff and customers—from a local businessman to an octogenarian kitchen-garden activist—we get a taste of the *panna* festival. One glass after another keeps coming. We don't just sample, we guzzle each of the eight celebrated drinks—a blood-red rhododendron cóncoction, a thick-as-oatmeal barley drink, sweet mango nectar, a light and tangy litchi juice, and more.

Heading back to the offices through Delhi traffic, with its onslaught of soot and billboards, vendors and stalls, hawkers and peddlers, we see Pepsi and Coke logos splattered everywhere. The well-intentioned *panna* festival tucked away in the back of an urban market feels like a drop, though a tasty one, in the proverbial bucket. But, then again, I remind myself, Navdanya is just getting started. They laughed at Gandhi, too.

Plus, still reveling in my *panna* gluttony, I remember the power of pleasure. Anna and I swear never to touch another soda as long as we live.

PLANTING "ZONES FOR FREEDOM"

The next day we take a packed train from Delhi to where Navdanya and the Research Foundation began, to Vandana's hometown of Dehra Dun, a city of almost 300,000 nestled in a Northern Indian valley in the foothills of the Himalaya.

Arriving at the station, we're swept into the crowd of passengers, wondering at first how our guides will find us until we realize we're the only Westerners here. Vinod Kumar Bhatt, a thirty-two-year-old Navdanya agronomist, greets us with a friendly handshake, saying, "You both look just like you do on your Web site!" We're surprised at first. We seem far from DSL connections and URLs, but then we remember how much the organization depends on the Internet to communicate with each other, tap information, and connect with a worldwide network. We're also met by Negi Darban Singh, a wiry man with a thin moustache and wavy hair. Negi is Navdanya's district coordinator and will be our interpreter and constantly energetic guide for the next week.

As we leave the station and drive into Dehra Dun in our open-air jeep, the din of motor scooters makes conversation almost impossible. Traffic is at a virtual standstill, and soot cakes every wall we pass—and our faces, necks, and throats, too. "Thirty years ago," shouts Negi above the commotion, "there were only two scooters here."

Luckily, we don't stay in the city long but head to the outskirts, to the Navdanya demonstration farm. There, farmers learn how to save indigenous seeds and grow food organically, and are encouraged to share knowledge and seeds.

The twelve-and-a-half-acre farm, Negi explains, was originally part of Vandana's family homestead. When Vandana told us that her first office was in her parents' cowshed, I was amused by the parallel in my own life. I, too, had converted an old barn to live and work in, just as Vandana had done with her cowshed, and in my case I'd left the horse stalls intact to hold books, not animals.

From Negi and Vinod we get the scoop. "We've converted fifteen villages in the region from conventional farming to organics. Now we're going to an additional twenty," explains Negi. I'm struck that Negi, like many people, uses the term "conventional" to refer to chemical agriculture, which didn't even exist here forty years ago. How quickly something becomes the "convention"!

As Negi explains what he does, I catch on that he's really the outreach worker, the circuit rider—the Johnny Appleseed . . . well, sort of. Instead of just taking seeds to villages, though, he's encouraging farmers to value and keep their own diverse varieties, and to revive the practice of seed exchange.

What we'd read on the plane now clicks in. Negi's talking about Zones for Freedom—Vandana's name for villages that pledge to reject chemical fertilizers and pesticides, genetically modified seeds, and patents on life.

As we near the Navdanya farm and pass through a mango grove, the quiet envelops us, a welcome contrast to the Dehra Dun bustle. Vinod describes what we're about to see—or at least imagine—since our travel dates in India may have been perfectly timed to hit the *panna* festival but *not* to see much growing in the fields here.

Standing on the cement porch of the small building that holds the seed collection, Anna and I look out over the soon-to-be-planted fields. "We grow fifty crops here, including four hundred different varieties. In rice alone, we have over two hundred varieties," Vinod quietly explains. "We're collecting more varieties from farmers and adding them every year."

The importance of this work to protect agricultural diversity sinks in when I think of the rapid loss of diversity worldwide, much due to industrial agriculture's pressure to standardize. The Green Revolution encouraged farmers, who for centuries planted a variety of crops, to plant the same seeds over large areas—think of all those manicured fields of corn or wheat that are the trademark of our breadbasket.

Historically, India's rice diversity was the richest in the world. It's home to roughly 40,000 varieties.[20] But here, as in more and more countries, farmers are adopting a small number of modern crop varieties. In the Phillipines and Indonesia, for example, four out of five farmers now plant commercial seeds, foregoing local varieties. In Indonesia, 1,500 local rice varieties have become extinct since the early 1980s, and one single variety has come to dominate the country.[21] Imagine the vulnerability to pest or disease.

LESSONS BRIDGE CONTINENTS

When Anna asks what Vinod's biggest surprise has been in this work, I expect to hear about a seed-breeding breakthrough, but instead he says simply, "What's most surprising is that people are joining us. People who didn't believe in eco-farming are now with us, after seeing our results. They see that the quality and the taste is much better, whether it's tea, milk, rice, onions, potatoes, whatever it is."

Here in India, for one of the few times in all my many years focused on food and hunger—but not the last time on this journey—we hear people talking about the importance of *taste*.

"We work closely with farmers in the area," Vinod continues, "learning and sharing how to make herbal pesticides and compost. Nature is balanced. What disease you have in the field, you find a solution in the field. Farmers are now coming to us, letting us know what they need. One wants vegetables well suited to dry conditions. Another, something responsive to irrigation; another, grains able to withstand high wind velocity."

The farm shows the value of diverse, often-overlooked traditional varieties, yes, but it's also demonstrating how a family of six can live and thrive on one half-acre—with not only food to eat but also crops to sell, even honey. (Bee pollination is essential to organic farming, Vinod explains, as Anna dodges the few bees buzzing near us.)

Vinod reminds me very much of a man I'd met years ago in Guatemala. (I was with Anna then, too, but she wasn't quite the partner she is now. She was only three!) At the time, development worker Roland Bunch was teaching indigenous people—pushed by big lowland haciendas onto steep, easily eroded hillsides—how to increase corn yields using erosion-retarding ditches. He did the best he could to help, but eking out much food at all was tough.

Two decades later, Roland is much more optimistic. He's worked with small farmers on poor soils in a dozen countries. Roland told me recently that we now know how to make the vast majority of soils highly fertile, without commercial seeds and with little or no infusion of chemicals.

The key, Vinod and Roland agree, is maximizing the soil's organic matter. Compost does the trick, of course, but compost can be a lot of work. So, Roland and his co-experimenters plant "green manure" and cover crops—like clover—to accomplish the same thing that compost does but without the hassle of building heaps and transporting compost to the fields. Through trial and error, four other principles emerged for Roland: keeping soil covered, leaving the soil untilled, maintaining plant diversity, and, in the acid soils of the humid tropics, feeding nutrients (phosphorus, for example) to plants through mulch.[22]

Like Vinod, Roland stresses that it's often the poor, illiterate farmers themselves who are developing this "cutting edge technology," as he calls it. They're experimenting, observing, and comparing approaches to transform infertile soil.

I make a promise to myself that when we get home, I'll hook up Roland and Vinod. Across continents and climates, they're arriving at similar discoveries.

Now, looking out into the mainly brown field of Vinod's demonstration plot, Anna and I see a farmer harvesting something. "What's she gathering?" I ask. We had been told nothing was harvestable at this time of year.

"Grass for cows," Vinod answers. "Green Revolution scientists call them weeds."

HIMALAYAN GRAFFITI

The next morning we pile into a jeep with Negi and his favorite driver, and we head off to see the villages Negi has drawn onto the Navdanya path. As we bounce along, my thoughts travel back to what Vandana said gave her courage to face harsh public attacks on her for her controversial opinions.

"My parents exposed my sister and me to things that modern, urban kids are made to be afraid of—forests, rivers, tribal people," she told Anna and me. "We were left to find our own way and to do things that generate fear. We were taught to be fearless."

I've been staring for hours at mile after mile of eucalyptus lining the roads, wondering whether these are the forests so important in Vandana's childhood, when Negi interrupts my musings by grumbling about what pests eucalyptus trees are. (Actually, eucalyptus, now spread to many countries, are a sad example of the production-fixation thought trap. Not native to India and introduced here because they grow fast, eucalyptus use a lot of water, depriving nearby plants, and are even said to cause soil erosion, not control it.)

But what really wakes me up is what's *on* the trees—not growing but written. Vertically painted down the trunks of an entire stand is the familiar Pepsi logo, turning these foreign implants into billboards advertising still more foreign implants!

After several hours of driving, we start climbing into the mountains, and the road narrows to a dirt lane cut into the mountainside. Winding up, up, up into the Himalayan foothills, I silently thank our dear driver for honking at every hairpin turn. I try not to look down, but it's too beautiful not to. Across the valley, the mountains are haloed with wispy clouds and carved with green terraces like chiseled steps.

By the time we arrive in Pullinda, it's well after lunchtime. The village's seventy homes cling to the hillside like the narrow road we've just climbed. On many of their whitewashed stone walls we notice the painted marks identifying seed savers and sharers who receive seeds from Navdanya each season. In return for the seeds, the farmers promise to give back after harvest as much as twice the amount of seeds they received, or to share their seeds with at least two other farmers and let Navdanya know. As Farida in Bangladesh would say, they're spreading seed wealth, seed diversity, and knowledge, like the hyacinth.

Negi ushers us into a small turquoise room with thick walls and windows the size of lunch pails. The village honchos—elders, including the chief—sit on the floor sharing a water pipe with a swanlike stem. We sit on low stools facing them.

"The government introduced chemical agricultural here twenty years ago," says Manoj Kumar, the village chief. "If we keep going this direction, in ten years the whole region will die."

As the gravity of his words sinks in, we hear the soft gurgling of the pipe and smell tobacco leaves burning, faint and sweet. Manoj continues, explaining: "Almost everyone in this area has had physical problems. Headaches, stomach problems, kidneys. People are weaker now. I'm sixty-three, but I can carry fifty to sixty kilograms. My son, he can't even carry twenty."

"So, we're bringing back traditional varieties—three to four rices, four to five millets, four to five legumes," he says. Pointing to the bulging bags stacked high in the corner, he adds, "that's the government rice we're still getting. We won't even plant it anymore, because our seeds are so much better."

We listen to the mixture of anger and hope in the voices of Manoj and his friends, realizing that, for them, reclaiming traditional seeds and farming practices is not a nice cultural exercise; it's a matter of life and death.

As we leave Pullinda for the next village, a hut catches Anna's eye. How could it not? Big Hindi letters cover virtually its entire side.

"Negi, what does that say?" Anna asks, shooting a picture.

"We reject Monsanto and gene patenting. We reject terminator technology."

Anna and I laugh in amazement. "Terminator technology" is the popular name for a seed type patented just a few years ago by the U.S. Department of Agriculture and the agribusiness giant Delta & Pine Land Seed Company.[23] Like a hybrid, this new type of seed becomes useless after one growing season, forcing farmers to buy new seeds every year and making them dependent on the companies. Other agribusiness companies are pursuing this technology, too. Reading the bright green words with new understanding, Anna and I wonder aloud what Americans would think of their government's resources going into technology that increases farmers' dependency and what terminator-technology patenters would say to the farmers whom we're meeting.

As we climb still higher, a nagging thought won't leave me. Vandana, Vinod, really all Navdanya staff, said this movement was based in the villages, but what can these villagers really know about biotechnology? Is the graffiti proof that they've been sold another packaged ideology, not the Green Revolution's, but Navdanya's? I want to ask Anna, but three villagers who hitched a ride, too, are pressed in between us, hanging on to bags of rice so the bags don't slip out of the open sides of the jeep. I hold my questions, but not for long.

What My Heart is Saying

"Here's where you'll sleep the night," says Negi, as we climb the steps to a small room in the center of the even tinier village of Ramani. "Soon the room will be Navdanya's storage space for seed saving. The earthen pots in the corner," says Negi, pointing, "hold the beginning."

Sheaves of grain decorate the mauve walls of an otherwise bare room with no water or other facilities. But, hey, I think to myself, we haven't lugged soft-plastic water bottles—always looking unsettlingly like intravenous feeding bags—thousands of miles from Boston for nothing!

That afternoon and evening, a steady stream of guests, all men, of course, come to tell us about village seed saving and why they reject chemical agriculture. The most memorable is Chandra Singh Nega, a striking man in his sixties, with a shock of white hair, wearing a pale-green pajama-like suit.

"This guy was the enemy," Negi says, teasing Chandra, who laughs, too. "He was the biggest seller of fertilizers and pesticides around. He made lots of money, but he went to the Navdanya demonstration farm and decided to give it all up."

"Why?" Anna and I ask in unison.

"I started having breathing problems and allergies," Chandra explains, "and learned it had to do with the chemicals I was selling. I knew I had to give that up or it would kill me, so now I sell tea and food." We learn he's sort of the local truck stop. People traveling between villages often stop to enjoy the meals he and his young daughter prepare. Later that night, we're treated to our own roadside dinner of rice, lentils, yogurt, and cucumber in their one-table eatery.

Chandra explains how farmers here got sold on chemical farming. "The companies advertised that you get better yields. At first, the government gave farmers the fertilizer for free, then they started charging more and more. It was hard for farmers to pay, but the soil had gotten so bad from all the chemical use that they *had* to buy fertilizer."

As proprietor of the local food shop and men's hangout, Chandra, I realize, must be a real asset to Negi. Having him "with the program" must stimulate a lot of emulators.

Later that night, over dinner, Negi tells us how he himself came to work with Navdanya. "I was in the export-import business when I met Dr. Vandana Shiva's sister, Mira. I started reading more in the newspapers about what Dr. Shiva was doing. I thought it was so good, I just went to her house and told her, 'I want to work with you.' That was in 1990, before we even had a demonstration farm.

"I'm not working for the money," he adds. "I'm working for what my heart is saying to me."

LIVING DEMOCRACY ON TWO CONTINENTS

Back in our room lit by a rickety lantern, we're hooking our mosquito net to the ceiling when I notice for the first time a Navdanya poster on the wall. It's a painting of a tree, with elephants, oxen, horses, fruits, and vegetables all nestled in its leafy branches and interlaced roots. In the center of the poster are only two words—the English translation pops out: LIVING DEMOCRACY.

I take a deep breath.

These are the exact words I'd chosen almost ten years ago to capture my own vision of democracy and to name my organization, the Center for Living Democracy. I used "living democracy" to remind us that democracy is *a way of life,* something we practice every day—not something done "for us" or "to us." Over the years, some who've followed my work seemed bewildered by my choices. To some, democracy seemed a diversion from my anti-hunger path. But I had learned that to get to the roots of hunger I had to look at democracy itself—who makes decisions, whose voices are heard. Here, Navdanya similarly uses "living democracy" to express a vision that goes beyond the manmade, the institutions. It's a democracy that embraces all living things. The fruit and fish and flowers of the poster are a celebration of this idea.

Finding these words here in this tiny village in the foothills of the Himalaya feels like a confirmation of the inner logic of my life's journey. As I crawl under the netting, I think about how living democracy has followed me to the other side of the earth.

With this comforting thought, I assume that I'm going to sleep especially well, and I do, until a mosquito assault on Anna leads to a desperate match-lit search for the attackers, and I end up burning a hole in the netting.

The next morning dawns misty but relatively mild, and we go by foot from here. Mercifully, we start by winding down. Across the valley, we see farmers doing their early-morning harvesting and women walking to collect the day's water. By midmorning we reach Uttirchha, a village whose eighty families live in whitewashed stone-and-mud houses perched on the mountainside and whose narrow stairways connect them to stone patios.

We have come to learn about living democracy, called *jaiv panchayat* in Hindi, but its full meaning in this context still eludes us. On one of the villages' wide patios, we're invited to meet the village elders. A bouquet of orange flowers set on a squat wooden table welcomes us, but the table's purpose is more than to display flowers. It's here so Darshan Lal Chowary can show us—not just tell us—what *jaiv panchayat* really means.

Darshan, whose strong angular features and deep-lined face give him a regal air, opens a large book, each page displaying a specimen—a leaf or a seed of the plants in this community. Below each are botanical information and details about how it's used.

"We're documenting our ecological resources, all our plants and animals," explains Darshan. "The book will describe what they are used for—food, tea, medicine. We'll have more than one thousand plants in here before we're finished.

"Now, no one can come into our community and claim a patent on these plants and tell us they've discovered the plants' uses," he continues. "Anyone who wants this will have to get our permission first." Gesturing to the kids who've gathered around us, he adds, "It's also a way to remember, to share our knowledge with the next generation."

I think back to Vandana's early insight—that, in India, the seed is the entry point for reclaiming one's culture and evolving something more life-serving than a global corporate order that reduces all life to commodities. Registers, like the book of specimens laid out for us this morning, will allow farmers to assert their rights to prior intellectual innovations. The goal, as Vandana had explained, is to limit corporations' ability to claim intellectual property rights to knowledge developed by Indian farmers.

Since most seeds grown in India are farmers' own varieties, not seeds sold by multinational seed companies, it's easy to see why farmers are concerned that what they've developed could be appropriated by others. With industrial countries' markets mostly saturated, it's also clear why multinational seed companies would be eager to penetrate the enormous untapped market here. What a sales opportunity! Just convince farmers their traditional seeds are inadequate, then develop new seeds that don't reproduce, so farmers have to buy them. Voila! Profits soar.

"We sent one thousand postcards from this area to the government saying that we reject seed patenting," Negi fills in. "We wrote to W. R. Grace about its neem patent, and we protested the turmeric patent, too."

The registries of plant and animal life are just part of what Negi encourages here. Uttirchha is also one of the villages that is learning from the Dehra Dun demonstration farm. Through the farm and these village visits, Negi is helping the entire village to shake chemical agriculture.

"Before, there were no serious pests in this area," explains Darshan. "We had only one problem—fungus. So the government said, 'Use this pesticide to kill it. You can have it for free.' We started using pesticides, but we must have killed many helpful insects, because many pests started coming. And the pesticide wasn't free anymore. We had to buy it. The food didn't taste good, either, and we didn't feel good—we had health problems, stomachaches, body pain, trouble with breathing."

As we talk with Darshan and other elders, the morning mist melts away and we can see beyond the ledge for miles and miles. It's hard to imagine these hillsides contaminated with chemical fertilizer and pesticides. They look pristine, and Negi is determined to make the land as healthy as it looks. He explains, "I told them it would take five to seven years to shift from chemicals and to rebuild the soil. We've been helping them for several years now, we've only got another year to go."

THE LAST HONEST MAN

After lunch we learn that what goes down must come up as we head out to Charekh, an even tinier village of thirty-five families, which Negi says has never had Western visitors.

As we navigate the narrow trails, I keep my eyes on Anna, ahead of me in her long brown plaid skirt, handy in a culture in which women don't wear pants or shorts. I'm wearing my black equivalent. Obviously, we hadn't packed for rocky mountain trails.

"REI, eat your heart out!" Anna laughs. "Those sporting-goods companies convince people they need high-tech gear—if they could only see us in our flip-flops!"

By the time we reach Charekh at dusk, the altitude has cooled the air and clouds have crept in, enclosing the village in white. Chilled, Anna wraps herself in our Grameen Check cloth. We sit on a stone landing to visit with the village head, Harenda Singh, whose poise and piercing green eyes convey an inner calm.

"Here is the only honest village head in this region," Negi says, putting his arm around his friend. Negi had already told us that most chiefs skim money off World Bank loans meant for local development projects, and that many accept bribes and otherwise mishandle village money. So I ask, simply, why is he honest when others cheat?

"Why should I compromise my principles now?" Harenda answers. "I'm fifty-six, I know I'll have to answer to God soon."

Statistically, he's right—the average man in India lives to be sixty-two.

Harenda is my age, exactly, but I feel my life is beginning anew—I have potentially decades more to learn and live. As I absorb the life-stunting reality of poverty, the evening's chill seems to penetrate even deeper.

That night, our tiny room packs with grandmothers, mothers, and young kids. We can't converse, but we joke, mime, and share songs. Anna tests her limited repertoire of shadow hand puppets, and with apologies to Pete Seeger she and I belt out a rendition of "This Land is Your Land."

In the rain the next morning, we hike out. Circling up, way up, behind the village, we look down and see almost all the villagers huddled beneath a stone overhang, babies on hips, toddlers held by one hand, umbrellas in the other, waving up to us. Their waves go on and on. We wave, too, until the village is finally swallowed by heavy, gray clouds.

Walking the rocky trail back to the road, Harenda tells us that his is one of the few villages in the region without road access. He hasn't been willing to pay the bribes to get one built, he explains.

In less than two hours, we round the last bend and see terraced mountains receding for hundreds of miles. Anna snaps a panoramic series of shots. Click, click, click. Then I hear her catch her breath.

"Look, Mom," she says, just before clicking the final picture. The only person we've encountered in our hike to and from the village has emerged from around the corner into the photograph. The woman's aquamarine sari trails along the ground, and one hand keeps a heavy gunnysack of rice in place on her head. She appears, it seems, as if to remind us: *Don't romanticize this scene,* and never forget—despite the fact that the official village leaders are all men—it's the women who do the heavy lifting here, figuratively and often literally.

THE PUNJAB LOOMS LARGE

From the Himalayan foothills, our next stop is the Punjab—it looms large as the testing ground for the Green Revolution as well as the hottest spot of our trip. Punjab highs have been known to reach above 115 degrees.

To catch our overnight train from Delhi, Jafri, the soft-spoken young Navdanya scientist, leads us through the crowded station on whose stairs the destitute sleep. We see no other westerners, few other women.

The next day, bleary from a four A.M. arrival, we meet up with Sumel Singh, our interpreter, who is a doctoral student in Punjab cultural history. His customary full beard and vivid orange turban make him seem older than Anna, even though they are the same age. Reaching the village of Bucho Khurd at midmorning, we see that Sumel and Jafri have gathered quite a number of farmers to talk with us.

Streaming with perspiration in the maroon-colored traditional garb that I've brought from Bangladesh, I'm determined to look dignified as "the American author." We're sitting in the middle of an open stone porch with peeling turquoise paint. Dozens of men, some sitting and others standing, most bearded, all wearing colorful turbans—apricot, cranberry, lavender, gold, pink, orange—fill the porch around Anna and me.

As Jafri and Sumel explain who we are and what we want to know, we can make out only a few words—soya, neem, Pepsi. The windup seems to go on forever, but the intensity of the men's expressions and their alertness despite the choking heat convince me that they're hanging on every word.

I search the faces, trying to imagine what they are thinking. We already know enough to realize we're looking at desperate men. They've just lost their war with the bollworm—a moth larva that feeds on crops and, unfortunately in this case, found this area's cotton balls quite appealing. Cotton, grown here for most of the century, took off in the '60s when farmers were sold on the Green Revolution notion that new seeds, chemical fertilizers, pesticides, and modern machinery would bring prosperity.

After Jafri and Sumel finish, the first to speak is a man with a long white beard, a plaid blue-and-yellow cloth around his waist, and a matching turban. "The bollworm appeared as early as 1973. We sprayed and increased spraying," he explains. "By the 1990s, it was still a big problem. We tried a lot of pesticides, but it was a total failure—and we were using up all our groundwater, too!" he adds.

"The Land Mortgage Bank has sent foreclosure notices to a third of the households here," explains a heavy man in a deep purple turban. "Other notices are due soon. You see, to promote the Green Revolution [to get farmers to embrace the industrial model], the government subsidized the price of the inputs. Now we have to pay the full price, and it's much higher than we expected. Plus, our crops are failing. Almost every farmer in this village is indebted five to seven *lakh*." This is roughly equivalent to between $10,000 and $15,000—more than three times what the average Indian in this region brings home *in an entire year*.

At one point, Jafri, who hopes this disaster will open these farmers' minds to organic methods, tries to get a reading on whether they would be tempted by another high-tech fix like genetically engineered Bt cotton, with pest resistance bred into the seeds. Pest resistance, that is, until the pests evolve new resistance.

"Sure, get it to us, we're ready to buy it," seems to be their response.

Anna and I look at each other. In some ways it is hard for us to grasp how people who've been so burnt by promises of quick fixes could be ready to leap at yet another one. Yet part of me recognizes that, of course, when desperate, *all* most of us can think of is quick relief. And we know the Indian press is telling them their salvation may indeed rest on genetic engineering. In a recent Indian news account, DNA discoverer James Watson lamented the country's "excessive and retrograde fear of genetics."[24] Get over the silly fears, the media is saying, Bt cotton seeds can be a solution to your tragedy. What a market Monsanto and multinational agribusiness companies seem to have sitting right before us!

As we end the meeting and gather our things, Sumel explains that the demise of cotton threatens economic collapse not just for farmers, but for the entire Punjab state. Agriculture is the base of the economy here. "The state may not even be able to pay its teachers next year," he says. Sumel reminds us that it's not just about economics. "The situation here is very volatile."

Decades ago, even officers within top U.S. foundations sponsoring the Green Revolution's introduction foresaw the socially explosive potential of the new technology. While in public they criticized people like Joe and me for questioning it, at least one high-placed foundation official noted at the time that increased output doesn't necessarily mean "positive social change."[25] His concern that the technology would destabilize communities turned out to be prescient. The Punjab has suffered some of the most widespread violence in independent India.[26] Terrifying economic losses are fanning the fire again.

SEEDS OF SUICIDE

Leaving the village, we drive back through the town of Bhatinda and see with new eyes. "Farmers are so desperate they are selling their tractors to pay off debts," Sumel says. Parts, too, Anna and I guess, as we pass a corner with heaps of tractor and harvester scraps.

Jafri tells us: "Two years ago, the bollworm and crop failures swept Andhra Pradesh. In one district I researched, pesticide use increased two thousand percent in just the previous three years, but the crops still failed. The bollworm had become resistant.

"Two years ago," he continues, "more than three hundred farmers in this district committed suicide, many by drinking the very pesticides that had so indebted them."

Jafri hopes this bollworm disaster can become an opportunity to prevent further tragedy. It can teach farmers to look beyond the next quick fix. "We're working on biological controls of the bollworm using tobacco leaves, ginger, chili, and neem oil," he explains. "If we can say that we've succeeded in controlling the bollworm organically, then we expect a large audience."

Jafri is also teaching composting and helping farmers convert to organic cultivation, particularly for wheat, both for eating and selling. After we get back to the U.S., we will hear from Jafri that well over one hundred farmers in the village we visited, plus one other, are now using Navdanya's traditional wheat varieties. Even though their yields per acre are 50 to 75 percent of what they had produced with Green Revolution varieties, the farmers are coming out way ahead: Without chemicals, their costs of production—which had put them in such debt—are only *one quarter* of what they had been spending.[27]

ON BEING A GIRL

Later that afternoon, in a small shadowy room, we talk with a group of Punjabi farmers about everything from suicide, to their sources of hope, to their opinions about the World Trade Organization protest in Seattle.

On the way back to our car, I notice tree branches artfully hanging from an archway. When I ask why they're there, one man says with pride, "Those are from the neem. We hang them when a son is born."

I flash to our morning arrival in Bhatinda, when I noticed dozens of signs for amniocentesis facilities hanging from awnings and sides of buildings. At first I thought this remote town just had remarkable women's health care, but then I remembered. Like in communities throughout India, there's an epidemic here: There are 1,000 boys for every 888 girls.[28] Even though naturally more males are born, for every 1,000 births at least sixty-two girls are still missing—either aborted, or killed at birth. Nationally, the problem has gotten so severe that laws have been passed to try to stop it. Vandana's sister told us it's now illegal for doctors to inform patients of a fetus's gender, determined by amniocentesis, for fear girls may be aborted.

These thoughts boil up, and I don't think about what I say next, "So if I were born here my mother wouldn't hang neem branches for me?"

The men laugh—these, the men who just spent hours talking with us and giving me, it seemed, the respect of an equal. "That's right," one says, and I can't tell if he's embarrassed or proud. —Anna

That night, waiting on the dimly lit railway platform in Bhatinda for our midnight train to Delhi, we chat with Jafri, whose quiet determination both Anna and I have come to admire. With the desperate farmers' voices still in our minds, and thinking too about the ecological disaster underway and the misery of the people who are sleeping at our feet in this station, we want to know what keeps Jafri going.

"It's not in spite of, but *because* things are so bad that I have to be involved," Jafri says with calm clarity, his face illuminated by the bare bulbs high above us. "When I see how terrible things are, I have to do something. It's the only way *I* can survive."

STILL SEEKING ANNAPOORNA

It's our last day in Delhi, and Anna and I flash back to our plane ride here, when we first learned that the goddess of food is *Annapoorna*. We moderns may find quaint the idea that gods and goddesses could be omnipotent over life's essentials, like food; but on this day Anna and I will meet a mere mortal with more power, no doubt, than was ever ascribed to Annapoorna.

We arrive at the Ministry of Consumer Affairs and Public Distribution to meet Shanta Kumar, who is in charge of India's food distribution and fair-price shops, which have been around since I studied the Indian food system thirty years ago. The shops offer basic food items at government-subsidized low prices for the poor.

We're ushered down labyrinthine halls—with the institutional quality of a hospital but packed with paper, not people—and enter what feels like a TV parody of a bureaucrat's office. Dark mahogany walls suck up what little artificial light there is, and row after row of brown chairs block the oversized, paperless desk at the far end of the room. When Shanta Kumar stands to greet us, his serious face with black-rimmed glasses is perfectly reflected in the spotless, shiny desktop. A small computer, with a screen the size of an old Kaypro's, blinks fluorescent green words.

After we squeeze awkwardly into the front row of chairs, we tell him we've just returned from the Punjab, where we saw warehouses overflowing with government-owned grain, protected from the elements only by thin black tarps.

"Oh, yes," he says proudly, "We now have the biggest surpluses in history—sixteen million tons above our twenty-four-million-ton buffer stock." (Not even counting the buffer, that's thirty-two pounds of grain for every man, woman, and child in the country.) Since we know that monsoon rains are expected any day, we ask what he plans to do with all this excess.

"We'd like to export it if we can," Kumar says matter-of-factly, as if the impending monsoon wouldn't make exporting moot. And as if the fact that hunger is rampant here had no bearing on what the government does with its food. Just before this meeting, a leading Indian nutritionist told us that half of India's children suffer from inadequate nutrition, and I've read that 60 percent of Indian infants would be placed in intensive care if they were born in California.[29]

So, we ask what seems to us the obvious question: "With so many hungry people in your country, why don't you just make this surplus available to them?"

He looks at us sternly, as if we've suggested he donate the Parliament building to the homeless. "Oh, no we couldn't do that," he says shaking his head. "We already give too many subsidies to the poor."

We realize at that moment that this office reflects his mindset—tragically trapped in a previous era, unaware of the solutions his own people are developing. We sit there searching. What would it take to free him from this failing framework? How could he become engaged with the creative edges of those communities addressing persistent hunger and poverty in their land? We barely challenge him, though. Sleep-deprived from our Punjabi night train and our five A.M. arrival in Delhi, neither of us can muster a proper comeback. But we know now, that the next time a biotech executive, or anyone else, claims our world's problem is inadequate supply, we can recommend they talk with Mr. Kumar. We'll suggest they ask how he dealt with his problem of rotting surpluses in a society where malnutrition stunts the lives of half the children.[30]

INDIA: AWAKENING OUR SENSES

Coconut-Ginger Curry

Serves
6 to 8

Indian chef Claire Datta, one of the few women chefs in New Delhi, inspired this light, pungent vegetable curry. Claire works closely with Navdanya Foods, turning their organic products into tasty breads and cookies and breakfast cereals.

This curry is a delightful medley of winter vegetables, bathed in a flavorful mixture of spices and coconut, whose scents will linger in your kitchen.

6 cups hot cooked basmati rice

4 tablespoons vegetable oil (preferably canola oil)

1 tablespoon cumin seeds

1½ tablespoons coriander seeds

2 tablespoons fresh ginger, minced

2 tablespoons garlic, crushed

½ cup shredded unsweetened coconut

1 15-ounce can coconut milk (low-fat or regular)

1½ pounds waxy potatoes (red, new, or Yukon—not russet), peeled and cut into 1-inch chunks

¾ pound winter squash, peeled and cut into 1-inch chunks

¾ pound cauliflower, cut into 1-inch florets

¾ pound carrots, cut into 1-inch chunks

¾ pound green beans, trimmed and cut into 2-inch pieces

¾ pound onion, sliced into half-moons

1½ to 2 teaspoons salt

2 teaspoons turmeric

up to ¼ cup fresh lime juice (about 2 limes)

crushed red pepper to taste (about 1 teaspoon)

1½ cups frozen peas, defrosted

While making the curry, cook the rice. Use enough to make 6 to 8 cups (depending on the number of diners).

To make the coconut-spice paste, heat 1 tablespoon of the oil in a medium-size skillet. Add cumin seeds, coriander seeds, and ginger, and sauté over medium heat until the seeds pop (about 5 minutes). Add the garlic and shredded coconut, and sauté another 2 to 3 minutes, or until coconut is lightly toasted. Transfer to small blender or spice grinder, and add about ¼ cup of the coconut milk. Purée to a smooth paste and set aside. (You can add a little more of the coconut milk if needed, to make the paste really smooth.)

In a large pot, steam potatoes and squash together until they are slightly tender (what I would consider about half done). Add cauliflower, carrots, and green beans, and continue to steam until all vegetables are done. (Make sure the potatoes and squash are thoroughly cooked, not al dente. The other vegetables can be slightly crisp.) Refresh under cold running water, and set in a colander to drain.

While vegetables are steaming and draining, heat the remaining 3 tablespoons of oil in a big deep skillet or large pot (big enough to hold all the vegetables). Add the onion, salt, and turmeric, and sauté for about 8 to 10 minutes over medium heat, or until the onion is translucent. Add the coconut-spice paste and stir together. Add the steamed vegetables, and stir until the vegetables are well coated. Pour in the remaining coconut milk (you can use the coconut milk to rinse the last of the spice mixture out of the blender, then add it all). Stir well.

Bring to a low simmer. Cover and continue to simmer gently for 10 minutes. Add salt to taste. Add lime juice, 1 tablespoon at a time, to taste. Add red pepper flakes, a quarter teaspoon at a time, to taste. Add thoroughly defrosted peas to top of curry, cover, and let sit for a couple of minutes to warm the peas.

Serve hot, over basmati rice.

WALKING TO NAIROBI

As for me,
I've made a choice.

GREEN BELT MOVEMENT SLOGAN

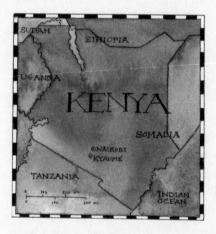

The minivan stops, and in the moment it takes to grab my backpack and climb out, Anna's already been swept away. All I can see of my daughter is her long, brown plaid skirt swaying, the same skirt that I'd followed two months ago over high Himalayan trails in India.

From a distance, I can see Anna dancing, hands held high, with women dressed in brightly colored grass skirts and white T-shirts. They draw Anna and the fifteen others pouring out of our minivans into their contagious welcome dance. KiKamba lyrics pierce the air, seeming to lift even higher the red dust circling up around us from our stomping feet.

I find myself holding back, though; partly, I'm just stunned. Sure, our Green Belt guide had warned us, repeatedly, before we left Nairobi to be prepared for a big welcome crowd. But I assumed he meant a crowd of silent onlookers, like the villagers we'd encountered in Bangladesh and India, not this. Certainly I didn't expect the hugs, the laughter, this openhearted greeting beyond anything I'd experienced even from old friends.

Singing and swaying, now all of us together, we weave our way, parade-like, down a dirt path into an open courtyard, where folding chairs are set out for us so that we can be properly welcomed by the dancers and dignitaries.

I take my seat, and when the dust finally settles, I look around. I see nothing but unadorned one-story buildings, roughly constructed of handmade mud bricks, bordering the courtyard. A blackboard propped against a crumbling brick wall reads: KYAUME SCHOOL WELCOMES THE GREEN BELT MOVEMENT, the village self-empowering network we're here in Kenya to learn from.

As the women celebrate our arrival with still more dancing and singing, I feel the strength of their spirits in their confident bearing and clear, strong voices. But part of me keeps asking, "Where does this joy come from?" All I can see is destitution. (And that's before we learn that only one in five kids can even afford this Godforsaken-looking school.) Is their apparent joy at our arrival a kind of denial, a way to hide the real pain they must feel?

After the chief welcomes us, the headmaster welcomes us, the assistant chief welcomes us, and parent leaders welcome us, we're invited inside one of the classrooms, where dozens of bowls piled high with food are laid out on a long table. At lunch, we're introduced to the family who will be our hosts during our stay.

I steal a moment to peek into the classroom next-door. I see nothing but broken-down desks. Nothing. No books, no supplies. The desks are so rickety that my immediate thought is "If the kids were better fed, the desks might collapse."

Afterward, back in the barren courtyard, I'm amused as one of our guides from Nairobi, Muta Maathai—the twenty-six-year-old son of Green Belt founder Wangari Maathai—gets a brief lesson in archery from two tall, thin men in blue. The arrows of the men in blue hit the classroom wall with force. Muta's dive pathetically into the red earth. I find myself a bit nervous, though, with all these kids around, when I realize they're shooting real arrows with long, sharp points.

Only later do we learn that these "instructors" are actually the school's guards showing Muta their weapons. "But what could robbers possibly steal here?" I ask Muta.

"They could take the flagpole," he explains. "They could take the doors off the hinges."

With his words, the depth of deprivation in this small village strikes more powerfully. Though Kenya is portrayed back home as a peaceful safari wonderland, the reality is a country ruled since 1978 by a president who banned alternative political parties and even made insulting him a crime. Donald Mumbo, a Green Belt employee and anthropologist who'd taken us around Nairobi on our first day, shook his head as we drove by the city's worst slums. For the first time, he told us, some desperate mothers are abandoning their babies out of hopelessness. Overall in Africa, household income has fallen by a fifth in the last twenty-five years. Two-thirds of Kenyans, he said, live in abject poverty, on two dollars a day or less; and, adding to the misery, the current drought, we're told, is the worst on record.[1]

It is in the midst of this hardship that we arrive to learn about the Green Belt Movement and Wangari Maathai. For part of our time here, we'll be in the company of fifteen other Americans who've also come to learn about the Movement firsthand. Here in the school courtyard, Anna and I see the first signs of Green Belt's impact. Sparsely dotting the ground are scrawny saplings, each painstakingly covered by a mesh of thorny branches to protect it from hungry goats. These thorny mounds will turn into what Anna and I soon come to see as Wangari's genius.

From a Messy House

On the drive from Nairobi to Kyaume, it had become clear why our Green Belt hosts had chosen to bring us here.

Past the smudged van windows, the vista is more lunar than lush. For most of the time we see no trees at all, and the few we do see seem truly sad. Not much higher than a tall man, their branches are barren except for spiky barbs sticking out every which way as if asking for help. For mile after mile, we see only vast stretches of pale, parched earth.

But as we approach Kyaume, we see something different. We see green.

As we enter the village, our van weaves down a road that narrows into a wide dirt trail. It's hard to guess how many people live here—we're told about 1,000—because so many trees block our view. Most of all, we see coffee—low and leafy trees lining the road in neat rows. Second to coffee are *grevilla*—known throughout Kenya as the "Wangari Tree," we later learn. There are many others, too: avocado, papaya, mango, orange, and more. Along with trees, we also catch sight of gardens of green.

We've left the world of brown and entered the world of green for one reason: Wangari Maathai. When we first met her in the living room of the Green Belt's Lang'ata Training Center on the edge of Nairobi, Wangari greeted us with her ready grin, which always makes her seem to be on the brink of a hearty laugh.

The origins of the Green Belt Movement date back to the early 1970s when Wangari—the first woman PhD in biological sciences in East Africa—was watching the Sahara desert creep south. "What was once flourishing agricultural land was becoming nothing but sand," Wangari says when we ask how the Movement began.

She saw Kenya's forests shrinking to less than 5 percent of what they once had been, lost to the same desertification that poses a problem in more than one hundred countries. Wangari knew that when trees go, so do the roots that retain topsoil and capture what little water does fall. When trees go, so does the protection from the wind that keeps soil from blowing away. She knew that this meant villagers, mainly women, were walking farther and farther to get water and firewood. She saw the vicious cycle of forest loss, desertification, and communities' growing inability to feed themselves.

Government foresters weren't much help. "I tried going to talk to them about what could be done, but they weren't interested," Wangari tells us. "The trees they were planting were exotics, trees that are bad for the soil—cedar, pine, and especially eucalyptus. Sure, those trees grow fast, but they use up huge amounts of water."

Wangari decided to act. On Earth Day 1977, Wangari, then thirty-seven, planted her first trees, an act that launched a movement whose impact has gone far beyond tree planting and has even rattled Kenya's most powerful political players.

I'd long thought of Earth Day as a nice thing invented by privileged Americans, but not—unfortunately for the earth—expressing the most pressing concerns of the poverty-stricken. I had always assumed that those facing day-to-day survival challenges often had to put long-term environmental concerns second. Now, here in Kenya, I see that it's precisely because the poorest bear the brunt of deforestation that Wangari saw them as being the most motivated to actually do something about it.

Early in our visit, Muta, Wangari's tall, relaxed son, described his mother's first attempt to create a tree nursery in their home. It was not appreciated by his father, who had just been elected to the Kenyan parliament. "Dad thought it made the place look too messy, so my mother put the idea on hold. But she didn't give up. She saw what her husband could not see when he saw only a messy house."

What Wangari saw is that it takes a village to grow a tree. Today, the village movement she launched from her "messy" home boasts 6,000 registered groups throughout Kenya, all with their own tree nurseries. And Wangari's vision has stretched well beyond Kenya, too, with groups from other African countries coming here to learn from what she ignited.

From her modest beginning over two decades ago, it hasn't been easy. Though tree planting may seem innocuous, the ripples here are revolutionary. Wangari and her movement have inspired tens of thousands of women in villages throughout the country to see themselves as citizens, and that has allowed them to perceive their country's forests as a public good, one they have a right and duty to protect from private land-grabbers. It has given women the strength to question everything from their husbands' control to President Daniel arap Moi's rule. It has challenged government corruption and blocked building on public parks. The Movement has proven so threatening that Moi's government has attacked Wangari's work and Wangari herself, who has even been beaten and jailed.

TWENTY MILLION AND ONE?

On our second day in Kyaume, Anna and I get a chance to try our hand at the art of tree-planting, with the help of local tree-nursery women.

With blue jeans rolled up and lamenting how dumb I was to wear a white T-shirt, I squat in dark-red dirt, gripping my seedling rooted in the cut-off bottom of a milk carton. How do I get the thing out without smashing it? I wonder. The dirt around the seedling feels as solid as a brick. I bang the sides of the carton, hoping to soften it up, until one of the village women, seeing my struggle, does the obvious. She pours water over it.

Finally, the seedling and its protective earth pop free, and a woman rushes to take the now-empty carton for an awaiting seedling. I gently pat down the earth, propping my little plant in place. The baby tree suddenly looks so vulnerable.

Another woman hands me a Coke bottle filled with water. Since it looks too dirty to drink, I realize the water is not for me, but for my tree. I'm shown how to turn the bottle upside down and place it next to the seedling so the water slowly seeps into the ground in a form of rudimentary irrigation, giving my tree-to-be a chance to fight the encroaching desert.

I stand up to survey my accomplishment. It doesn't look too impressive, I admit, but then, one tree isn't the point here. This little bit of green may in fact be tree number 20,000,001 planted by the Green Belt Movement in the last twenty years.

Twenty million trees all planted by women in villages with such scarce resources? The number is so striking that, even though I'd heard the figure before, it had never stuck. I always feared I had misremembered it. I just couldn't imagine a feat of that magnitude: a movement generating thousands of nurseries scattered across a country the size of Texas, with mostly illiterate members and using few of the organizing helpers which we take for granted—like the telephone.

Now, surrounded by women villagers—the *de facto* foresters—and standing above one hundred seedlings in tidy ten-by-ten rows—their fragile toothpick-thin stems holding the promise of shade, firewood, and food—the number becomes more believable.

WHO PLANTED YOUR FORESTS?

One evening in Kyaume, Anna and I stay up late talking with Ramana, Regina, and several other Green Belt women hosting us. Ramana—close to my age—is a large woman, commanding but warm. Regina, twenty-five, whose radiance never dims during our entire stay, caught my attention from our first Kyaume moment. As we exited the vans into the dancing entourage, her voice penetrated the air above the others. In the women's call-and-response, it was Regina who called.

Now, we sit together on couches draped with embroidered white cloth that honors the arrival of guests. A kerosene lantern hangs from the high ceiling; its loud hissing making us all lean in close as we talk. In the corner of the living room, a black-and-white TV, connected by a tangle of wires to a car battery, rests precariously on a nearby shelf, showing Brazilian soap operas.

We want to find out what has changed because of Green Belt.

"It's much more green, even nowadays when there are still no rains," Regina tells us. "My house is so beautiful, surrounded by trees. Others passing see my trees and ask, 'How did you get so much green?' Then I tell them about the Movement and help them get trees for themselves."

In the past, the Green Belt nurseries gave away trees for free, and the Movement paid nursery women the equivalent of three cents for each tree that survived. Green Belt now plans to sell seedlings at affordable prices and use that money to pay for some of the Movement's costs.

Green Belt groups meet weekly to encourage tree-planting and information-sharing. Anna and I have always thought of these meetings as logistical, but when we ask what the women discuss, Regina and Ramana mention personal problems just as frequently as they do tree-planting. Alcoholism among husbands, for instance, is common here. Back in Nairobi, Wangari told us that the Movement has started a campaign targeting village bars. In some villages, it's easier to buy a beer, Wangari lamented, than it is to buy beans. Domestic violence is rampant as well, she said. In a country in which most married women report that their husbands beat them, I see how a place to gather strength outside the home is critical.[2]

"In Green Belt I have the freedom to be with other women," Regina adds. "If you have no friends, your husband can keep you in the house all day, and you do all the work. Now I am so happy."

As we talk, I'm struck by the irony of what my eyes catch on TV. The Brazilian *telenovela* flashes between a man giving his girlfriend several hard slaps and a woman screaming at her boyfriend, who is wildly brandishing a gun.

Anna then asks the very practical question, "Before Green Belt, where did you get your firewood?"

"We would walk to the nearest forest," Ramana tells us. "It's about fifteen kilometers."

"Round-trip?"

"No, each way."

Once reaching the forest, we learn, the women are sometimes chased away by land-grabbers—the term here for land speculators illegally logging or building on public land. On these days, they would come home empty-handed.

I try to imagine walking almost nineteen miles round-trip several times a week, even without carrying an unwieldy load of firewood, and frankly . . . can't.

"There were hardly any trees here before Green Belt, and they all belonged to our husbands," another woman sitting with us chimes in. "To get wood, I had to ask my husband. He could refuse. Now they are my trees."

"The movement also taught us to plan ahead," she adds. "If I need to cut down a tree, I plant two others first, and I wait to make sure they grow."

When we ask how many trees the women have planted, Regina becomes almost apologetic. "I just started, only twenty." Ramana, an obvious leader, reports with a proud grin, "Two hundred."

I start doing the numbers in my head, guessing at averages and multiplying the number of members by the number of nurseries. It's easy to see the genius of getting tree-planting know-how to the people.

As my head fills with calculations, a half-dozen women come dancing and singing through the open front door and Ramana, Regina, and Anna jump up to join them. In the middle of the concrete-floored living room, amidst the shadows from the crackling lantern, their voices ring out a welcome song for guests, and the cheering and dancing continue for a good half hour.

By the time Ramana and Regina bid our visitors goodbye, it's late and Anna and I are both exhausted. But they have questions for us, too. Sitting down again, Regina asks, as if she's been waiting all evening to pop the question, "How many trees have you planted?"

Anna and I look at each other. It's our turn to feel apologetic. When Anna says, "Uh, none" and I say, "One . . . yesterday." Their faces fall. They look genuinely confused.

"But we've seen on TV the big forests in your country. Who planted all those trees?"

We try to explain, but we're both stuck. I've always taken for granted that forests recreate themselves. But, of course, once humans create deserts, forests depend on us—on Green Belt Movements and on people like Ramana and Regina.

FORESTERS WITHOUT DIPLOMAS

The next morning, I get up early and walk down the narrow dirt road near the house. Looking at the trees lining the road and surrounding the homes, I think to myself: How could it be that it never occurred to villagers, before the Green Belt Movement, to plant trees if they needed firewood? Why did it take a movement to create this near-oasis?

I think back to our similar questions in Bangladesh. How could it be that in such a fertile land, villagers had to be taught to grow vegetables?

Ruminating, I return to work that I read over a decade ago by University of Pennsylvania psychologist Martin Seligman and his studies of what he calls "learned helplessness." Seligman shows how easy it is, in the "right" conditions, for any of us to be made to believe we are incompetent, that we don't have answers and must depend on others—to feel that, since nothing we do makes a difference, why bother trying? Though Seligman told us he never applied his ideas to colonialism, I see now that there may be no better case study.

Under British rule, Kenyans were told that their religion was immoral and their traditional crops were backward. From a priest friend of Wangari's we learn that, upon discovering that the local word for "prayer" meant something akin to celebration, the colonialists were appalled. They taught the Kenyans a new word which carries a meaning closer to "beg." Suddenly prayer shifted from celebration to supplication. And traditional foods? Africa's cereals were often relegated to categories with pejorative connotations, referred to as "coarse grains," "minor crops," or "famine foods."[3] Later, multinational companies, eager to unload Western grain surpluses, sold Africans on the notion that crops unsuited to Africa, like wheat, were superior. One ad directed at parents read, "He'll be smart. He'll go far. He'll eat bread."[4]

Add to these defeating messages Kenya's decades of dictatorial and corrupt government, combined with Western aid agencies and development programs pumping their solutions into the country, and I see the value in the Green Belt Movement's working to "unteach" helplessness, to redeem indigenous knowledge, and to strengthen villagers' sense of their rights as citizens.

When Wangari began, the Kenyan forestry service, established under the British, believed that villagers, especially women, weren't capable of creating tree nurseries. That was the work of the experts, the foresters.

"We were breaking the code," Wangari tells us, once we get back to Nairobi. "We were trying to show that planting trees can be a commonplace thing. Anybody can plant a tree. You may need a degree to be a forester, but you don't need a degree to dig a hole, plant a tree, water it, and take care of it.

"We told the women: 'Use the methods you know, and if you don't know, invent.' They would use broken pots. They would put the soil and seeds there and watch as they germinated. If they germinated, well and good; if not, try again.

"We demystified forestry. In the beginning, the foresters were not amused. They said I was adulterating the profession. I told them, 'We need millions of trees and you foresters are too few, you'll never produce them. So you need to make everyone foresters.' I call us foresters without diplomas."

COFFEE, COFFEE EVERYWHERE BUT NOT A DROP TO DRINK

Wangari tells us, "The colonists made people believe they had an answer for everything." One answer was cash crops. As one African writer describes: "Colonialism programmed African countries to produce what they do not consume and to consume what they do not produce."[5] And, once independent, Kenya didn't change direction.

The economists' rationale, which I'd first read ad nauseam decades ago, is that specialization in export crops like coffee makes sense because countries should grow what best suits their climate and soils, and then—according to the hallowed theory of "comparative advantage"—sell on the international market and use the profits to buy what they need that grows best elsewhere. Anna tells me that thirty years later her university economics textbooks still argue that David Ricardo, the father of comparative advantage, was right.

And, even though Ricardo's prerequisite conditions hardly hold in today's world, comparative advantage remains a central tenet of the globalization religion sweeping the planet. Indeed, by the mid-1990s, the export focus had been taken so far that forty-four countries worldwide were deriving from 60 percent to almost 100 percent of their foreign exchange revenues from a *single* commodity.

In the mid-'70s, Joe Collins and I—writing *Food First* in our cramped office above the A&P grocery in Hastings-on-Hudson, New York—questioned an overconfidence in export crops that makes a people dependent upon imports for basic food survival. "Food self-reliance doesn't necessarily mean producing everything the nation eats," we wrote, "but producing enough of its basic foods to be independent of outside forces."[6]

Once on the cash-crop export path, the "outside" forces to which one becomes exposed include decisions by other countries suddenly to produce *your* export crop. In a recent case, the Vietnamese government jumped on the globalization bandwagon and began subsidizing its farmers to grow coffee. Out of nowhere, Vietnam rose to become the world's second-largest supplier—helping push coffee prices down to their lowest level in decades. Now, this little village on another continent is feeling the effect.[7]

Also, when David Ricardo extolled the benefits of comparative advantage, "capital" couldn't move—couldn't pick up and leave, say, Flint, Michigan, and head to Tijuana, Mexico. Now that corporations can and do, Ricardo's arguments no longer hold. In fact, a country's comparative advantage may lie in nothing "natural" at all; it may only be that its businesses are willing to exploit their workers more heartlessly.

Despite our piles of evidence, international development experts still dismissed critics like Joe and me as naïve and impractical. We were chastised for advocating approaches that could only lock "developing" countries in poverty. Without cash crops, how could poor countries earn the foreign exchange to buy themselves into the modern era?

If cash crops were the answer, Kenya should be proof. By the mid-1980s, just three crops—coffee, tea, and oil—made up three-quarters of Kenya's export earnings. But poverty was still rampant, and was made worse by the continuing weak prices for exports of raw commodities worldwide.

I remember how hard it was in the '70s to believe what we had written, given its dismissal by the dominant voices. Of course, I didn't know then that twenty-five years later I'd be here in Kyaume witnessing for myself the consequences of the rush to cash crops.

Today, everywhere in Kyaume we see coffee trees—row after row after row. But we never see anyone actually drinking coffee, though there is powdered stuff put out at breakfast, apparently because Americans are presumed to drink it. Kyaume coffee, like most of Kenya's coffee, is shipped off to Nairobi for export.

One morning, we chat with Mumo Musyoka, a thirty-one-year-old coffee grower and Green Belt leader in Kyaume. We want to know about coffee, and Mumo graciously obliges. From the classroom where we sit I can peer through large holes cut into the mud walls for windows, and all I see is acre after acre of coffee. The crop that—along with tea and other exports including cut flowers—was supposed to put Kenya on the road to prosperity.

"Coffee came here in 1963," Mumo tells us. "We used to be able to make a lot of profit growing it. But last year, my family produced four hundred kilos, and after subtracting the cost of fertilizers and pesticides, we got nothing. We didn't get a single cent." This year the return was almost as bad.

Mumo tells us part of the problem is the middlemen who cheat small farmers like herself. Costly chemical inputs are also a big financial burden. When Anna says that small producers are also not protected from international coffee prices that fluctuate wildly, going way up and way down, Mumo laughs.

"Here there's no up and down. It's just down and down." (I will later wish we'd known enough to explain what fair-trade coffee—described in the next chapter, *Stirring the Sleeping Giant*—might mean for Kyaume.)

Mumo and others are so fed up with coffee—with world prices now one-third lower than the average cost of production—that many are ready to cut down the plants that have dominated this village for almost forty years. "We've already replaced some coffee trees," Mumo tells us.

"Without coffee, what would you do for cash?" Anna asks.

"We'd grow corn, beans, peas. We could sell those," she answers confidently, "and if they didn't sell, at least we could eat."

GREEN SPRINGS FROM GUNNYSACKS

So I'm not surprised when Mumo exudes enthusiasm for the Green Belt Movement's expanded work beyond tree planting. In the last few years, Green Belt has taken on "household food security," encouraging members to reclaim the best of traditional African mixed-food farming. The Movement has been teaching how to farm free of chemical dependency, and distribute seeds for long-neglected foods, like sweet potatoes, arrowroot, pigeon peas, cassava, millet, sorghum, and more.

I recall asking Wangari during our long chat back in Nairobi what sparked Green Belt to add food security to its work.

"Hunger" had been her simple answer.

We listen to Mumo to better understand why. In part, the Kenyan government had continued the colonial focus on cash crops. Besides coffee and tea, now some of the best farmland in the country is being used to place Kenya near Holland as one of the world's top cut-flower exporters.[8]

Neglected by government agronomists and development agencies, more than 2,000 African native grains, roots, fruits, and other food plants have now dwindled so much that some scholars call them the "lost crops of Africa."[9]

In working to revive these "lost crops," Mumo stresses that it's not just sentimental pining for the past. And, as she talks, I think back to Negi in India and Farida in Bangladesh; of their parallel efforts to reclaim and spread their seed heritage. "Over centuries, Africans had learned to cultivate food that worked in this environment," Mumo says. "We grew root crops such as cassava, arrowroot, and sweet potatoes, as well as groundnuts [peanuts]. We grew pumpkins, all kinds of things.

"These were all crops that could be kept a long time, either because you could store them underground, or, like pumpkins, you could keep them and they wouldn't rot. As long as you don't break the pumpkin's neck or puncture the skin, it can survive a long time.

"Many root crops will last for years in the ground, where they are naturally protected from insects and the sun. These crops are the ones that bridged the harvests and fed us during droughts," Mumo explains. "Now we're getting seeds from Green Belt, seeds for groundnuts, sweet potatoes, millet—foods that won't dry up and die if we don't get rain."

Mumo also tells us about a Green Belt workshop where she learned ways to help her get out from under the chemical agriculture burden.

"Some, like composting, my parents always did, but the practice was forgotten because modern fertilizers grow things so quickly."

She also tells us about "double digging"—reversing soil layers because the deeper soil, as she says, "has more minerals, so crops grow bigger. We learn to put leaves between the layers for air, too."

Later in the day, Anna and I are eager to try our hand at some of these new (old) practices. Under the bright midday sun, surrounded by coffee trees, we learn, for example, how to fill a gunnysack with earth, and then plant seedlings in the soil on top; how to poke holes and stick seedlings into the side of the sack as well. The process is easy, and for a drought-stricken region, brilliant. The sacks prevent water from draining out into the thirsty ground.

When we get home that evening, I notice for the first time just outside the kitchen door three gunnysacks exploding in green leaves. Fresh food literally within arm's reach of the pot! Obviously, Ramana has had the same instruction we just had.

WE MEET A THUG

Our teacher in creating gunnysack gardens was Joseph Karangathe. A soft-spoken man of thirty-two, Karangathe sits with us after our lesson. When we ask how he became involved with Green Belt, he takes us back to when he was a teenager and found himself with no money to fulfill his dream of college.

"I turned to hawking fruit on the streets," Karangathe tells us, "and then I became a shoemaker."

But in the early '90s, his life changed radically. The "tribal clashes," in which thousands were killed and tens of thousands displaced throughout Kenya, tore apart his community in the Rift Valley.

"Homes were burned and looted. My family and I felt insecure. What future do we have here? I was told to return to my ancestral lands, but I didn't even know where that was."

During the tribal clashes, Karangathe lost all of his livestock, and he and his community faced serious hunger. So a group coalesced—thirty-five men and women in all—with the goal of rebuilding the local economy. Using solar power, they began saving energy and created their own kitchen gardens to become food-secure. Then, the whole group decided to take a course in sustainable agriculture.

"Even though I didn't have land," he tells us, "my community said I should be part of it anyway. When it was over, the group said I should be the promoter—the one who oversees and reminds everyone of what we learned.

"The government agricultural agent was pushing inputs—pesticides and fertilizers—that people didn't have money to buy. So the group paid for me to go to college to learn organic farming. I went for two years." Listening to Karangathe, I weigh the likelihood back home of neighbors teaming up to put a friend through college: slim.

Once Karangathe's training was complete, Wangari offered him a job in the Green Belt Movement, and his Rift Valley community encouraged him to take it. All they asked in return for having supported his education was that, from time to time, he help them with their organic-farming efforts.

"I started with the pilot phase of the Green Belt food security program. My belief came from the practice. I believe people can sustain themselves once they understand how everything relates to everything—how the animals and crops and trees all relate and contribute to each other so you don't need chemicals."

His approach seems so commonsensical, so useful to people with almost no cash—so appropriate in a country where half the people live on less than one dollar a day. But we quickly learn that talking common sense is not without risk.

At one gathering to which Karangathe invited villagers to learn about organic farming, a local government farm agent called the police. "Pointing at me, the farm agent said, 'There's a thug here. He's invading my jurisdiction with unproven technologies. Arrest him.'

"They wanted to disperse the meeting, but I protested, 'I don't think this is an illegal meeting,' I said to the chief. I told the government agent that what is lacking is communication, dialogue between the conventionally trained and the organic. 'We don't have to fight. Let's join hands. You can disperse the group, but I want to go to your boss and sort it out.'

"The next day, I went to the divisional agricultural officer," Karangathe tells us calmly, and I see his soft-spoken, gentle demeanor as a real asset.

"'One of your staff didn't understand and tried to stop my meeting,' I explained to the officer. He then confessed that no matter how hard he'd tried using chemical inputs, he'd not been able to make farmers sustainable. 'We don't have the skills,' he told me. 'We can join together and learn from you.' So we made friends."

"But why did they try to arrest you in the first place?" Anna asks. "Why are government officials so wed to chemical agriculture?"

"Because conventional farming is promoted for the benefit of those who produce the inputs. See, the government training package for farmers is not determined by the government—it's designed by the companies who sell the chemicals.

"Now I say to the government agents, 'You've promoted chemical fertilizers and pesticides for thirty-five years, and people are still hungry. So what's your solution—more fertilizers and pesticides?'"

Knowing what Karangathe has faced—from tribal clashes to being told that his teachings are crazy, even criminal—I'm curious about what sustains him.

"I felt I had to do this. Before, the business I was doing didn't give me satisfaction. I wanted to do something that satisfied my heart. If you just get money, it only makes you disturbed.

"It's like walking to Nairobi," Karangathe says, leaning forward on the edge of the couch.

"It's a long way to Nairobi. A very long way. I don't know how I'm going to get there, but I just start walking. And someone comes along who is going the same direction. Someone picks me up on a bicycle and takes me part of the way. I get off and walk. Then maybe in the next town I meet someone who picks me up and takes me a bit further. Then I walk some more.

"The most important thing is that I know where I want to go—and that I just keep walking."

"What We've Lost, We're Getting Back."

The next afternoon, Lea Kisomo agrees to tell us about her much longer-cultivated perspective on food security here. In a faded green, yellow, and blue dress, her head wrapped in a white floral cloth, Lea has the calm bearing of a Green Belt elder. At the age of seventy-two, she has lived more than two decades longer than the average Kenyan woman.

We sit together in a tiny living room, with army certificates of the man of the house hung at odd angles on the bright yellow wall behind her.

"I've given birth to ten children," she begins through a Green Belt translator, "but only four are still alive today." I take a deep breath, trying to register what that one fact would mean in a woman's life.

But Lea moves on, reminiscing about the fruits, vegetables, and grain that she and her family ate fifty years ago. "Somehow they've been forgotten," she sighs. "Now our children are getting funny diseases. They're getting sick with things they never had before. They're a lot weaker now."

"What food do you miss the most?" Anna asks.

She pauses pensively and then says with a smile as if she's tasting it again, "Porridge made from millet. It's sweet and strong." And I flash to the lifeless white bread we'd been served that morning.

The pleasure these memories bring her is evident, as Lea talks about the hope Green Belt's food security program has given her for her village and her family.

After our thank-you's, Anna and I begin to get up, but before I do, Lea takes my forearm.

"When you go home," she says, looking me straight in the eyes, "tell your people that we Kamba people had lost our culture, especially our food security, but now we are going to regain it. What we've lost, we're getting back."

DANCING FOR BREAKFAST

On our last morning in Kyaume I want to get all the final photographs, tidy our room, and express our heartfelt thanks. I have an agenda. But, to tell you the truth, all I remember of that morning is the singing, which again turns into dancing. In the living room, on the porch, in the yard under the mango tree, Ramana and her children, Regina and the other women who've come to say goodbye dance with us as casually and comfortably as if we'd known each other all our lives.

Never before in my life have I danced at breakfast.

I think back to just a few days earlier, when I climbed out of the van and watched the dancing. I remember thinking, while not wanting to: How can they be so happy when life is so bleak?

It takes me several days before I get over myself and join in the dancing and singing. Over time, I stop questioning and find my answer. I let myself simply feel what these women, despite circumstances that could be called grim, are expressing: joy in discovering their power to transform their village, joy in the strength they've found together, joy in being perfect hosts to their far-flung visitors from America, joy in being alive. I now see that our new friends are not denying suffering. They're celebrating life—with all its pain.

As I'm heading outside to join the dancing, I see a large calendar on the wall. It's a promotional piece from Eli Lilly Pharmaceuticals. How odd, I think. Then I catch what it's selling—it's an ad for Prozac. I smile, pass through the door, and join the dancing with new vigor.

Pitfalls of Not Solving for Pattern #2

I'd been popping the fluorescent malaria pills with diligence for weeks, aware of the epidemic sweeping the continent. It hit closer to home when Regina told us that her sister had just died of the disease, and when we learned of the other people in Kyaume who have lost family members. Across the continent, malaria is killing more than one million people each year, mainly children.[10]

So when Hans Herren, a 1995 World Food Prize winner and a scientist here in Nairobi, tells us he's working on malaria, my ears perk up.

"I just submitted a forty million dollar grant for malaria prevention," Hans tells us over dinner in Nairobi, "but it's a long shot. Most of the money is going to vaccine development, though no one knows when or even if a vaccine will be discovered.

"In the meantime, we've developed simple prevention tools that are so cheap they could be in every village, now. If I had the money, in ten years I could reduce malaria here by fifty percent. But promoting 'non-sciency' things like teaching people to protect themselves from exposure or disseminating cheap products that disrupt the mating patterns of mosquitoes or kill the larvae and adults, is not as sexy as researching a vaccine—and not as full of profit potential."

Listening to Hans, I think again about the cost of dissecting our problems down to assumed solutions. In this case, a cure-all vaccine. Even if we had a vaccine, would those who most need it be able to afford it? Plus, malaria is not simply a symptom of a growing number of infected mosquitoes; it's a symptom of poverty. If we improved economic equality and health care, giving people tools to help themselves, we would reduce deaths not just from malaria, but from the dozens of other preventable illnesses, from dehydration to diarrhea to dengue fever.

After dinner, Hans drives us back to the Lang'ata guesthouse through Nairobi's now-deserted streets. He promises to be in touch with Wangari. While the science establishment focuses on a vaccine, Wangari's Green Belt women might just be one of the low-tech, people paths to saving lives from malaria.   —Anna

THE "WRONG BUS SYNDROME"

With only a few days left in Kenya, we're back at the Lang'ata guesthouse, Green Belt's training center on the edge of Nairobi, a recent gift from the Austrian government. We're tickled to have Wangari to ourselves for an evening, and we begin dinner together at a long table covered with a bright yellow tablecloth. Through steel security gates, we can see in the twilight the parched grounds where, that morning, monkeys had entertained us.

Wangari, radiant in a deep-green head wrap, focuses on us with her contagious energy. The flickering lights powered by a humming generator—a now-familiar sound of the city-wide power ration brought on by the drought—make the room feel cozy.

In Kyaume, Anna and I saw what a powerful trigger tree-planting can be. Women—isolated and intimidated by their husbands, spending a big chunk of every week in the exhausting search for firewood—have come together and found new energy, hope, and direction. So I'm taken aback at first when Wangari begins our dinner conversation by telling us that, while planting trees is one entry point of the Green Belt Movement, "civic education is *really* the entry point."

Civic education? I think to myself. Could anything sound less appealing? I recall civics in high school as a total yawn in which nothing stuck except "checks and balances" and some 19th-century president's campaign slogan. Really pretty useless. Definitely not an "entry point."

Here in Kenya, we quickly learn, it's different.

"Even if you enter with trees," explains Wangari, "until people understand their rights, especially their environmental rights; how to stand up for their rights and have the courage to stand up—until then, even the planting of trees is not safe. People can always be intimidated. They can always be pushed back."

In Kenya, planting trees and protecting trees are not neutral acts. They mean confronting authority. Wangari knows. She herself has been arrested many times for protesting the tearing down of public forests. In her successful fight to save a downtown Nairobi park, she was beaten so badly by government police that she had to be hospitalized.

For Wangari, civic education is not about learning abstract, distant power structures and procedures, it's about gaining confidence in one's self, confidence in being able to stand up for one's rights and one's community.

"We call civic education 'self-knowledge,'" Wangari explains, and I realize she is describing what I call "living democracy."

"The turning point for people who join the Green Belt Movement is often in a workshop we call the 'wrong bus syndrome,'" she says, pulling out a little handbook with that name on it. More than 15,000 people have gone through the workshop, at least one from each of the communities in which Green Belt's nurseries are based.

Over steaming plates of rice and vegetables, Wangari reminds us that everyone has taken a bus at some point, so "we start there. We begin with the obvious.

"Now, if you're supposed to take a bus, then you must make sure you get on a bus going your direction so you can get to your destination. Most likely, if you take the wrong bus, you'll encounter a lot of problems because you were not prepared. You may get to the place and you don't know anybody. You won't know where to sleep. You might get arrested for loitering," she says with a grin.

"So we say, but if you go in the direction you have planned for, you are likely to enjoy it. When you get there, you'll meet the people you expected. Life is likely to be pretty good!" We laugh along with her.

"Now we ask the question: Why on God's earth would anyone get to the bus station and get on the wrong bus?

"Sometimes people say, 'Oh, if you cannot read'—because many people here cannot. What do you do? You ask people who can read. But people can mislead you. A dishonest person can tell you this bus is going in your direction. Much, much later you discover that you went in the wrong direction.

"We can spend a whole day talking about how people have been misled, by books, by preachers, by teachers—many times . . ."

Listening to Wangari, I feel I'm in the seminar with her. I like her emphasizing that we can all be misled. It spares one feeling like a total loser if one's life is not what one wants it to be. Yet it doesn't take us off the hook, either, because we've allowed ourselves to be misled. It's a gentle avenue into people's hearts.

"Then we ask, 'What are all the problems you have—in your own life, in your family, in your community, maybe even in your own nation?' Very quickly they give all the problems: hunger, lack of water, no transport, poor education, no books.

"'Where do you think these problems come from?' we ask. They give all kinds of answers—the local chief, the husband, the pastor, the wife, the children.

"Then we ask, 'What do you think the solution is?'

"They may say, 'Vote out this government.' 'Have a revolution.' 'Pray.' 'Cultivate more food.' But when we ask where the solutions are, they rarely mention themselves.

"Without denying the big obstacles we all face, especially these villagers, we do create many of our own problems—either through omission or commission. Many problems we have a capacity to change. So, I tell them, 'We can change our lives. We can change our destiny. If you've been misled—and many people are in that category—and you discover you were misled, you have a choice. You can decide to continue in the wrong direction and take a chance wherever the bus will lead you. Or you can decide to get out of that bus.'"

Wangari mimics herself talking tough: "'You yourself don't know that the forest controls the river flow? That without the forest we will not have river flow? If you don't, then you see the forest being destroyed, and you do nothing. You see the forest being privatized, and you do nothing. You see a school that does not have a windbreak, and you do nothing—and then the winds come and blow down the school and your children are killed, and you say it's the will of God? Excuse me, that's stupidity.'

"Now that can take two days discussing, and that's when the personal transformation takes place. That's when people realize, yes, they may have been misled, but they have brains and also can think. That's when we make a break, and from then on we are dealing with a different kind of person—very motivated, self-conscious, willing to make decisions, willing to go back to their communities and make a difference.

"After we've taken people to this point, we talk about how to channel their energy," Wangari continues. "Now we can tell people, 'You planted trees and started a tree nursery on your land and your neighbors' land, so now you take part in reforesting public lands.'"

What Wangari is describing is what Anna and I have seen throughout our journey: those precious moments of dissonance when people see themselves and the world with new eyes. I imagine the energy released in the seminar room when people first realize they are not simply victims. I feel a rush of excitement as Wangari renews my hope that this inner awakening is possible for every one of us, no matter how swamped and trapped we feel.

As for Me, I've Made a Choice

Anna and I ask Wangari about the origins of the slogan we'd seen adorning Green Belt T-shirts. AS FOR ME, I'VE MADE A CHOICE. It stirs us each time we see it.

"When you go through the wrong-bus syndrome, you discover you've been misled," Wangari explains. "Then you have to ask, 'Am I going to continue no matter where this bus leads?' That's a difficult thing. You have to make a choice! There are some people who say, 'I guess I'll continue going until it stops.' I tell them, the bus may never stop; you may find yourself in Cairo. Then it would be even worse because you can't speak the language!'"

At this point Anna and I crack up, and Wangari brings home her point: "To be out of that bus, you have to make a choice."

As we listen to Wangari describe empowerment, Green Belt style, my earlier ruminations on human malleability return. I think about how delicate our little psyches are; how we think of ourselves as such intelligent creatures—we Homo sapiens—and yet our common sense about what we need to do for ourselves is so easily overridden by fear of those in authority; overridden by messages that we are not competent. Yet, precisely because we are so malleable, this lost sense of self can be regained in new circumstances—as I myself am learning this year.

Wangari has helped us see the ways in which Kenyans have been misled and made not to trust their own knowledge, but what about the rest of us?

Corporate globalization is great, we're told, only a few kinks to work out—never mind that greenhouse gas emissions are creating global climate chaos or that we're losing to extinction one species every twenty minutes. Our food system is terrific, ads remind us daily—never mind that almost half the world's grain goes to animals while thousands die each day for lack of food.

If we're all on the wrong bus globally, how do we get off? I desperately don't want to end up in Cairo.

Who's Paying for the Ride?

We move from the dinner table to more comfortable seats by the fireplace. Wangari sinks into a beige armchair, and Anna and I sit cross-legged on the floor. The generator is still purring, but the lights have dimmed even more. One of our hosts brings us candles. The evening chill is cut by burning charcoal, and by hot cups of tea that just keep coming.

Wangari, always able to make something abstract become real, shifts our conversation to the impact of her country's foreign debt. Wangari is a Kenyan leader in the global organization Jubilee 2000, which takes its name from the Biblical jubilee year in which slaves are freed, land redistributed, and debts forgiven.

Jubilee 2000 and Wangari are getting the word out about the weight of the debt burden for poor countries—now at roughly $2 trillion.[11] With debts so large and interest rates climbing, Wangari tells us, many heavily indebted poor countries are ending up paying rich ones more each year than they receive in aid. Much more. Each year, we learn, Kenya pays over $4 in debt servicing for every $1 it receives in development aid.[12]

During the '80s, commodity prices dropped worldwide, devastating countries like Kenya that are dependent on export-crop income. Yet, under pressure from the World Bank and the International Monetary Fund to pay off debt, the Kenyan government pushed even more of its economy onto the export treadmill to earn foreign exchange, even encouraging the export of natural resources, like wood. No wonder Wangari is as motivated by her Jubilee 2000 work as by her work with Green Belt; they are integrally linked.

She reminds us what this has meant for Kenyans. Servicing its foreign debt eats up almost half the country's GNP and amounts to $20 million each year *more* than the government spends on health and education combined.[13] Kyaume's school principal told us school fees increased without warning this year—more than doubling for secondary schools—so now, many more families can't afford to send their kids to school. When we'd asked people in Kyaume why school fees went up, no one could explain. Now, Wangari tells us that the government hiked the fees to finance the debt.

Cutting government funding for schools, Wangari reminds us, is also connected to the International Monetary Fund's "structural adjustment programs." Though the term has always sounded a bit like a chiropractor's helpful realignment, what it really refers to are strict conditions a country must meet to receive loans from the Fund. They include cutting government spending, mainly by shrinking subsidies and services such as education and health care.

Even though evidence mounts that structural adjustment, by requiring governments to cut back on public services, hurts those already suffering the most—the poorest and the youngest—strict conditions continue.[14] School-fee hikes here in Kenya are just one symptom.

I think of the young men we met in Kyaume just a few days earlier who told us of a particularly ironic consequence of Kenya's high school fees: At a recent Green Belt action to save public land from illegal logging, student demonstrators were attacked by other students, by government-paid youth desperate for money to cover the skyrocketing costs of their education.

"When we ask for debt relief," Wangari continues, "donors say our debt should not be canceled because African leaders are corrupt. They say, even if you cancel debts the benefits will not go to the poor. So, it's no use canceling it. Meanwhile, the corrupt leaders are cutting off social services to pay off debt.

"Do you realize we've repaid the original amount borrowed several times over?" she asks us. "But high interest rates make it impossible for us to ever pay it all off.

"Debt is no longer totally an economic issue. It's no longer a business issue. It's a moral issue. Lenders are asking people who never saw the money, who never received the money, to pay it back. I'm one-hundred-percent sure that the White House knows, or could find out easily, how much money President Moi has outside this country. So why don't they freeze that stolen money, and make Moi pay them back rather than make innocent peasants suffer?

"Sometimes the lenders say, 'Okay we could consider that it's a moral issue, we could accept that the money never reached the poor people, and that the people who ought to repay this money are the elites who misused or stole it. But even if we did, how do we ensure that in the future the politicians are going to be more accountable to their people?'

"That's when I tell them: That's why we're doing civic education. This is why I'm in the pro-democracy movement!" Wangari says, letting her frustration show. "While rich nations were supporting our dictatorial leaders, people like me were being thrown out of universities for speaking out, some became refugees or were sent to jail, some even were killed.

"This is why I'm telling our people we must get out of this bus. It's the wrong bus and we must learn to elect the proper people into government. We haven't gotten there yet, and as long as we're carrying these debts, we never will. We will get so poor we won't be able to raise our voices anyway."

THE HORNS THAT HOLD UP THE SKY

Listening to Wangari, I reflect on my own fears, which despite my best efforts, I still feel: fear of loneliness, of criticism, of ineffectiveness. These fears seem puny next to hers, yet I've struggled with varying success to overcome them. So I'm curious to know what has made her able to face the life-and-death fears that she has.

"I have paid a heavy price, which is sometimes what people fear. When you step forward, you get exposed. Sometimes you get criticized, sometimes you lose friends—I lost a friend called a husband.

"Sometimes people say, 'Why do you take that kind of a risk that makes

IN GOD'S IMAGE

On our last night in Nairobi, Wangari invites Reverend Timothy Njoya, a priest and friend in the pro-democracy movement, to speak with us. We sit together in the Lang'ata living room, Njoya at one end, his small frame sinking into an armchair, his stiff white priest's collar striking against a midnight-blue shirt. Njoya's voice is animated, peppered with jokes and wily insider winks to Wangari.

He tells about his life, the life of a radical priest. Years ago, he was de-frocked for claiming that Jesus was an advocate of social justice. When he was finally "re-frocked," Njoya decided to write a sermon that would question the reality of democracy in Kenya. This was a nervy thing to do in a country in which the president has ruled since 1978, has decreed that insulting him is a crime, and has imprisoned, attacked, and even murdered his critics.

With the help of friends, Njoya broadcast the sermon live on the radio. He tells us that everyone who knew him believed he would be killed, as did he. So, when he finished the sermon, he went home and, as he tells us, waited to die.

That night nine men arrived at his house.

"When I opened the door," Njoya says, "I was struck across the hand with a long spear. Three fingers were severed. Another attacked and I put up my hand to block. The blade came down, hard." Njoya holds up his hand, stretching his fingers, pointing to a thumb with a raised, telltale scar: "Here, right here."

He jumps up to demonstrate his block from the other side. "One you lose certain things?' But for me it has never felt like a loss. I always feel like I'm walking. When I get to a point where I have to make a jump, then I make a jump. Sometimes I get burnt, sometimes I get crushed, but I cross over." Wangari smiles, adding, "There's always another promise on the other side."

The whir of the generator has stopped, and the lights are bright again. The power is back on, which means it must be past eleven P.M.—the ration shuts off the city's electricity from six in the morning to eleven at night. I'm

hacked this finger completely off. I was using my left hand to protect my heart. I had lost three fingers. I started to use this hand, but I thought I don't want to waste my right hand, too, so I better use my legs."

He drops to the ground. Njoya on the floor, laughing, loafer-clad feet in the air, looks like a dad launching his toddler in a game of airplane. I'm imagining the absurdity of it: The attacker held up by Njoya's thin, short legs.

"One of the men was holding his sword above me," Njoya says, still on his back, feet in the air, still laughing. "I said, 'Yes, my brother, I have forgiven you. You should also forgive me for hitting you with my feet.'" All of a sudden, to his attacker Njoya became human again—flesh, like him.

"Then he bandaged my hand and took my fingers and returned them, and returned them, and returned them," Njoya says, gesturing with each of his fingers.

"I told them, 'Now, since you have done this, you, take my Bible and you, take my camera from America. You take my suits.' I was dying anyway, my intestines were about out here," he says sweeping his arm wide. "I told them, 'You, you take care of my family and you take my library.'

"The men said, 'We didn't know you were such a good man. Those who sent us to kill you didn't tell us that truth.'

"I lost consciousness. I woke up several days later my fingers sewed on, but poorly, sticking out in funny directions. That was the first time I was almost killed," Njoya says, smiling.

I have mixed feelings about my own faith, but meeting Njoya—sensing his dedication to democracy, seeing his humor and downright sprightliness, learning of his brushes with death and his survival—I think, if there is a God, truly this man is created in his image. —Anna surprised Wangari wants to continue, given the hour, but she seems determined to help us understand.

"I grew up in the Rift Valley," she tells us, "and on either side there were ridges. On all sides I could see the limit. I believed that was the whole world. I believed that the ridges—where the sky or, quite often, the clouds would reach the mountains—were where the world ended.

"I remember asking my mother, 'Why doesn't the sky come down, because everything else comes down, but not the sky?'

"My mother told me, 'Up on the ridges are big, big buffaloes, and these buffaloes have big horns and these are the horns that hold up the sky.' For a long time, that's what I believed.

"Then one day we set out on a journey, the longest of my life. For the first time I came to the ridge, and I discovered there was something beyond. I was so happy to know that the whole world was not in that valley; that there was another world.

"That little journey reminds me of the many, many journeys I have made since. Before you go, you think that the world is just here, and then you go to the ridge and you see there is another world. There are so many ridges in life, and if you are willing to go to the top of the ridge, you will see another world beyond. But if you don't go—if you don't take the risk—if you only stay where you're safe, then of course you never see past the ridge."

DROUGHT, DÉJÀ VU

It's finally time to leave Kenya, and we get to the airport early—maybe it's a premonition about Ethiopian Airlines.

The check-in line is long, so we grab a paper. Suddenly, I'm thrown back in time once more—to the 1970s, when famine in West Africa triggered my decision to write *Food First*. Our research on the West African famine at that time showed that, even in the worst years, many of the countries were producing enough grain to feed everyone. Some were even exporting food.[15]

Now, the headlines again are screaming: Eighty percent of Kenya hit by drought, 30 million Kenyans at risk of starving. One reads: "Famine, it looms again, over Horn of Africa." We're told that Kenya faces famine because—in three years—it has barely rained.

I want to scream back, but instead grumble only to Anna, "It's not that drought isn't a problem, but why can't these writers see what we've just seen, what Wangari sees: It's *people* who make deserts, who turn drought into disaster."

It's not hard to grasp how this disaster has been created. Coffee trees we saw everywhere in Kyaume are only part of the sacrifice of traditional crops that evolved in Africa precisely because they could withstand periodic drought. This disaster also reflects a legacy of colonialism and lost culture that has left villagers cutting wood for decades without the wherewithal to replace it; the land-grabbers illegally cutting down forests on public land; corruption in government that drives decisions on dams and water projects more than sound engineering does; and government and development-aid agencies promoting crops unsuited to this climate.

In the '70s, I learned the sad truth that human beings, not nature, make famines, but I see this fact is also hopeful. I see it in the seedling I planted back in Kyaume. I see it in the joy of the Green Belt members we met. I see it in Wangari's life. We *can* choose.

So, when Ethiopian Airlines tells us they can't locate us in their computers, though we hold our tickets in our hands, Anna and I discover Green-Belt-style chutzpah. We have a mission; we must get home to tell our story. We don't budge, and mysteriously our reservations pop up.

KENYA: AWAKENING OUR SENSES

Celebrating Root Vegetables Soup
ADAPTED FROM MOLLIE KATZEN'S *Vegetable Heaven*

Serves
6 to 8

Rutabagas, turnips, and parsnips don't normally get a whole lot of attention, but this delicious soup, at long last, provides their fifteen minutes of fame. I never thought something so earthy could be this beautiful: pale sunny yellow with spots of creamy white, gold, and bright orange peeking through. It's naturally sweet, too, and slightly hot from the ginger and the optional horseradish. This takes about an hour to make, only 20 minutes of which is work.—Mollie

1 tablespoon butter or vegetable oil

1½ cups onion, chopped

1 heaping tablespoon minced garlic

3 to 4 tablespoons ginger, minced

2½ teaspoons salt

1 medium rutabaga, peeled and diced (about ½ pound)

2 small turnips (about ½ pound), peeled and diced

1 medium sweet potato or yam (about ¾ pound), peeled and diced

2 medium-small potatoes (about ¾ pound), peeled and diced

1 8-inch parsnip (about ¾ pound), peeled and diced

2 large carrots, peeled and diced

6 cups water

1 cinnamon stick

optional garnish: a fine sprinkling of grated fresh horseradish (go easy)

Melt the butter or heat the oil in a soup pot or Dutch oven. Add the onion, garlic, ginger, and ½ teaspoon of salt, and sauté over low heat for about 10 minutes.

Add the remaining vegetables and another teaspoon of salt. Stir, cover, and cook over medium heat for 10 to 15 more minutes.

Add the water and the cinnamon stick. Bring it to a boil, then turn the heat way down. Cover and simmer for 10 minutes. Remove the cinnamon stick, cover again, and continue to simmer for about 5 more minutes, or until the vegetables are completely tender.

Place about a quarter of the vegetables and some of their cooking liquid in a food processor or blender, and process briefly to thicken (but not necessarily to smoothly purée). Return the processed batch to the rest of the soup, and stir it in. This treatment gives the soup a delightful, varied texture.

Serve hot, with a very light sprinkling of grated fresh horseradish on top if desired.

CHAPTER

8

STIRRING THE SLEEPING GIANT

The most important thing is dignity.
We got back our dignity.

ROSARIO CASTELLON, NICARAGUA

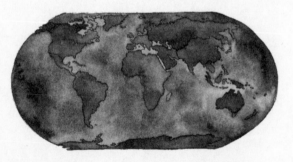

Far from Africa, we're on the move again—this time by train, heading north from Paris to Holland. My seatmate looks friendly, so I ask if he'd like coffee before I head off to the café car. As I'd hoped, my offer ignites conversation, and I'm surprised to learn the slightly-built, bearded man next to me is actually a Dutch cargo-ship captain, Jan Den Daas. He's on his way home to Rotterdam.

We whiz past the Holland of postcards and in-flight magazines—green fields flat as a dance floor, small houses tucked behind fences. Only the occasional square concrete structures seem off in this picture.

"Those are bunkers," Jan explains. "This was an important battleground where we fought against the Germans in World War Two."

Pointing to a high mound, he adds, "That's a dike that keeps the water back. In the early fifties, this was all under water." He gestures out our window. "I can still remember in 1953 when two thousand people died in the flooding."

As the fields speed by, his two points of history seem more than chance remarks; they seem designed just for me at this moment. What I now see from my window as placid farmland and charming villages, with little girls running hand in hand, was just yesterday a gory battlefield and the site of tragic drowning. This landscape is a reminder not to take "what is" for granted.

At the Utrecht station, Jan keeps me company until I'm handed off to Kees Elgershuizen, a Dutch friend who has offered to drive me to my destination: the heart of the fair-trade movement in Europe.

Fair trade—the simple notion that producers are assured a fair price—has long seemed to me an obvious centerpiece of any strategy to end the poverty and powerlessness at the root of hunger. Half the world's population still lives on less than $2 a day, and the majority of them are small farmers.

Shortly after *Diet for a Small Planet* was published, I decided to learn about the coffee trade. After all, I thought, coffee is the second most valuable commodity traded in the world. If I could understand the dynamics of how coffee trade traps in poverty more than 20 million small coffee farmers in eighty countries, I figured I could grasp the more general pattern showing up in the harsh lives of small producers of other commodities like bananas, tea, cocoa, and spices.

Learning more about small coffee producers, I saw that they face two huge problems. For one, coffee prices swing wildly as Mumo's experience so vividly personalized in Kenya. Graphs of world coffee prices always looked to me like Pinocchio on a lie-detector test—the spikes and dips both extreme. Between one year and the next during the '90s, there was a threefold price fluctuation. Today, farmers are getting less for their coffee than at any time in the last one hundred years.

Plus, small coffee producers receive only a tiny share, about 5 percent, of what consumers in the North pay for their product. Most of them work all day to earn less than $3, or about what consumers here spend on just one Grande Café Latte at a Starbucks. Imagine if coffee growers were compensated like the producers of the world's first-ranked commodity traded—oil!

Though the problems became clearer and clearer, I still didn't have a clue about what one might do to solve them.

THE GHOST OF MAX HAVELAAR

I've come to Utrecht to learn more about the origins and the vision of the fair-trade movement—a strategy that has been growing for decades. I'm hoping it might hold promise for increasing the return to poor farmers, cushioning the blows of market volatility and easing hunger. And as Anna and I learn more about this strategy, we begin to see the implications of fair trade as even more far-reaching. The fair-trade movement becomes for us additional evidence of how people around the world are evolving capitalism, and how our actions, even small ones, make big ripples.

Walking—almost running because we're so late—along the tree-lined canals and narrow brick streets of Utrecht, Kees and I rush to meet Hans Bolscher, director of the Max Havelaar Foundation. Entering breathless, we're escorted into an inviting room with high ceilings, butterscotch walls, and windows crowned with stained glass. Hans, an energetic man in his forties, seats us at a large, dark-wood table.

Kees laughs when I'm asked what I'd like to drink and say, "Coffee, if you have some." The "if" is hardly appropriate here. Behind me is a glass cabinet full of colorfully wrapped coffee, samplings of the brands carrying the Max Havelaar fair-trade label.

Curious, I start with the puzzle of the name and ask the obvious, "Why Max Havelaar?"

"Our name goes back over a hundred and forty years to Eduard Douwes Dekker," Hans explains, "a colonial official in the Dutch East Indies, now Indonesia. [Ever wonder why we call coffee Java? Java was the center of Dutch coffee growing.] Appalled by the abuses of the colonial coffee plantations and by colonial policies causing local food production to stagnate, Dekker wrote a part-exposé, part-autobiography called *Max Havelaar of the Coffee Auction Houses of the Nederlandse Trade Company.* The 1859 book is a passionate protest. Its main character, Max Havelaar, champions the rights of local farmers.

"Everybody in the Netherlands knows this name," Hans continues. "It's part of our culture, so Max Havelaar was an obvious choice—not just because of name recognition but to remind ourselves that millions of coffee farmers still suffer from the extreme abuses and unequal balances of power that Dekker described." As I listen to his story, Eduard Dekker becomes for me a Dutch Upton Sinclair.

FROM CHARITY TO FAIRNESS

Fair trade has come a long way since Max Havelaar started in the late '80s at the urging of coffee farmers in Mexico, who said they would prefer fair trade instead of charity aid. Then, Hans tells us, fair trade still meant little do-good shops scattered in cities around Europe, selling products—from rugs to carvings to placemats—bought at fair prices directly from small producers abroad.

"It was nice, but it didn't amount to much," Hans admits. "It was just a closed circle of well-meaning people. But in the mid-eighties, coffee growers in Mexico started pushing us. 'If we are going to get anywhere,' they said, 'we must have access to real markets.' At first, we thought we could go to the CEOs of big food companies and convince them to pay better prices to producers. It was pretty naïve, but we had hope. The CEOs said, 'Oh no, we can't pay more to the producers; we operate in the free market. What if we pay a higher price and other companies don't?'

"A year of talk produced nothing. That's when we realized we had to focus on consumers first. Without consumers willing to pay more, and without consumers putting pressure on companies, fair trade could never work."

As Hans fills me in on the history, I recall the basic picture of fair-trade coffee that Paul Rice—Hans's counterpart at TransFair USA (the U.S. fair-trade certifier)—painted when we visited his warehouse-like offices in Oakland, California, earlier in the year. I hadn't seen Paul since the '80s, when I worked with him on a book about land reform in Nicaragua, where he'd spent eleven years helping to develop farmer cooperatives before returning to U.C. Berkeley to get a business degree.

Paul explained to us the way fair trade works: Importers and roasters pay a fee to a fair-trade certifier—in the U.S. it's his organization—and a premium per pound of coffee, allowing Paul's group to put a fair floor under prices coffee farmers receive—no matter what the zigzag of the world market. Like certifiers in Europe, TransFair USA ensures that coffee with the "Fair Trade Certified" label meets specific criteria—that, for example, the coffee is produced by democratically organized small farmers with full knowledge of market prices.

"Right now," Paul told us, "world coffee prices are extremely low, and most small farmers are only getting twenty-five cents for a pound that retails here for eight dollars or more. The fair-trade network assures a floor of a dollar twenty-six a pound, and we make sure it goes directly to farmers, pushing their annual incomes up from five hundred dollars a year to around two thousand dollars on average.

"That still may not sound like much, but the difference in the lives of coffee growers is huge," Paul said. "In practical terms for many farmers it means being able to stay on the land, keep their farm, and feed their kids."

Hans tells me that thanks to efforts like his—and Paul's in the U.S. as well as dozens of other organizations working on fair trade worldwide—half a million coffee farmers are now benefiting from fair trade in more than twenty countries in Central and South America, Africa, and Asia, and millions more could potentially benefit.

In Europe I'm amazed how fast this idea has caught on. It's been just twelve years since Max Havelaar launched its label, but its coffee is now carried in almost all the country's supermarkets. From coffee, Max Havelaar has expanded to certify other fair-trade products like cocoa, honey, bananas, and tea. I see that their Max Havelaar intuition paid off, too. Its name recognition in Holland is now 92 percent. (In my own little test, I learned my train seatmate was quite familiar with the Max Havelaar brand.)

The idea is spreading, and not just in Holland. Hans tells me that fair-trade products can be found in 40,000 supermarkets across Europe, and fair-trade certifiers now offer products in seventeen countries worldwide. They've created their own umbrella group, the Fair-trade Labelling Organizations International, whose goals include a common fair-trade label recognized around the world.[1]

ROAST STARBUCKS?

Here in the U.S., fair-trade efforts started much the way Max Havelaar's did—small. One of the first fair-trade coffee importers, Equal Exchange, was founded in 1986 by three men in their early twenties with little knowledge of business or international finance and a $700 loan from a relative. Over the years, Equal Exchange built a business importing fair-trade coffee, developing ties with farming cooperatives around the world, and generating consumer interest. Now, their Boston-based, worker-owned organization has over a dozen trading partners in ten countries in Latin America, Africa, and Asia.

While Equal Exchange's importing efforts started fifteen years ago, it took longer for fair-trade labeling to swim the Atlantic. Our own fair-trade certifier, TransFair USA, only opened shop in 1998, but it's already making a big splash. Today, coffee drinkers can enjoy fair-trade coffee in city-council lunchrooms on the West Coast, in supermarkets across the country, and in Exxon/Mobil gas stations on an interstate near you.

The movement started by enlisting specialty roasters and sellers, and by mobilizing consumers nationally to demand fair-trade coffee—just what Hans knew they had to do in Europe. Starbucks was an early, obvious target—the company boasts one-quarter of the country's coffee shops. Global Exchange, a grassroots organization with a fair-trade coffee campaign, approached Starbucks in 1999 asking it to carry fair-trade coffee in its more than 2,500 stores across the country. Starbucks claimed interest but ultimately said there was no way the bottom line could handle it.

So Global Exchange organized what was going to be a thirty-city "Roast Starbucks" campaign, with consumers demanding that Starbucks offer fair-trade coffee. Then, in what the *Financial Times* called a "remarkable coincidence," Starbucks signed an agreement with TransFair USA—Paul's certifying group—just days before the launch of the campaign and one day before the April 2000 anti-World Bank-and-corporate-globalization protest in Washington, D.C.

Global Exchange called off its consumer action.

As Global Exchange's fair-trade organizer, Deborah James, explained to us, "Starbucks had seen Kathie Lee Gifford's clothing line exposed in anti-sweatshop campaigns and had seen the consumer backlash against the apparel industry. They didn't want to be the Nike of the coffee industry."

Returning from Europe, we marched into the nearest Starbucks and, sure enough, there it was: packages of Starbucks' new line of fair-trade-certified coffee beans in their own display rack near the counter. But consumer demands didn't stop. As our book was going to press, citizens demonstrating in more than 200 cities across the country called on Starbucks to sell brewed fair-trade coffee, not just beans. Unless the company brews fair-trade, how could its use amount to more than a token? Consumers also called on Starbucks to ensure that none of its products contain GMOs or are grown under terms unfair to farmers. After protests and news conferences and letters to the company, Starbucks finally agreed to serve fair-trade coffee, but that's it—so far.

Besides Starbucks, TransFair USA has signed certification contracts with 160 companies, who are now selling fair-trade-certified coffee in more than 12,500 cafés and supermarkets—up from several hundred a few years ago. We learned that Safeway supermarkets even made it company policy that all its 1,600 stores stock fair-trade coffee—because customers demanded it.

To put this movement in perspective, though: Most coffee isn't traded by small importers, but by a few mega-companies. The biggest coffee roaster and seller in the world is Philip Morris, known more for its cigarettes than its coffee. Its Maxwell House brand controls a quarter of the coffee market in the U.S. and, relevant to Max Havelaar's challenge, a staggering 65 percent of the Dutch market.[2] But there's no reason awakened consumers cannot push the mega-companies as well.

RIPPLES OF FAIR DEALS:
MAMA TALK-TALK LOSES HER MONOPOLY

Reflecting on these U.S. victories, Anna and I think we're catching on to the scale and importance of fair trade. But something Hans said back in Max Havelaar-land, and what we will learn from two farmers actually living the experience—one in Guatemala and one in Nicaragua—show us how much we still have to learn.

Before I leave Max Havelaar, Hans tells me a story to make sure I get it.

"There's a region where we work in Sierra Leone with a middleman they call Mama Talk-Talk. She had a monopoly on the coffee trade there and would pay farmers only twenty percent of the wholesale price. A group of farmers started a coffee cooperative and found out about Max Havelaar. When they sold their first container—a standard measure of thirty-seven thousand five hundred pounds of green coffee—to the Dutch fair-trade market, we gave them information about market prices and paid them several times more than they were used to getting. Suddenly, prices in the whole region shot up. Mama Talk-Talk lost her monopoly.

"Fair trade is not always about cutting out the middlemen," Hans explains. "Part of the problem has been that the middlemen have a monopoly on information. That's why they've been so dangerous. We end that information monopoly."

BALTAZAR'S BETTER-BUSINESS STRATEGY

Later, at home in Cambridge, we have a chance to talk with a Guatemalan coffee farmer—thanks to long-distance phone service and the translation help of a friend, Thomas Fricke, cofounder of the largest U.S. importer of organic spices—Vermont-based ForesTrade. Through its on-the-ground projects, ForesTrade helps farmers in Guatemala, in Madagascar, in Grenada, and throughout Asia to enter the global fair-trade market. The company also helps farmers shift to organic methods and diversify their crops. The presence of ForesTrade in these communities, Thomas tells us, also often stimulates the kind of competition that Mama Talk-Talk would hate, which ends up increasing prices for farmers.

Baltazar Francisco Miguel—the fellow on the other end of the line—is one of them. He lives a bumpy thirteen-hour drive from Guatemala City in the rugged mountains near the Mexican border in the town of Barrillas. Together with 600 families, twenty-four-year-old Baltazar is part of a decade-old coffee-and-cardamom growers' association now selling to Equal Exchange, ForesTrade, and another major fair-trade importer, Royal Coffee.

"Before," he explains across the crackly phone connection, "because we are so remote, we were completely dependent on the coyotes [a common Latin American term for middlemen]. Some years the price we got for our coffee was even less than our production costs. We made nothing."

"Now," he continues, "with stable and better prices, nutrition is better, and I just visited a nearby village where I met forty families who were able to improve their houses in the last year. Children are able to go to school, too."

I ask, not expecting what is to come, "How does better, more stable income relate to children being in school? Do parents have to pay for school?"

"Our association is not just about money. We do a lot of training, including adult literacy," Baltazar explains. "So parents here now appreciate the importance of education, and many more want to send their children to school. It's a big sacrifice to send your children away every day, because they help on the farm, but what parents learned gave them a lot of encouragement."

At the end of our conversation, Baltazar wants us to know: "Our training is not just business strategy, it's about values. We talk with our members about the values of fairness and of common purpose with other small farmers here and around the world."

ROSARIO DREAMS THE FUTURE

While we're working on this chapter, we invite Rosario Castellon, age forty, to my home, knowing that she'll be able to tell us firsthand what fair trade has meant for coffee farmers in Nicaragua. She was general manager of a leading coffee export cooperative there for years and comes from a long line of coffee farmers.

On a sunny fall afternoon, Rosario, now based in the U.S. working for Equal Exchange, and fair-trade promoter Deborah James sit with Anna and me between their appearances on a campus tour to enlist student energy for the fair-trade movement.

We want to know what difference Rosario has seen in Nicaragua because of the fair-trade movement. Patiently answering our questions, Rosario is remarkably enthusiastic, giving no sign of discomfort, though her leg is propped up in a cast from a car accident.

"For us," referring to a Nicaraguan cooperative association of almost

3,000 farmer families that Paul Rice helped establish in 1990, "the big difference was that farmers could plan for their own future for the first time.

"In most of our fair-trade export contracts, sixty percent of the money comes six months in advance. This is very important. Before, the creditor had a stranglehold on us, we could never plan anything. Now that we get money in advance and get a fair price for our harvest, we can create a strategy. We can use that money to invest in production, or we can decide, 'Yes, we'll invest in a school this year.' Next year we know we'll have money to build a health center."

As she talks, I think back to the Landless Workers' Movement in Brazil (*Chapter 3: The Battle for Human Nature*), and how people in the Movement came to see that securing land is only the beginning. The deeper challenge is creating communities. So we ask whether what Rosario experienced in Nicaragua is typical.

Her answer is an emphatic "Yes."

"I've visited seventeen coffee cooperatives in ten countries, and it's not just better family income, it's overall community development. I know one Mexican cooperative in the fair-trade movement created the first public bus line in the region, built the only secondary school, and opened the first community health clinic."

Echoing our feelings, Rosario says, "I had no idea how deep and long-lasting the effects of fair trade would be. What I see is a shift of consciousness in farmers, from being just producers to becoming entrepreneurs who look at every aspect of farming. Before, their only concern was high yields without thinking about the environment. Now farmers know that quality is most important. We grow shade-grown coffee, which is of higher quality, and we don't use chemicals."

In fact, Rosario tells us, most fair-trade-certified coffee available in the U.S. today is also certified organic, making the movement a powerful force for environmental conservation in addition to fairness for farmers.

Before we bid them good luck for the rest of their journey, Rosario adds a parting thought: "When we started, the object was getting the most money. But fair trade is not just that. Before, we had no idea how much traders made from our coffee. Now, we have marketing people who give us full disclosure. We operate more as equals, as partners with foreign traders. We can be real players now.

"The most important thing is dignity. Fair trade gave us back our dignity."

PITFALLS OF NOT SOLVING FOR PATTERN #3

In the early 1970s, international development agencies advised Latin American coffee farmers to "get technified."[3] Toss out your antiquated production equipment! Replace traditional coffee varieties with faster-growing ones! Cut down forest overhang and let those trees grow fast and strong in the sun! The U.S. Agency for International Development even provided a lot of the training and money—$80 million across the continent. Over the years, more than 40 percent of coffee throughout much of Latin America has been converted to sun coffee.[4]

While technification required more inputs, like fertilizers, pesticides, and water, its supporters pointed to immediate, irrefutable results: Coffee yields nearly quadrupled. Overall, the one-third increase in global coffee yield since the '60s, experts say, can be attributed to technification.[5] Problem solved.

But what sun-coffee backers don't see is what happens when you narrowly focus on yields. The chemical inputs and huge amounts of water end up destroying the fertility of soil in coffee-growing regions. The costly inputs burden already struggling farmers with big debts. Plus, all those pesticides have ghastly consequences for farmers' and their families' health. Another unanticipated consequence: Cutting down the canopy over millions of acres of coffee farms has disrupted an entire ecosystem, disturbing a crucial stop-off point for migratory birds that perched in the overhang. Not so coincidentally, these bird species have been declining throughout North America ever since.[6]

But even more basic, what the "technify experts" didn't see was that yields weren't the problem to begin with. The problem was, and is, as our fair-trade friends show us, an entire system that prevents coffee farmers from getting the price they deserve for yields they *already* achieve. With the help of fair trade, many farmers are now returning to traditional growing methods, including shade-grown coffee, and finally getting the prices they deserve.   —Anna

FARAWAY FAIRNESS

In exploring the fair-trade movement, Anna and I were unnerved to realize the arbitrary lines in our own minds. Of course, small farmers in the third world need and deserve a fair price. Finally, a movement is beginning to ensure it. But what about those who produce food in our own country—farmers and farmworkers? "Fair trade" evokes faraway images. How can we erase the divisions that keep us from seeing unfairness to producers as a world crisis, not just "over there" somewhere?

Whenever I think about farmers here in the U.S., what always comes to mind is a farm auction I saw near Walthill, Nebraska. It was a summer day in the mid-1980s, and grain prices had fallen so low that farms—many in business for generations—were folding fast. I felt like a witness to an auction at a funeral. Farmers, many of them longtime neighbors, swarmed the property like vultures, inspecting harvesters and bed frames, tractors and teapots. The family stood by silently watching all their possessions being sold to the highest bidder.

Now when I think about the decimation of farm communities, I don't just think about Walthill. I think about Bhatinda, India, or Kyaume, Kenya, where prices paid to farmers continue to drop and bankruptcies like the one I saw that day persist.

Here at home, farming resembles ever more closely what Americans have always associated with the "third world"—not family farms but increasingly big estates using hired labor. Every year, we rely on roughly a million farmworkers planting and harvesting our food, and, depending on the season, several million more undocumented migrant workers.[7]

The lives of these laborers hardly differ from the Brazilian landless "cold meals." Often, migrant farmworkers live in quarters little better than the black plastic shacks we visited in Brazil. And many of the laws we think protect all workers fail to shield farmworkers. In some states, farmworkers aren't guaranteed collective bargaining rights or the federal minimum wage.

As part of their work, our farmworkers also face the life-threatening hazard of industrial agriculture: pesticides, daily exposure to which has been linked to cancer, brain damage, hormone disruption, and birth defects.[8]

Most farmworkers live well below the official poverty line, and the average life expectancy for our farmworkers is just forty-nine years.[9] That's more than two decades less of life than the general population enjoys. Ironically, it's also significantly lower than that of people living in Costa Rica, Nicaragua, or El Salvador—countries from which many of our migrant farmworkers come.[12]

A Sixth-Grade Memory

When I was twelve, I went with my mother to Ohio on a trip the Farm Labor Organizing Committee planned so that a few dozen people—from church leaders to journalists—could talk with farmworkers face to face. If people could see for themselves the lives of our farmworkers, FLOC believed, they would be motivated to demand fairness and help end their invisibility here. At the time, I just thought it was a cool way to get out of school for a few days. I didn't know that it would forever change the way I looked at my world.

On our first day, we arrived at midmorning at a migrant farmworker's home near the fields where she worked. The house was a small wooden shack, barely big enough for her and her three children.

While her kids played quietly nearby, we sat by her bed talking. She told us she was dying of cancer. Like thousands of farmworkers every year, she'd been poisoned, we believed, by the pesticides she was surrounded by every day in the fields.

Later, as we were getting up to leave, she asked my mother and me with a tone of genuine bewilderment, "I don't understand. What could be more important than what we do? We put food on your table. Why don't people value our work?"

—Anna

Five Cents

If consumers paid only three cents more for a cup of coffee and it went directly to producers, that tiny sum from each of us would be enough for coffee-cooperative members to build decent lives and livable communities. Three cents. Here at home, we read a study from the United Farmworkers Union that just five more cents per pint of California strawberries would increase by half the pay of strawberry workers, significantly improving their living standards.[10] Five cents.

Personally, I can't imagine anyone already willing to pay a few dollars for a pint of strawberries who wouldn't pay five cents more. The challenge isn't getting Americans to be more generous, more caring. It's about creating opportunities for people to express their sense of fairness by letting them know the real impact of their purchasing power. Ultimately, it's about getting consumers to mount enough pressure so corporations see there's no choice: If they want our business, they must pay decent, living wages. In the process, we as a society create new norms of what is acceptable.

So a vital question for Anna and me is: Can we bring the fair-trade movement home? Can we erase arbitrary lines between fairness "over there" and fairness to those who grow and harvest our food here?

As we learned from people in the fair-trade movement, when consumers are given the choice to act on their values, they do, and their lives are richer for it. "We give consumers a way to join forces with farmers," Paul Rice had told us, describing the role of fair trade. "We're seeing a groundswell of consumers who feel good about spending a few cents more for a cup, or a pound, of fair-trade coffee, knowing it means they're ensuring that farmers get paid fairly.

"Church groups are used to boycotting products from companies doing things they don't like. Now they have a tool for saying what they *do* like, for a 'buycott.' In the San Francisco fair-trade coffee campaign, stores saw a big increase in sales of coffee stickered with the fair-trade label. We can explode the myth that Americans are not willing to pay for values," Paul told us, exuding the same buoyant optimism he brought to helping build successful coffee cooperatives in Nicaragua. "We can show that the consumer is a sleeping giant."

It may just be this awakened giant that will make a stronger call for fairness at home. For decades, consumers have been able to "buycott" products made by companies known to be farmworker-unionized. With the Internet, we're also entering an era of marketing possibilities that directly link conscientious consumers and small producers. And now, new labeling schemes give consumers other opportunities to voice their values. In the past several years, the Oregon-based Food Alliance has pioneered a label so that consumers can see which companies have met their criteria, and it is now encouraging similar locally based labeling efforts across the country. Before receiving the Food Alliance seal of approval, companies must prove, for instance, that they are working to protect the environment through erosion control, cutting back on chemical usage, and reducing water use. Those raising animals must prove that they're doing so humanely. And the companies must also show that they treat their workers fairly.

All this sounded so helpful. We were sobered, though, talking with people working with farmworkers themselves. A Northwest-area farmworkers union cautioned that, at the moment, the Food Alliance label has more bite when it comes to protecting the soil than protecting workers. The union's caution was an important reminder that, as powerful as we consumers can be, we also must be savvy. As corporations catch on that we care—about fair trade, worker rights, chemical-free products, and more—many will claim to be jumping on the bandwagon. We must ensure they really do jump, and stay on.

THE PC POLICE GET A VACATION

Political correctness has gotten a bad rap. Americans have become leery of preachiness, whether it's Jerry Falwell's or Jerry Brown's. But I'm coming to see conscious choices we make as consumers not as some politically correct performance. What we choose to buy, where we choose to shop, even whether we choose to be part of campaigns to pressure companies like Starbucks to buy fair-trade coffee—all this is not an homage to some weighty obligation; it's a celebration of the world we want.

Finally, we have real choices, ways to know where and how our products are made. And honestly, it just feels good.

Just like I bet dozens of student groups around the country involved in Global Exchange's fair-trade coffee campaign feel good when they succeed in getting fair-trade coffee stocked in campus cafés. Recently, Columbia University students even convinced Starbucks to retract its "no fair-trade coffee on campuses" position.

Like these students, I'm happy to know when I buy my cup of coffee in the morning that I haven't participated in exploiting workers thousands of miles away. It's good to know that when I buy union strawberries I'm not encouraging the slow killing of a farmworker from pesticide exposure.

Now, when I shop, I walk through aisles differently. When I buy fair-trade coffee, I picture Mumo in Kyaume, Kenya, and Rosario's family in Nicaragua. When I buy locally made cheese, I picture Bob in Plain, Wisconsin (you'll soon meet him, too).

My choices as a consumer used to feel so small, but now I'm convinced they have real power. Together we are a sleeping giant and, awakened, we can really stir things up.

—Anna

As Anna and I are finishing this chapter, we think again about Hans Bolscher. "The challenge," Hans had said, "is creating a link in the minds of consumers between fair trade and an intangible that makes us, as consumers, feel good about ourselves. Our message is that this is how it ought to be—this is trade of the future. Buying fair-trade goods means being part of a world where people treat each other decently; part of a shared value of a desirable future."

WAS IT EVER OTHERWISE?

Just before leaving Max Havelaar headquarters, I asked Hans why he chose to devote his energies to fair trade. He explained by describing his work with Doctors Without Borders, an international group that sends doctors and health-care workers into third-world countries. He enjoyed the work, he said, but realized he wanted to be part of preventing wounds, not just putting on bandages.

His choice to help make sure people are fairly paid for their labor, through fair trade, can stop some of the wounds poverty causes. It seems so obvious, but how long will it take the obvious to become the norm?

Returning home, I'm struck by a news account noting that coffee drinkers can now "appease their social conscience along with their thirst."[14] Hmm. We Americans don't think we're appeasing our social conscience when, for example, we allow women or African-Americans to vote. And, doesn't basic survival rank above voting for most of us? Why is a choice to ensure that producers can feed their families and live in dignity something especially righteous?

When will the "click in perception" come, the moment when we take for granted that producers get a fair price, and not just coffee producers but all the millions who work the land to put food on our tables? A moment when, as a people, we think, "Of course, of course. You mean it was ever otherwise?"

Just like on the train ride to Utrecht. Then, watching the tranquil scenes flash by, I couldn't imagine it any other way—certainly not that in my lifetime, right here, right where happy girls are now playing, was a bloody battlefield. So, I think to myself, there is no reason that within my remaining lifetime, it won't become unimaginable that those who labor to feed and clothe us would ever have been treated with anything other than the respect and gratitude they deserve.

THE WORLD: AWAKENING OUR SENSES

Indra and Sylvie's Chai

Makes
6 cups

Chai, an Indian tea, is made with spices that have various healing effects according to the Indian Ayurvedic tradition. The black pepper is believed to be a blood purifier. The cardamom helps digestion, and cloves are good for the nervous system. The cinnamon is good for the bones, and the ginger helps with physical weakness, increases energy, and assists digestion. The milk is soothing to the stomach. This recipe comes from Sylvie Blanchet, cofounder of ForesTrade, and her friend Indra Khalsa. For the richest taste, use organic spices like the ones Sylvie and Thomas bring us through ForesTrade.

5 cups water

15 whole cloves (approximately 1 teaspoon)

20 cardamom pods, crushed

35 whole peppercorns (about 1 teaspoon)

5 sticks cinnamon

16 slices fresh ginger (a 2½-inch piece, peeled)

½ teaspoon nutmeg

6 teaspoons whole black tea, loose

¼ cup honey

3 cups milk or soymilk

In a large pot, bring the water to a boil. Add all the spices and cover. Allow the spices to boil gently for 30 minutes; the mixture will boil down to about 3 cups.

If you want to drink it right away, add black tea and steep for 3 to 5 minutes. (Be sure not to leave it in any longer, as the tea can become quite bitter.) Strain the tea and spices as you pour the liquid back into the pot. Add honey and milk while stirring, and bring almost to a boil. Serve.

If you would like to drink it later, allow the mixture to cool with the spices in it. Strain and refrigerate. When you are ready, heat the Chai, add the loose black tea, honey, and milk. Let tea steep 3 to 5 minutes, then strain and serve.

CHAPTER

9

THE LAST TASTE
OF PARIS

En marche vers l'agriculture de demain.
(We are walking to the agriculture of tomorrow.)

THE ALLIANCE:

FARMERS-ENVIRONMENTALISTS-CONSUMERS

FOR SUSTAINABLE AGRICULTURE

AND FOOD CITIZENSHIP

The last train to Paris left five minutes ago. (Hannes's watch was slow.) So I'll spend the night in Brussels. Not so bad. I'll call Anna so she won't worry, and I'll have more time with Hannes— our conversation over dinner was hardly enough to re-weave the threads of our lives that were dropped twenty years ago in Rome.

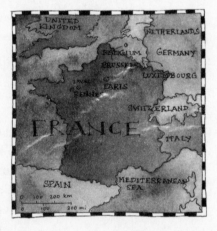

We walk the dark streets from the Midi station searching for the hotel the train attendant recommended. I realize I shouldn't have worried about being steered to luxury beyond my expense account, as I squeeze past furniture stored in the hotel's stairwell and into a room so small the bathroom door hits the bed. I leave behind my heavy laptop, and Hannes and I head out again.

I'm here hoping Hannes, a German, can help me grasp the European paradox Anna and I want to unravel.

Since I wrote *Diet for a Small Planet,* Europe has taken the fast track toward American-style farming—bigger and bigger farms that are more and more dependent on multinational suppliers of seeds, chemicals, and machines. The Europe of small, quaint villages surrounded by family farms is vanishing. During the 1990s, a quarter of a million European farms disappeared from the land.

In France, a single-minded production focus has placed this relatively small country among the world's top agricultural exporters. At the same time, food, always a source of national pride for the French—as for many Europeans—has become a cause of anxiety. Scares about mad cow disease, unsafe poultry, and contaminated drinking water have shattered many Europeans' faith in the people entrusted to secure their food.

But in the past thirty years, a very different story has emerged as well, one challenging industrial-style farming and reconnecting communities, farming, and economies.

It's these two contradictory paths that Anna and I want to learn about—and Hannes, I know, is the man to ask.

I last saw Hannes Lorenzen in 1979, the year he and I helped lead an international band of renegade young people to stage a counter-conference to the United Nation's World Conference on Agrarian Reform and Rural Development, in Rome. While the officials pontificated next door, we hosted, in a stately one-time monastery, peasants from Latin America and Africa who spoke about the real impact of American and European policies on their lives.

As Hannes talks to me now, still with a boyishness and just-below-the-surface laugh, he seems every bit the outside-established-channels visionary whom I remember. But in the twenty years since we last met, he's become a voice *within* the structures of power, too—he's now advisor to the head of the European Parliament's agriculture and rural development commission.

THE PELLWORM POSSIBILITY

The bar we find is hardly ideal, with its smokers and video games only feet from our table, but I scarcely notice. I'm intrigued by what Hannes says next. After he orders a traditional Flemish brew made from cherries, telling me I'll never find *this* in America, I expect him to launch into the nitty-gritty of European policy. Instead, he asks, grinning, "You mean I never told you about Pellworm? It's an island where I spent my holidays as a child on the farm of my father's family. It's three feet below sea level, so you have to climb the dikes just to see the sea."[1]

I'm wondering how Hannes will connect this tiny island with the European-wide policy he's knee-deep in as I take my first gulp of beer. I choose not to mention that it reminds me of cough syrup I grudgingly swallowed as a kid.

"Twelve years ago," Hannes continues, "our regional government threatened to convert the island into a national park. People were worried that it would destroy our farming way of life. At first, the islanders just said 'No, absolutely not.' Our slogan was 'Freedom for Frisians!'"

I'd never even heard of Frisians before, and now they want freedom! I chuckle to myself, but Hannes clarifies. Teasing me about Americans' paltry knowledge of European geography, he tells me, "Frisians are islands along the coast of the North Seas."

He continues. "We decided to bring together farmers, fishermen, shopkeepers, the doctor—people I knew from my childhood. I said, 'We don't have to be *against* this. We can use this as an opportunity.'

"Inviting visitors to tell us what they loved about Pellworm, we started to look with different eyes at what we had."

Neighbors began working together to rethink ways to farm and to develop island tourism, Hannes explains. To meet electricity needs, they created wind power, solar energy, energy derived from animal waste, and even geothermic storage. They also found ways to reduce the amount of energy they used. To their surprise, they discovered that tourists prefer organic, local dishes and are even willing to pay more for them. Now a significant part of the farming is organic, and farmers sell directly to local shops and restaurants.

"A new spirit emerged," Hannes says. "We started exchange visits with other economically disadvantaged islands and communities in what we call the Eco-Islands Network.

"On one of those visits, farmers from the Estonian island of Hiiumaa noticed that farmers on Pellworm weren't using their wool. For us, prices were so low it wasn't even worth clipping the sheep. So the Estonians said, 'Let us use your wool, and we'll make sweaters to sell in the region.'

"Together, we created what every economist is looking for—value-added. Estonians, who aren't part of the European Union, got access to the EU with wool that, *within* the EU, had no value. See, it's networking like this that can kick off a new kind of economy!"

I'm hoping that Hannes can't read my mind. Pellworm and Hiiumaa are charming examples of possibility, but each is barely a speck on the map, literally. They hardly seem harbingers of global economic change. For the rest of the evening, though, we leave Pellworm and drift across Europe, and I begin to see differently.

After his Pellworm experience, Hannes began to uncover similar efforts elsewhere in Europe—people bringing economics back into community life. He found many.

Out of these examples, Hannes and a French colleague created a Europe-wide sustainable development network of forty communities to spread Pellworm's and their own hard-earned lesson: that when you re-embed new, sustainable economics in community life, you can create viable local answers to globalization.

After describing this network, Hannes adds, "This is no romantic, European dream," raising his mug of cherry beer. "It's real, it's happening."

UGLY WORD, BEAUTIFUL CONCEPT

The next morning, I do make it to the sleek, high-speed train to Paris on time and, zipping along the tracks through Belgian farmland, I think more about the shift in thinking that Hannes described.

Now, I can see the network as Hannes does, as a real glimpse of the possible and as larger than the sum of its parts: an emergence of communities finding solutions not through a "take it apart" mentality and piece-by-piece problem-solving, but through knitting their local solutions together. They seem to be going beyond "us-against-them" thinking—remember the "Freedom for Frisians" starting block? They're modeling a different way of interacting, one that's more like the natural world, in whole systems.

Thanks to Pellworm, and now this network, Hannes is no longer a fringe, wishful thinker. He's got the material to back his moxie, and he's using it to advise the European Parliament and other policymakers.

Hannes is working with others in Europe to shift EU policy from the current "productivity model" to a "quality model." That means changing the focus from generating the maximum tonnage of grain or meat or milk to caring for landscapes, protecting diversity of wild and cultivated plants and animals, and ensuring that the economy works for the community, not the other way around.

There's a buzzword for it, Hannes told me. It's being used from the halls of the European Parliament in Brussels to the World Trade Organization's headquarters in Geneva. The term is "multifunctionality," and while it may sound just about as dry and uninspiring as a word can be, in its own clunky way it conveys agriculture's *multiple* dimensions. Agriculture is never just about quantity. It's also, and always, about providing safe and nutritious sustenance, preserving the environment and a rural way of life, and keeping people from crowding into already stressed cities.

Multifunctionality—this shift in focus from quantity to quality—is also about respecting the history and culture that root people to a place—whether it's Bordeaux produced in Bordeaux or whether it's olive oil in Greece, where, Hannes says, farmers are convinced *they* produce the world's finest.

This rootedness to the particularity of place is the opposite of attitudes in the U.S., where our drive toward uniformity promises that the hamburger we bite into in Boston will taste the same in Billings.

Sipping coffee from the train's café car, I continue to mull over the meaning of quality. My coffee, rich and delicious, was individually brewed just for me in its own mug, and isn't burning my fingers through a paper cup. Is that quality—although of a trivial sort? The publicly supported high-speed rail sparing me the hassle of driving—and saving the planet from another gas-guzzling car—that's quality, and not at all trivial.

But how do we measure it? Economists assure us we can measure quality of life by rising living standards . . . and then they take a very narrow view of what that means. Rising living standards are measured in per-capita income, or consumption rates, or GDP. Defenders of corporate globalization argue no nation can enjoy rising living standards unless it lowers trade barriers and encourages business investment unfettered by public policies like those Hannes and his allies are pursuing. But I've never been convinced. Rising living standards, as captured by economists, have always seemed to me a dubious measure of well-being. Income can rise, and right along with it can come worsening pollution, longer commute hours, deteriorating health, and ever-more-contaminated water.

Making rising living standards—defined in narrow economic measures—our goal reflects a locked-in focus on production. So I'm pleased we're meeting people who are letting go of this fixation and stirring public debate about richer, more accurate measures of our well-being—such as those embedded in multifunctionality here in Europe or in living democracy in India.[2]

A Clunky Term Goes to Poland

I expect endless blocks of drab public housing, gray skylines, plumes of smoke from tired factories. Instead, driving a tiny rental car through Poland's country roads, I find families harvesting hay, boys selling baskets of strawberries, and kids picking flowers in golden fields. Visiting small farms that dot this landscape, I meet farmer after farmer living off the land and tending it without chemicals.

I came to Poland to learn about the network created by Jadwiga Lopata to preserve the Polish countryside and help the small farmers, whose families have been here for centuries, to become certified organic.

When I meet Jadwiga, birdlike and blond, she breathlessly tells me about the conference she just organized on "revaluing" countryside values—those that respect non-consumer culture and view farmers as stewards of the earth, not as technicians measuring outputs in tons and crossing fingers for the next technical fix.

Poland, she explains to me, is one of the last vestiges in Europe of small-scale, nonchemical farming. Under communism, farmers here had little money to buy chemicals and, cut off by the Iron Curtain from U.S. exports, they were not inundated with our agricultural chemicals like much of the rest of the world. So today, in a country the size of New Mexico, two million farmers—more than there are in the entire U.S.—are farming organically for the most part, almost by default.

As I listen to Jadwiga and visit the farms she has drawn into her ecotourism network, the wooden "multifunctionality" comes to life. I taste it in the wild strawberry cake farmer Helena Kobiela makes for me. I sense it in her daughter when she tells me she comes home from Kraków every weekend to spend time on the farm. I hear it from Marian Wegryzn when he tells me he gave up chemical farming after he watched his animals and himself grow sicker and sicker. I see it in the land I walk with him, still with a limp because of his illness, in the dairy cows grazing on his dark green pastures, and in the thick grove of trees where he harvests his honey.   —Anna

THE BUYING POWER OF THE FRENCH DAIRY COW

Wanting to bring multifunctionality to life, we head out early for Brittany and the farm of Jean-Yves Griot who is part of Hannes's network. But we quickly discover that departing Paris at five A.M. is not nearly early enough. The word for traffic jam—*bouchon* (cork)—is our morning language lesson, and I think back longingly to my peaceful train ride the day before.

In our French interpreter Eric Reiffsteck's tiny red Twingo, we finally escape Paris traffic and fly west past cornfields as big as those we'll see in Wisconsin and past hog operations almost as huge and foul-smelling as those in our Midwest. A farmer in Hannes's network here seems to me about as likely as a vegan at a barbecue. We're driving through a stronghold of large-scale industrial farming with all the markings of this claim to fame: severely polluted groundwater, increasing unemployment, and fewer and fewer farmers.

Several hours later, we're lost. Winding through the little village of Laval, searching out Jean-Yves' farm, we can't spot a single person to help us. We finally make it to *chez* Griot and are greeted by blossoming roses and blue hydrangea wrapping his 18th-century farmstead even before we see the five-language welcome sign in his foyer.

At fifty-seven, with gray hair and wearing a pale-blue Oxford, Jean-Yves looks to me more like a congenial college professor than a farmer, and, sitting down at his wooden-plank table that's at least twelve feet long, I learn I'm not entirely wrong. In the '70s, Jean-Yves was a teacher at a national research institute in Paris.

"I wanted to work with my hands," he tells us, "but I was worried that farming might mean I'd be too tired for anything else. So I decided to find a partner to farm with me so each of us could have more time.

"In the beginning—we arrived here in 1977—we planted corn and bought soy meal from the U.S. and Brazil to feed our dairy cows. We used fertilizers and pesticides on all our crops. We did exactly what everyone else was doing."

But two moments in his life—his moments of dissonance—forever changed how Jean-Yves thought about farming and himself.

"During the late '70s," Jean-Yves explains, filling our glasses with bottled water, "we began hearing more and more about hunger in the third world. Meanwhile, I knew we here in Europe had mountains of butter and rivers of milk. I thought, how wonderful—we can ship surpluses to those who need them more.

"But I started learning that giving away or selling our surpluses at low prices to the third world ends up making prices *so low* that small, local farmers in those countries are destroyed. I was shocked. What I thought was helping was actually part of the problem.

"I wanted to do something. So a group of us contacted other milk producers in France and started educating them about the impact of exporting our surpluses."

Sitting in this old stone farmhouse, I couldn't feel farther from the Mission District in San Francisco, but back when Jean-Yves was having this revelation, we at Food First were having similar aha moments. Through our research, we were discovering that—counter to what one might assume—chronic food handouts (as opposed to disaster relief) were actually harming local economies, driving the prices of basic foodstuffs down and pushing local farmers out of business. Food aid was also shifting tastes away from locally grown foods, setting the stage for long-term import dependency.[3]

But we sometimes felt like lonely voices. All around us, church groups, aid agencies, the U.S. government—everyone, it seemed—saw poor countries as incapable of feeding themselves and our exports as the answer. Many American farmers took comfort, believing that, even if they were struggling, at least they were helping to "feed a hungry world." Despite this drumbeat, we in Food First's funky offices in the Mission and Jean-Yves in his picturesque French farm kept questioning.

"Once I saw how exporting our surpluses could be damaging," Jean-Yves continues, "I started seeing how our *importing* feed for animals was also contributing to the problem of world hunger.

"It was immoral to me that Brazil would be exporting feed for livestock in Europe while hundreds of thousands of its own people were starving. I was shocked when I realized that the French dairy cow has more buying power than a hungry person in Brazil." (As you hear Jean-Yves talk about his 1970s revelation of the clout of a French dairy cow, remember that today in Brazil *two-thirds* of that country's grain goes to livestock, not to people.)

"We wanted Europe to stop buying soy from countries like Brazil and stop sending dairy exports that were hurting their farmers," Jean-Yves continues. Jean-Yves' worry seems as appropriate now as it was in the '70s. We just learned, for instance, that 60,000 small dairy co-ops in India—mostly run by women—may not survive recent World Trade Organization rules requiring their country to lower its barriers to milk imports.[4]

"We were just a small network of milk producers talking to each other, but we decided to do something. So we started in our own small way. We changed the one thing we could: how we farm. Together we decided to become less dependent on imported feed, instead raising our cows more on the pasture."

A RETURN TO THE MIDDLE AGES?

Something closer to home triggered Jean-Yves' second moment of dissonance.

"By 1990, the water in our town was undrinkable," Jean-Yves tells us quietly. "The farmers in our network, about eight hundred of us, wanted to understand why and find out if there was anything we could do.

"Looking at the data on the nearby Mayenne River, we saw that nitrate levels had remained steady until 1977, but at that point they had started rising. We noticed that, ever since, they've been climbing at *exactly* the same rate as corn cultivation."

Worldwide nitrate levels—largely from nitrogen fertilizer—have doubled in the past 200 years and could double again in another fifty, with widespread impacts. Scientists say that nitrate runoff from Midwest farms is already a big reason why as much as a 7,000-square-mile area in the Gulf of Mexico suffers oxygen levels so low that it's been called a "dead zone," with sea creatures at the bottom of the food chain dying.[5]

Using nitrogen fertilizers, farmers have been able to boost corn yields dramatically, making cheaper grain available for export and for animal feed. But there's a major drawback. Roughly half of all nitrogen applied by farmers never makes it into the harvested crops.[6] Corn, one of the worst offenders, uses nitrogen for just a few months of the year, leaving many months for nitrogen to make mischief by leaching into groundwater and then into waterways.

"The water crisis was touching everybody here—the schools were even serving kids bottled water," Jean-Yves says. "We had to carry our own water to our houses. It was like we were returning to the Middle Ages."

Seeing the connection between what was happening to the community's water and how they were farming, Jean-Yves' farmers network volunteered to test alternatives. "As a farmer, I felt responsible," Jean-Yves says. "So we halved the chemicals we were using for corn."

At the end of five years, an independent office tested whether they had reduced nitrates in the river, Jean-Yves explains. Of course, Anna and I are expecting the punch line to be that these farmer-experimenters triumphed over pollution.

But Jean-Yves says solemnly, "We found no difference.

"That was the real turning point. We realized we couldn't just cut back on chemicals; we had to change our *entire system*. The real problem, again, was relying on corn feed for our cows. So we had one more reason to choose more pasture, less corn," Jean-Yves says with a professorial matter-of-factness.

It's too soon to know whether this redirection—looking at the whole picture, not just the pieces—has made an impact, but it just may help move his little community back into the 21st century and out of the Middle Ages.

EDUCATING THE SLEEPING GIANT

Walking through the long shadows of the late afternoon past a midnight-blue wooden wagon and flowering hydrangea, I remind myself not to romanticize farming. I know it's all-consuming work. So, I wonder, did Jean-Yves's original plan to work with a partner really end up giving him more time for other pursuits?

As we stand at the edge of his pine-green pasture, Jean-Yves explains what he does in his "farm-free" time—and my question is answered. He talks with passion about his work with a sustainable agriculture network, and I see how critical Jean-Yves' early choice to farm with a partner was. It gave him *time*. Time to look beneath the surface. Time to see with new eyes—to hatch a new, healthier vision.

As soon as Eric tells us that the name of Jean-Yves's group, Réseau Agricole Durable, means "Sustainable Agriculture Network," I'm delighted. I prefer "durable" to our softer-sounding "sustainable." In English, of course, "durable" suggests toughness. I like that. Sustainability isn't wimpy. It's tough-minded. It's realistic. It's the strength to stand up and admit that industrial farming isn't working.

Jean-Yves tells us the network's latest project is to launch a Sustainable Agriculture food label—in many ways like the Food Alliance's in our Northwest, mentioned in the previous chapter. Consumers across Europe would recognize the label as a seal of approval, a stamp showing that the product was made with care for the earth, for workers, and for small farmers. Farmers certified with the label wouldn't be required to forego all chemicals, but instead would have to limit chemical use and take other steps, like planting trees to prevent soil erosion and ensuring workers are paid a living wage.

The label would enable European consumers to choose products grown sustainably and reward farmers by honoring their efforts. It sounds good,

THE HIGH COST OF CHEAP

Passing through Jean-Yves's village, with its towering church and tiny stone homes, we see no places to stop for lunch. So we end up at Leclerc, a sort of French Wal-Mart. In a parking lot big enough to rival any American mall's, I wait in the Twingo. I have my notebook on my lap from our hour-long drive here, with its 135 tally-marks—one for each of the trucks we passed that was loaded with the goods of "productivist" Brittany and bound for Paris.

Musing about how out-of-place the giant trucks seem on quiet country roads, I watch a scene unfold like a silent movie. Women park, take empty carts, and walk into Leclerc. Others return with carts of food, load their cars, fasten seat belts, pull away. They're all alone, faces listless. They remind me of myself on my own shopping trips—under an overpass, along the East River, and the long walk home.

Megastores, like the one I'd go to in Harlem or the one here in Brittany— these are what we're told are more "efficient" and give us more choice and cheaper food. This is what we've traded for the local shops and village stores.

but, I ask Jean-Yves, "Won't consumers look at the price tag and think, 'This is too expensive. Why shouldn't I just buy food produced without chemicals when they're cheaper?'?"

"Many consumers now do think that way," Jean-Yves says, "but that's why we're educating them.

"Today, consumers don't realize we pay for our food not just once, but many times. We pay at the store, yes. But we pay again in taxes going to subsidies for the biggest producers, who don't need them. We pay a third time in the costs of pollution we endure from large farms destroying our soil, water, and air. Then we pay again in social services for those squeezed out by factory farms. And we pay *again* in the costs of urban crowding and sprawl.

"So, sure, you can say the price tag of our network's food is often a little higher—producing sustainably costs more in labor, for instance—but conventional foods are not really less expensive. It's just that their costs are hidden.

"The future of sustainable agriculture is in the hands of the consumer— as consumers, we must literally start seeing price differently," he says ada-

On some level, I guess I'd believed the tradeoff necessary, inevitable. But I see differently now. Is a food system really efficient when the average American buys food that's already traveled more than 1,500 miles to get to us?[7] Or when more than $10 billion a year—of the money we pay for food and drinks—goes to pay for companies to advertise to us, while overeating is one of our biggest health problems?[8] Or when for every dollar we spend on food, farmers are getting the equivalent of two dimes?[9] Or when for every job a mega-company like Wal-Mart creates in a community, one and a half are lost?[10]

The loss of the local *boulangerie* is happening fast, and the trend is being repeated worldwide. At home, in the less than ten years that Wal-Mart has entered the food-sales business, it has become our second-largest food retailer.[11] It likes to boast "super selection at everyday low prices." But when I hear that now, I'll think of searching for shops in tiny Laval, and what John Robbins writes in *The Food Revolution:* "Sometimes the price of cheap is very, very high."[12]

—Anna

mantly. Here in Brittany, Jean-Yves is reminding Anna and me that the sleeping giant must wake up and get educated. And Jean-Yves's challenge may not be as daunting as one might assume. Already, one recent opinion poll has found that two-thirds of Europeans are willing to pay more for organic food.[13] And when we get home, we will discover that in the U.S., too, the giant may be more awake than we'd thought. Four out of five New Yorkers polled recently say they'd pay extra for food grown in ways that safeguard water quality.[14]

ANOTHER AWKWARD WORD

We first heard about the French farmers' union, Confederation Paysanne, reading about the rabble-rousing, Roquefort-producing farmer José Bové and his dismantling of a McDonald's under construction. His was a hometown protest against trade policies that he and the Confederation see driving French farmers to ruin.

In the U.S. press, he's often portrayed as a lone Don Quixote figure, a handlebar-mustached caricature of the food-obsessed Frenchman—as if the Confederation Paysanne of which José is a leader were a mere curiosity.

Actually, his union represents one-fifth of French farmers and is growing fast, so we're eager to hear from one of its spokespeople about this movement that has taken its voice international, not only through activism like José's but through policy campaigns with farmers from Brazil to India.

The Twingo pulls into the drive of René Louail ("Mr. The Garlic," as Eric tells us the name sounds to French ears) and we're welcomed by a broad-shouldered man with a reddish five-o'clock shadow and a worn yellow polo shirt. As we walk down a stone path between tall hedges, René's apology for a tight schedule that gives us only a couple of hours reminds us that he's in high demand. His colleague José—appealing the three-month jail sentence for his McDonald's attack—is in India for a protest with Vandana Shiva against seed corporations, and that means René is even more constantly on call.

The four of us sit around his kitchen table, barely fitting into the small room, and René launches right in. He reminds us that the Confederation Paysanne is just thirteen years old, born in 1987 when it split from the mainstream farmers' union. René joined in the early '90s.

"I felt the mainstream union only benefited wealthy farmers," René explains. "I didn't feel comfortable. I didn't recognize myself in it.

"The Confederation, like me, believes we must focus on quality, on food safety, on taking care of the environment, not just on quantity." (Hannes's sentiments exactly.) "Since the early nineties, we've tried to shift the European community toward this approach and away from productivism."

Okay, these Europeans may not be the most poetic—"productivism" sounds about as clunky as "multifunctionality"—but the term works for me. To René, it means a narrow focus on production that ignores, for instance, consequences for the environment or whether what gets produced ever gets to those who need it. I think back to our effort at Food First to awaken people to the danger of a narrow production focus, but I had to wait decades to be in René's tiny kitchen and learn there's a word for it.

As Jean-Yves did, René reminds us that the real cost of productivism to the consumer is masked in part by the high subsidies the EU countries' taxpayers provide to their biggest farmers. Like the U.S., the European community bases subsidy levels on volume, so the biggest farmers get the most subsidies. In Europe, 80 percent of subsidies go to the largest 20 percent of farmers, and in the U.S. it's just as concentrated—these subsidies are now targeted more narrowly than ever to those at the top.[15] Meanwhile, it's the biggest farmers whose impact on the environment is the worst.

"One of our first campaigns was to make these subsidies fairer. We wanted people to understand that without paying any more taxes than what now go to large farms, we could have a different agriculture, one that helps small farmers and keeps more jobs in farming."

It's clear why the employment emphasis is so important in René's life and to others here. Jobs on farms in Europe dropped dramatically during the '90s, and Europeans losing farm work face a tough time finding it elsewhere. Unemployment rates in the double digits are not uncommon in Europe.

To the Confederation, job loss is just one symptom of productivism. René underscores that the Confederation works to protect not only farm jobs but also the environment, crop and animal diversity, and culture, too.

Oh, I think to myself, fitting these lessons together: Post-productivism meets multifunctionality.

CITIZEN FARMER

René didn't come to these realizations on his own. He had a little push—his own moment of dissonance. Until 1990, he operated a productivist farm. Like his parents, he relied heavily on machines, chemicals, and feed. But that year, a nearby agribusiness needing more space convinced the city to expropriate his land and sell it to them.

"René became one of the landless," Eric chimes in, reminding Anna and me of the Landless Workers' Movement members we met in Brazil.

"That was when everything changed for me," René explains. "I got this farm, and I started thinking differently. I'm now practicing the farming my parents rejected for the industrial model. It's my life's irony that I had to break with my family to go back to the way my parents farmed years ago.

"Before, I had no independence from agribusiness and the bank. They determined everything about how I produced, from what chemical combinations I had to use to what kinds of machines I could get loans for.

"Once I got out of the productivist trap, I had time to reflect. I realized I was part of the pollution problem here in Brittany."

As he speaks, René sits up straight in the wooden kitchen chair with his fingertips touching, his elbows resting on the table. Sounding much like Jean-Yves, René continues, "The level of nitrates in our water is more than twice the safety standard. I realized I was partly to blame. It was the kind of chemicals I was using to farm that was causing the pollution. Everyone is affected by what farmers do, and I didn't want to be part of the problem. I'm a farmer, but I'm also a citizen."

As René talks, my eyes wander out through the tall windows to the rain falling on the hedge's waxy green and yellow leaves, and farmers' voices move inside me back and forth across the Atlantic.

Even though René is in a hurry that's been made worse by our late arrival, he insists on giving us a tour of his farm. We walk down a slight hill to see his chickens and an alternative to the industrial-style poultry farm.

René's chickens range freely in and out of a long, low barn, its sides cut away to give them access. No neck-pecking like we'd seen among the chickens of Dahlia, the "Perdue Lady" in Bangladesh, nor stocking densities of the kind we're used to in the U.S., where some birds live on farms with more than 100,000 others and on average have as much living space as a page in this book.[16]

Rene also proudly takes us to see his hogs, all on beds of straw, not on concrete as in factory hog operations. The straw makes it easier to later use the hog's waste as fertilizer, and the composting straw keeps the animals warm, I learn later. (What a contrast to the virtual lakes of hog manure near giant hog operations polluting waterways both in the U.S. and Europe!)

Walking back to the car, René adds his final thoughts about his new way of farming. "When the Confederation talks about quality," he tells us, "we include respect for animals and for the relationship between the health of the animals and our own health. It's all connected."

But only as we climb back into the Twingo does what we're seeing really begin to sink in. René's vision, Jean-Yves's vision, is not fringe. The Confederation represents a growing portion of French farmers and is a member of Via Campesina, a movement launched in 1993, which includes small farmers' organizations in almost forty countries—including the Landless Workers' Movement in Brazil. All are pursuing a similar redirection—from the uniform, productivist model to farming that respects the farmer, the consumer, the land, and our distinct cultures. Already, efforts like theirs in Germany, for instance, have moved that country to set a goal of making one-fifth of its farmland chemical-free within the decade and of shifting farm subsidies away from simple production and toward rural community health.

As we start back to Paris in the encroaching twilight, I silently reminisce about the handful of young critics of industrial agriculture—none of us farmers—gathered twenty years ago at the counter-conference in Rome where I met Hannes. We were trying to draw voices of people from the countryside into the official debate on agrarian reform. Two decades later, it is farmers themselves, millions of them, who are leading the redirection.

THE ATLANTIC DIVIDES—GUINEA PIGS REVOLT

Back in Paris, my mind moves across the Atlantic again. At home, it's telling that no group representing a significant portion of American farmers is a member of Via Campesina, or aligned with what René might call a "post-productionism" approach to agriculture.

There is a big divide separating the continents, and it hits us powerfully when we learn about the European reaction to genetically modified foods. Years before Americans expressed concern about the safety of genetically modified foods, European consumers were actively questioning their use. While European companies have been among the leading developers of genetically engineered seeds—Novartis was a major innovator in GMOs—many of Europe's citizens have questioned their wisdom.

Are Europeans just skittish consumers and veiled protectionists, looking out for their own business interests, or are they forward-thinking and appropriately cautious?

To learn this part of the story, everyone tells us we must head to Greenpeace France. We're surprised. Our images of Greenpeace are of tiny boats in rough seas trying to block mammoth whaling ships, and of one called Rainbow Warrior sunk by the French secret police in 1985 for its protests against nuclear testing.

But when we're ushered into a conference room, the Greenpeace literature makes it clear just how behind the times we are. The group's GMO campaign now uses a quarter of the group's budget, second only to its antinuclear efforts.

Welcoming us into his small office, Bruno Rebelle, forty-two, the understated head of Greenpeace France (who has, I think with a smile, the perfect name for the job) is surprisingly relaxed despite the interruption of ringing phones and the fact that it's the end of his long day.

Thinking we're making small talk before getting into the *real* reason we're here, we ask Bruno why he came to Greenpeace.

Bruno says, with only a hint of a French accent, "I had been working with Veterinarians Without Borders, traveling for more than thirteen years throughout Africa. I was helping poor livestock-herders, which I knew was important, but I also wanted to go deeper. I saw firsthand how European policies were creating hunger in poor countries, and I wanted to get to the roots. That's why I came to Greenpeace.

"When I joined in the mid-nineties, my colleagues here had identified biodiversity and biotechnology as the key environmental challenges in the coming years. At the same time, France was a leader in biotech. Greenpeace decided to start gathering scientific evidence about the safety of GMOs. They saw potentially irreversible negative outcomes and risks that can't even be evaluated, such as introducing novel proteins into plants, which could cause allergic reactions if eaten, or inadvertent harm to animal life connected in the environment's web.

"We decided to focus on bringing to light the potential risks. Our first action was in 1996—one of the first against GMOs in the world. Our message was simply that we don't want to be lab animals," Bruno says. The scene he describes is vintage Greenpeace: protestors dressed as guinea pigs and lab rabbits to make the point amusingly graphic.

Out of costume, Greenpeace started talking to big companies like Dannon, Unilever, and Nestlé about their use of GMOs.

Meanwhile, in the U.S., most of the public was in the dark about genetically modified organisms. By 1997, 20 million acres of American farmland had already been planted with genetically modified seeds, and yet there was barely a news article about it.[17]

The next year was the turning point for Greenpeace, Bruno explains. In 1998, the French Conseil d'Etat, comparable to our Supreme Court, suspended authorization for the cultivation of genetically modified seeds. To arrive at this decision, the Conseil convened a group of ten laypeople—called a Conference of Citizens—and exposed them to a wide range of evidence and expert opinion, and then weighed their views heavily.[18]

I'm struck by the difference from the U.S., where the department of agriculture has for years been *helping* to introduce GMOs while devoting only 1 percent of its biotechnology research funds to assessing risks[19]—with no significant public deliberation at all. So, in the U.S., we never got a chance to weigh the risks of GMOs. These risks, in the view of some scientists, include a worsening of the trend toward genetic uniformity across wide areas, which heightens vulnerability to disease and pests. Or of GMOs transferring traits to wild plants, creating "super weeds." Or of the possibility that a toxin genetically engineered into a seed could be passed to beneficial insects that feed on crop pests or passed to insect herbivores.[20] Such are risks the French citizen panel must have reviewed.

"This group of citizens said, 'We must use the precautionary principle.' They weren't against all GMOs, but they felt each should be evaluated case by case," Bruno explains. A "guilty-until-proven-innocent" attitude toward safety in the food supply is how Anna and I see it.

"There was a lot of media coverage and public debate," Bruno continues. "We used this time as a chance to put pressure on companies to choose voluntarily to forego GMOs."

THE BITE OF THE BLACK LIST

To explain, Bruno hands us a pocket guide with lists of dozens of processed foods. Items in the black list contain GMOs; the white list is GMO-free.

"When we released the guide, it was actually quite funny. Corporations didn't jump on Greenpeace; they jumped on each other! They tried to prove products in the white list actually contained GMOs. They tried to expose the other companies," Bruno says, grinning. "Our Greenpeace consumer network also generated more than twenty thousand letters telling companies they don't want GMOs."

(When we get home, we will learn that Greenpeace USA is circulating a similar guide to GMO foods so American consumers have a choice, since our Food and Drug Administration does not require labeling. It has ignored clear public demand—including a half-million signatures on pro-labeling petitions submitted to Congress—and made the U.S. one of the only industrial countries in the world without mandatory labeling.[21])

"As soon as a small number of companies were GMO-free," Bruno continues, "others started to change their minds. Even Carrefour, whose recent merger with Promodes makes it the second-largest food retailer in the world, came to Greenpeace and said it wanted to be GMO-free." We learned later that the Swiss giant Novartis, at the time one of the world's biggest producers of GMO seeds, banned them from its own food brands.

"Remember, this was in the aftermath of the first mad cow disease scare and HIV contaminations in French blood supplies. The French were saying, 'You said to trust you once, trust you twice. Not a third time.'"

"We won a great victory," Bruno says, smiling. "Eighty percent of human food products in France are now GMO-free; the only country left in Europe cultivating GMOs is Spain." As Bruno talks of an almost-GMO-free Europe,

I'm jolted with the thought that three-fourths of all GMO-planted acres in the world are in the U.S, making us Americans the *real* guinea pigs!

But what to Bruno is an exciting victory is to others a failure in reason— evidence of the downside of democracy: political pressure and layperson paranoia, rather than science, driving decisions. They believe it's possible to create hermetically sealed environments where unbiased experts sit, deliberate, and decide, with no external influences acting on them.

But the unbiased expert is a fiction. We all function within a context of values, assumptions, and rewards. Every one of us has a mental map through which we perceive our world.

And, as we try to understand our own government's stance on GMOs, it helps to keep in mind that executives of biotechnology companies and the government officials charged with regulating them often work so closely together that they share one way of perceiving; they function in the same world. A former Environmental Protection Agency official responsible for pollution prevention and pesticides, for example, became a vice president of the biotech giant Monsanto. And Michael Taylor, the very person whose job at the Food and Drug Administration it was to oversee matters relating to GMOs, had earlier been a partner in the legal firm handling Monsanto's concerns related to government regulation. While an FDA deputy commissioner, he set guidelines that were tough on those dairies wanting to announce that their milk is free of a genetically modified growth hormone, but favorable to Monsanto. Later, Taylor went back to work for Monsanto.[22] Monsanto's stake in GMOs led the General Accounting Office to investigate Taylor for possible conflict of interest. They found no breach of the law, but that's not the point. These folks don't have to break the law, or be greedy, cynical patsies for corporate interests. They can simply be doing their job, to which they bring a frame of orientation—as Erich Fromm called it—to problem solving. That frame sees production as *the* goal and accepts our current institutions as givens not to be questioned.

True, many of the "experts" forging policy decisions do have a little more than a particular worldview influencing them. They have a direct financial stake in policy outcomes. Think, for example, of how the livestock industries—especially dairy—have shaped what Americans are told is good for us to eat. A group of medical professionals and others deeply troubled by the way the public has been misled by "experts" with clear vested interests recently won a lawsuit against the U.S. Department of Agriculture and the Department of Health and Human Services. Of the eleven members of the Advisory Council on the Dietary Guidelines for Americans, six currently have or recently have had financial ties to the meat, dairy, or egg industry.[23]

Before we leave, Bruno emphasizes that the challenge is much larger than finding the best way to make decisions about GMOs. With his enthusiasm building, he adds, "We must develop a more holistic understanding. Farmers have been told that to survive, to be competitive, they have to produce more, and that means more pesticides or new technologies like GMOs, they believe. But in my work in Africa I saw how European surpluses destroyed the local markets for meat produced by herders there. To me, productivism is the root. GMOs are only a symptom."

And to find that "holistic understanding," I think to myself, we need a genuine mix of perceptions, hopefully including those not so locked into the prevailing mental map. And that's why the Conference-of-Citizens approach Bruno described appeals so much to Anna and me.

Stuffing my notebook into my backpack and bidding adieu to this energetic, thoughtful man, I feel lighter. Bruno doesn't know René Louail in Brittany, or Hannes Lorenzen in Brussels, or the farmers we met in Brazil, India, or Kenya for that matter. But they all seem lit with the same flame, each in a unique way dissolving the thoughts traps that have so long constrained us.

A Tiny Tax

When I wrote *Diet for a Small Planet,* I was appalled by the sharp skewing of world wealth, but I could never have imagined then that thirty years later the gap would be even wider, much wider.

Today the richest 20 percent of the world consume 86 percent of world output, while the poorest 20 percent consume just over 1 percent.[24] The assets of just one company, Philip Morris, for example, are larger than the economies of 148 countries.[25]

While strides are being made in both the North and the South—thanks to efforts like those we chronicle here—there's still one bald fact: Without greater financial resources in the South, hope is hard to sustain for healing the growing misery of the majority of the world's people, who now lack essential resources.

It seems that two things must happen at once. Movements like Green Belt in Kenya, the Landless Workers' Movement in Brazil, and the Confederation Paysanne in France must continue to build the confidence and skills of citizens to stand together to strengthen democratic ways of life. At the same time, additional money must become available to relieve the stress of poverty—disease, early death, lousy or little education—so that more and more people will have the strength to build better lives. (I think of the schoolhouse in Kyaume, Kenya, with nothing but broken desks, and of Regina telling us that her sister had just died of malaria because the local clinic had no medicines to treat her.)

So, where will the resources come from?

Wangari Maathai in Kenya and the Landless Workers' Movement in Brazil stress that the forgiveness of burdensome foreign debts of the less-industrial countries—now standing at $2 trillion—will be one important source. With many countries paying their debt service by robbing social services, surely Wangari and the MST are right. (So far, even the debt relief promised is well under 10 percent of the total, and what's been granted is a tiny fraction of that.)

Now, here in France, we learn about another way to shrink the widening gap between rich and poor that has turned our small planet into two worlds. So it seems fitting that we should end our stay in Paris by talking with a woman pioneering a novel strategy to do just that.

We walk north from the Metro stop at St. Placide and enter a shadowy courtyard. At the door of her apartment, Susan George greets us with a cordial reserve I recall well. Sixty-six, tall and slender, with thick, cropped light hair, she looks just as I remember her when we shared dinner in San Francisco twelve years ago.

I've long been an admirer of Susan, seeing her as a gutsy woman with laudable persistence and a powerful mind. When Joe Collins and I teamed up in 1975, Susan, born and reared in Ohio, was already a longtime Parisian beginning her own book on world hunger, *How the Other Half Dies*. Since then, she has written on subjects ranging from third-world debt to international trade. I've always seen Susan's path as parallel to my own. If, in a sense, I have tried to dive beneath hunger to get at its roots in the scarcity of democracy, Susan has gone beneath hunger to its roots in economics—roots that we both know are inseparable.

Surrounded by French antiques in her living room, Anna and I sit on a small mustard-colored loveseat and Susan wastes no time—the big idea.

"You've heard of the Tobin Tax, haven't you?" she asks, and I nod with faint recognition, though in truth I've heard little about it.

"It's a simple idea—national governments levying tiny taxes on the foreign currency transactions occurring every day, transactions whose total value reach one and a half to two trillion dollars."

My hand stops above my notebook: $2 trillion . . . every day?

The number is almost inconceivable. But think of it this way: That's roughly equivalent to the entire *yearly* federal budget of the United States. It's seventeen times larger than the amount of *yearly* stock-market exchanges, and 85 percent of these transactions are purely speculative, having nothing to do with trade of real goods or services.

And think of how fast this all has happened. When I wrote *Diet for a Small Planet*, the technology for instantaneous global transactions didn't even exist. Only with the advent of rapid-fire twenty-four-hour-a-day trading have we seen the jump in volume that Susan describes.

"The tax," Susan says, "is named after the Nobel economist James Tobin, an advisor to President Kennedy, who came up with the idea twenty years ago." Susan tells us she is now a cofounder and vice president of a growing citizens' movement to make these tiny taxes real.

She explains the potential impact. "Even at ten cents to twenty-five cents on every hundred dollars, these taxes could generate one hundred to three hundred billion dollars each year. The money would then go to the poorest people in the poorest countries." Just imagine: Only a fraction of this, $40 billion a year, according to the UN, is enough to provide universal access to basic social services in all poor countries—and is less than the net worth of one man, Bill Gates.[26]

Susan's group, the Association for the Taxation of Financial Transactions for the Aid of Citizens—known by its more memorable acronym, ATTAC—is spreading quickly. With more than 25,000 members in France alone, it has chapters in seventeen countries and dozens of cities around the world. In Brazil, São Paulo adopted resolutions endorsing the tax, and supportive legislation has been introduced in the French Parliament, the European Parliament, the Canadian House of Commons, and even in the U.S. Congress.

I'm moved that ATTAC is thinking so big—a tiny tax, yes, but a huge idea. But I catch myself. Why does it seem so revolutionary? After all, progressive taxes—taxes to redress gross inequality and give us all a chance—were taken for granted in our culture until recently. Now, mind-boggling changes in the world economy open the door to the type of tax Susan is backing, one that falls on those most able to pay it, and one that is easy to assess, since these transactions are all electronic.

But such a tax is not just about generating revenue; it's also about slowing speculative trading. That was Tobin's original goal. Unseen to most of us, speculative trading—whether in financial markets or commodity markets—affects *most* those who are least able to cope with the instability it causes. Just think of Rosario and her family in Nicaragua. Before they joined the fair-trade movement, an entire year's work harvesting coffee could turn on the weather in Brazil, or rather on someone's hunch about the weather in Brazil.

As I learn more and begin to fathom the potential of the tax, I'm even more disturbed we've heard so little about this strategy at home—that it's not being covered seriously in the news. James Tobin even joked that there are more members of ATTAC in France than people who know his name in the U.S.[27] I'm sure he's right.

We know Susan has a meeting to get to, so we start gathering our things, mentioning that we just visited Brittany and a Confederation Paysanne leader.

"Oh, yes, the Confederation was a founding member of ATTAC," Susan tells us, "and I was a witness for José's defense in his McDonald's trial [at which some say as many as 50,000 people turned out in support]. I told the judge the World Trade Organization is making rules that are undermining French farmers and culture, and it is an illegal mechanism in a moral sense, so José's actions were justified. I said he'd exhausted all other recourses to protest."

As we rise to leave, she adds, "We're not against globalization, we're against *this type* of globalization." Susan's not against trade per se, or against technology, or business, necessarily. She's against a system whose design allows trade, technology, and business to enable something as unproductive and downright frivolous as speculative currency trading to advance as fast and as unimpeded as it has. She's against a system that allows a handful of people, virtual gamblers in our markets, to damage the well-being of millions.

Her criticism is of a system of globalization that takes the decisions about how our international economy is structured, and how our trade is managed, out of the democratic fold. Susan and many of the others we met this year are trying to bring it back in.

WHAT'S THE BEEF?

It's exactly this type of globalization that drives José Bové wild. (You'll hear more from José in the next chapter when we tour Wisconsin farms with him.) Through him we learn more about another big divide that separates the continents.

Toward the end of our stay in Paris, we pick up a popular weekly and immediately identify the signature pipe on its cover as José's. Inside, we learn that

16 percent of the French say that, if given the choice, they'd likely vote for José as their next president.

So what has José done to capture the hearts of the French?

In part, they identify with José's disapproval of corporate globalization and the consequent trade system governed since 1995 by the World Trade Organization. It was WTO-imposed trade sanctions that got José, a breeder of ewes whose milk is used in Roquefort cheese, ransacking McDonald's. The link? The WTO allowed the U.S. to slap a tariff on a range of European imports, including Roquefort, to retaliate against Europe's ban—in place since 1989— on U.S. beef raised with growth hormones, which is just about all of it.[28]

The U.S. had accused Europeans of using the ban as a way to protect their domestic beef producers, and had brought the case to a three-person WTO Dispute Resolution Panel. The panel sided with the Americans, concluding that there was no provable risk in hormone-raised beef. Also, Europe couldn't prove that its own beef was hormone-free. Thus Europe's ban wasn't justified. The WTO estimated its cost to the U.S. at $117 million in lost exports and gave the U.S. the go-ahead to recoup with tariffs adding up to this amount on a selection of European imports—from truffles to electric hair clippers to José's Roquefort cheese.

"It's undemocratic!" José would say to us about the WTO's ruling when we were with him in Wisconsin. To critics like José, the beef ruling proves that the WTO can block nations from protecting local food traditions and setting their own quality and safety standards.[29]

But for me, well . . . while I shared Jose's take on the WTO, I wasn't entirely sure about what was behind the beef ban. After all, in the U.S. we've had no debate about hormone-fed beef. Beef is simply—as the industry loved to repeat—"what's for dinner." None of our national research institutes have publicly questioned hormones in our beef. Although I've long chosen not to eat beef for a host of reasons, including health, growth-promoting hormones had never been a focus of concern. Could there be, I wondered, an element of economic self-interest hiding under the Europeans' "safer-than-thou" veneer?

Then Anna and I saw the one-hundred-plus-page report for the WTO on beef hormone safety from a twenty-member panel of European scientists. The group raised a host of concerns. They list possible neurobiological, reproductive, and immunological effects among them, as well as the possibility that the hormones could contribute to cancer. All this, they conclude, warrants hormone-fed beef wariness.[30]

Now that reputable scientists were raising concerns, I wondered why the WTO ruled that the evidence was inconclusive and disallowed the ban—and why did evidence have to be conclusive, anyway? After all, the guilty-until-proven-innocent principle has long been a widely accepted rule of thumb in approving pharmaceuticals here at home. So why not with food?

Then it hit me what was at stake. What would have happened if the WTO *had* condoned the Europeans' ban? The U.S. is the world's largest beef exporter. When I wrote *Diet*, we were exporting only 40 million pounds of beef; today it's sixty times that—almost 2.4 billion pounds of carcass-weight hormone-fed beef spreading around the world.[31] Any WTO action reinforcing doubt about the safety of U.S. beef could have caused millions of consumers to rethink their diet, throwing the beef industry into chaos.

As this all sinks in, Anna and I come back to what seems to be lost in the controversy. The hormones in question are used to add more weight to cattle faster—and this in a world in which overconsumption of meat is a growing health hazard. What's missing are opportunities for broad public debate on the best use of our precious food resources, venues where we can ask such questions as: Do we as citizens want the same precautionary principle that we use with drugs also applied to our food? And, regardless of the safety of hormones injected in cattle, in this case, do we want to encourage the production of feedlot-fed meat?

The WTO has not proven to be a forum for such democratic debate. No wonder so many, like José, look at the WTO and see corporate power protecting its interests, not a democratic body pursuing the broader public interest.

DEMOCRACY IN MAKING ECONOMIC AND CULTURAL CHOICES

For José and others critical of the WTO, a crisis for democracy is the WTO's power to shape new trade policies that push everyone to see the world through the same eyes. Virtually no national health, food safety, or environmental law challenged by a trading partner has withstood WTO scrutiny; they've been declared barriers to trade. And we'll never know the effect of the simple threat of sanctions. Even a relatively well-off country like South Korea felt it had to back down rather than risk WTO-sanctioned retaliation when the U.S. challenged its meat-shelf-life rule. South Korea tripled the number of days that meat is allowed to sit on the grocer's shelf.[32]

The WTO brags that its decisions are made through consensus, but is consensus attainable when many stakeholders aren't at the table? One-fifth of the member countries have never had permanent delegations stationed at Geneva headquarters; many simply cannot afford to.[33] And, how many countries could afford, for example, the $117 million price Europe is now paying to keep doing what it wants to—refuse American beef?

Being in Europe around people whose attitudes about food safety are so different from those of American policymakers, it is even easier for me to see the inappropriateness of an unelected global trade body, whose primary advisors come from business, setting a single standard for the globe.

The chasm between U.S. and European attitudes became clearer to us as we learned about mad cow disease (BSE), acquired in cows by their eating what had for years been common: feed that included ground-up animal parts. Mad cow disease, which can be fatal, is passed on to humans who eat meat from infected cows. Such feeding to cows was banned in the U.S. and Britain in the early 1990s, but hundreds of U.S. feed manufacturers and rendering companies—those that grind up animal body parts—aren't complying with BSE-prevention rules designed to make sure that feedstuff with animal parts doesn't get fed to cows, the Food and Drug Administration reports.[34]

Nonetheless, the U.S. media has portrayed European BSE concerns as over-reaction. In France, the first ten months of 2000 brought almost one hundred confirmed cases of mad cow disease in humans—three times more than the entire preceding year. When the French drastically reduced beef consumption, the American press dismissed the response as a "frenzy based more on fear than fact."[35]

U.S. officials and media pooh-poohing the European stance see the world through a different lens. For Hannes, José, and other farmers we met, saying "No" to hormones in meat and to the feeding of rendered animal parts to livestock is only a piece of rejecting an entire way of life, one that treats animals not as sentient beings but as nothing more than "units of production"; that focuses on production as *the* end in itself without regard to its consequences for the natural world or other people's cultures and economies.

What could feel more removed from daily life than trade and something called the WTO? But all this goes to the heart of how we define meaning in our lives. It's about whether the people of a community or a nation can define what quality and safety mean to them.

THE LAST TASTE OF PARIS

On the final Sunday morning of our visit, we rush around the corner from Eric's apartment to one of the nearly fifty open-air produce markets in Paris to buy provisions for brunch with his family.

Rue d'Aligre is closed to traffic, as it is every day except Mondays, and crammed with stalls teeming with produce and packed with people of all ages. We buy fresh thyme, tender tomatoes, onions, dates, figs, melons, and more. Lining the street are a *boulangerie* and a cheese shop, where we buy locally made goat cheese and baguettes baked hours before.

On the yogurt we buy, Eric points out the label: "AB" for Agriculture Biologique, the French organic label. After the government arrived at national organic standards and launched the label in the late '80s, he tells me, interest in organic food has grown fast in France. And this is true throughout Europe, where now half of all organics are sold in major supermarkets, not just specialty stores.[36]

Back atop four flights of old stone stairs, we lay out our catch on a small wooden table—the cheeses, bread, melon, and salad color the surface. When the Reiffstecks arrive, Madame Reiffsteck, a striking woman with endearing dimples, bears the *pièce de résistance,* a just-baked apple tart. The apples, she tells us, she picked that morning from a tree in her yard. (You can enjoy her tart, too. The recipe follows this chapter.)

As we sit down to the meal, I think of our conversation several days earlier with Anthony Jacobsohn, a French-American whom we met on advice from Alice Waters. Among his jobs are creating a national registry of local fruits and vegetables in France and advising similar projects in Hungary and other European countries. Anthony had told us that productivist agriculture is not only quickening the loss of small producers, it's destroying food diversity and wiping out distinctions among cultures around the world whose traditions and memories are grounded in the food they eat and share.

Biting into a tangy slice of tart, I wonder if through efforts of those we've met on our journey we might just save the abundance and bursting flavors that nature and farmers have evolved. I'm convinced that if everyone had the opportunity to enjoy the kind of food we're savoring this morning—not more expensive than a typical trip to my local supermarket—more of us would see Anthony's work and others' like it not as quirky or marginal but as vital to our happiness.

I remember reading about Washington apple farmers saddened that the taste they remember in their Red Delicious is gone. One marketer lamented

LISTENING TO THE SUGAR

I'd been reading about José Bové in the news for months, and I was looking forward to impressing him with my knowledge of France's food concerns. I'd just learned about his country's "Week of the Taste," celebrated with chefs going into schools to remind the young what something other than McDonald's tastes like. I picture French kids, tongues outstretched for another piece of Roquefort. I imagine their gleeful chorus: *C'est magnifique!*

I expect José to be pleased when I tell him; pleased that word had gotten around. After all, in my mind it's Roquefort cheese that the Week of the Taste is getting kids to remember. But, with an amused look, José informs me that the Week is actually the brainchild of the sugar industry.

The Week was created in 1990, and the sugar industry explains in their PR material that, at the time, "artificial sweeteners were seen as very fashionable, very low-fat and tasty. The idea was to launch a teaching campaign about the 'good taste of French food' signed by 'The Sugar.' The Sugar sent hundreds of chefs to schools to teach kids 'taste.' Those kids were seen as the consumers of tomorrow."[38]

What I thought was a celebration of French culture is actually a marketing tool . . . yes. But still, there's something to it. Maybe The Sugar and José have one thing in common. They both know it's easier to lose memory than to conserve it, and that preserving memory might take nothing short of a national campaign. Stick out your tongue, taste, and remember. —Anna

that farmers made "apples redder and redder and prettier and prettier" because that's what the big buyers wanted, and "they just about bred themselves out of existence."[37] I hope the flavors of Madame Reiffsteck's slightly discolored apples stay with me, and that these farmers' lament forecasts a trend—the return to diverse varieties, bred not for cosmetics but for taste.

KEEPING THE MYSTERY

On the plane ride home, I return to my conversation in Brussels over cherry beer with Hannes. That night, he had handed me a booklet called "Letting the

World Feed Itself"—pointedly not the typical "how to feed the world" framing. It opens with a trick picture, which looks at first like a fuzzy pointillist painting until you stare at it and move it away from your face. Instantly, a cow emerges in 3-D. Opening the book again, I excitedly show Anna the trick. She gives me that you're-behind-the-times look and informs me these pictures were all the rage years ago. So it's not new, but she does concede that it's a neat way to get people thinking about seeing beneath the surface.

Hannes had told me about his Europe-wide "Sustainable Mystery Tour" of community initiatives like those on Pellworm, which weave together sustainable economics and alternative farming and energy practices. He asked if I knew why "mystery" was part of his tour. I guessed it was an attempt to make sustainable development sound more palatable and, for those in my generation, a wink-wink takeoff on the Beatles' Magical Mystery Tour.

"It's because sustainability *is* a mystery," he said emphatically.

"We all come to it through different doors. Some see sustainability as protection against something, as protecting nature. Others see the heart of sustainability as people: 'If there are no villages left, you can forget about sustainability.' For others, the door is history and culture: 'If you don't respect your cultural and historical roots, forget it.' To some, like people I work with in Eastern Europe, the door is democracy: 'First of all, we have to be able to participate. If people try to tell us what to do, forget about sustainability.'

"I try to let people unravel the mystery for themselves. What is quality of life to them? Otherwise, they can't go forward. They'll think someone else will deliver the solutions. When people discover for themselves, they realize they have the potential to find solutions."

Still hours from landing in Boston, I flip to the end of Hannes's booklet. There again is the trick picture with the hidden cow munching happily on grass and flowers.

Hannes writes: "If with the naked eye it were easy to recognize a new dimension of food in the world"—what Anna and I are discovering on our journey—"then people wouldn't have to trouble to look beneath the surface. But many people from all walks of life are ready to bring together a new food culture, and yet this is not visible to the naked eye."

I love Hannes's playful reminder that to look at the world with new eyes we must challenge our perceptions—and that it's a plus, not a drawback, that we'll all come through different doors.

EUROPE: AWAKENING OUR SENSES

Madame Reiffsteck's Apple Tart

Serves 6

If you can, pick organic apples fresh from an orchard. Reine des Reinettes or Belle de Boskoop are superb, but the Granny Smiths we use in this tart keep their texture and taste as good and are easy to find. The French recipe called for brown sugar cane, which isn't available as such in American superstores; the closest we could get was brown sugar crystals. If you can't find the crystals, use regular brown sugar. This very simple recipe lives or dies on the taste of the apples. To add an American touch to the tart, serve with vanilla ice cream. Or, in keeping with the French, have it for Sunday brunch, as we did.

PASTRY BRISE

1½ cups unbleached all-purpose flour

9 tablespoons (1 stick plus 1 tablespoon) unsalted butter

½ teaspoon salt

¼ cup water

FILLING

3 to 4 (1½ pounds) Reine des Reinettes, Belle de Boskoop, or Granny Smith apples

2 tablespoons lemon juice (about 1 small lemon)

¾ cup brown sugar crystals or regular brown sugar

1 tablespoon butter, cut into quarter-inch cubes

TO MAKE THE CRUST

Preheat the oven to 350° F. Put the flour in a big bowl. Cut the butter into half-inch pieces. With the bottom of your fingers, mash the butter into the flour very roughly until the butter is incorporated into the flour.

Make a well in the flour mixture. Add salt. Slowly pour the water into the well as you mix everything together with your hands. The pastry must not be too sticky nor too soft. Sprinkle with flour as necessary, or add droplets of water if needed to get the right consistency. Make pastry into a ball and leave it for about an hour at room temperature.

Transfer pastry to a piece of wax paper big enough to roll the dough. Spread out the pastry with the ball of your hand until it's big enough to fit in a 9-inch pie pan. Use a rolling pin to flatten at the end. Carefully pick up the wax paper with the dough and flip the dough into the pie pan. Adjust crust to fit into the pan, and trim and crimp edges. Place the wax paper you just used on top of the crust and cover with dried beans or similar weights, so the crust doesn't shrink during baking.

Partially bake the crust in a 350° F oven for 10 minutes. Remove wax paper and beans, then bake for 10 minutes more. Take out crust. (You can make the crust ahead of time to this point and let stand for a few hours until you are ready to complete the recipe.) If you are making the tart right away, turn oven temperature up to 375° F.

To Make the Tart

While crust is baking, peel and core the apples and slice thinly. As you work, place slices in bowl and mix with lemon juice so that apples don't brown. Add the sugar and butter chunks to bowl of apples and mix gently.

When crust is ready, pile the apples into the crust if you are pressed for time. But if you want to follow in the French spirit, arrange apple slices on the partially baked crust in concentric circles, starting on the outside and working toward the center. This doesn't take much time at all and looks lovely. Tuck butter pieces throughout filling.

Bake in 375° F oven for 35 minutes, or until apples are golden. *Et voila!*

Frisian Oat Curry

Serves
6 to 8

What an unusual dish this is! Even after tasting it, we're still not sure whether to suggest it for breakfast, lunch, or dinner—which means it is as versatile as it is savory. The curry, nuts, and apples add flair to the oats, which contribute a delightful heft. It's a favorite recipe by Silke Zetl, a Pellworm farmer.

2½ cups oat groats

4 cups vegetable broth, divided

4 cups diced apples (about 1 pound, or 3 medium)

4 cups diced onions (about 1 pound, or 3 medium)

3 tablespoons lemon juice (about 1 large lemon)

2 tablespoons butter

3 tablespoons curry powder

¾ cup raw, unsalted cashew nuts (4 ounces)

1 teaspoon salt

½ teaspoon pepper

¾ cup raw, unsalted almonds (4 ounces)

Rinse the oats. Put them in a heavy-bottomed large Dutch oven while still damp, and heat, stirring, until the grains begin to burst. Add 3½ cups vegetable broth and bring to a boil. Let oats and broth simmer on low for 30 minutes. Turn off heat, cover pot, and let oats steep another 10 minutes.

Peel the apples, core, and dice them into ½-inch cubes. Sprinkle them with 2 tablespoons of lemon juice.

Dice the onions into ½-inch cubes. Heat the butter in a large pot. Add the onions and cook on medium-low heat for about 5 minutes, until softened. Add the apple cubes and stew together for 5 more minutes. Sprinkle the curry powder over apples and onions, stir, and cook briefly.

Add the cashew nuts. Add remaining ½ cup of vegetable broth and bring to a boil, then turn heat to low. Add salt, pepper, and more lemon juice to taste.

Toast the almonds lightly in an ungreased skillet or in a toaster oven, watching them carefully so they don't burn. Let cool, then chop into fine pieces.

Stir onion mixture into the oats and apples. Cook on low heat for 5 minutes. Sprinkle with toasted almonds and serve.

TAKING OFF THE COWBOY HAT

You know why we're so successful?
Because we love what we do.

JIM MILLER, FARMER, ORGANIC VALLEY

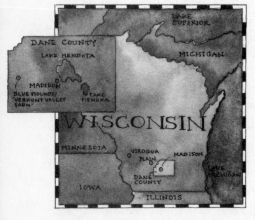

We turn on our heels and duck involuntarily. Has he seen us? Will I try to explain later? I've spotted José Bové just across the street—remember, he's the French farmer who gained his country's admiration, and international fame, for dismantling a McDonald's construction site.

In moments I'm slated to speak with him at a Madison, Wisconsin food festival, and here Anna and I are—exiting a McDonald's in his full view! Just minutes ago, as I was scribbling an outline of thoughts I wanted to share with the audience gathering nearby, my concentration was broken.

"Ow! Ow!" Anna exclaimed. A yellowjacket had just made a nosedive for her hand. Desperate for ice to dull the sting and slow the swelling, we spotted a nearby McDonald's. Within minutes Anna had her hand in ice in the biggest cup in the place, and for at least one motherly moment I was grateful for the golden arches. That is, until we walked out the door and saw the trademark handlebar moustache of Monsieur Bové.

Looking up beyond José, Anna and I see Wisconsin's capitol with its stately steps and towering dome. On this warm Saturday morning, as on every

Saturday from late April to early November, a festive collar rings the building. Forming a circle the size of eight city blocks, it's the country's largest farmers' market. On an average Saturday, more than 20,000 customers throng the streets, and more than 200 farmers sell everything from berries and beans to pickles and popovers. Here, you have to grow it or make it to sell, no middle-men allowed.

At the nearby Food for Thought Festival, the atmosphere is celebratory and light. Its displays offer a preview of what we'll absorb during our Wiscon-sin stay. We see tables heavy with locally made cheeses and books about sus-tainable farming and gardening. We walk past stalls with face-painting and carrot-necklace–making. We meet kids—who, we learn later, come from low-income neighborhoods—cradling golden chickens on handmade leashes and cheerfully telling passersby about their gardens.

It's sunny, just warm enough. It's fun being here with Anna. Yet I know that behind these displays and stalls is terrible pain. Wisconsin is losing three family farms a day on average, faster than most any other state in the nation. Bankruptcies. Farmer suicides. Drug-linked murders up threefold in a decade in rural areas. Pollution caused by farm chemicals scaring both farm and city people. All this plus intimidating threats by a mega-corporation to sue farm-ers and processors for doing what they think is right. Yet the festival reminds us that something else is emerging. People are finding their courage to change. Community is overcoming fear. And from this courage, tantalizing elements of renewal are taking shape—a story that will unfold for us day by day.

Not Swallowing Their Line

Under the white festival tent, I share the microphone with José—and get a chance to explain that, really, we were only in McDonald's for ice cubes.

I can easily see why these Wisconsin folks love him. His crusade—that of the Confederation Paysanne, the farmers' union in France we learned about from René Louail—dovetails with their vision of an agriculture that honors the earth, farmers, farmworkers, and eaters.

José tells our audience that thousands rallied at the French village court-house during his sentencing for his McDonald's vandalism, a symbolic protest against trade policies but also against the global push toward sameness. In this case, McDonald's sameness—the same variety of potato fried in the same way, with the same type of feed-lot hamburger from the same kind of beef fed the

same increasingly bioengineered corn and soy, and treated with the same antibiotics.

There's something that bugs José about the brutal sameness of it all. It's
"totalitarian," he tells us. I think I get what he means. It's totalitarian because
it's "totalizing"—my word, not José's—in the sense that these trade policies
don't allow countries, or people, to be different.

It's totalizing in the way that, once you start using antibiotics, resistance
develops and can transfer to humans who had no voice in the choice to take
the antibiotic route. Once genetically modified seeds are planted, they can
contaminate fields, robbing farmers of the choice to avoid them. (That's what
farmers are discovering across the country. A farmer in Canada was just
successfully sued by Monsanto for illegally growing Monsanto crops—even
though he said he'd never bought Monsanto seeds; the wind had blown the
pollen onto his property). Once GMO grains enter the distribution chain, it's
impossible to segregate them. That's what Gerber found out when it tried to
avoid GMOs in its baby foods and discovered it had to remove corn from its
mixed cereal. Despite the company's efforts to avoid it, GMO corn kept turning up. We're all affected, whether we like it or not.

The standardized approach to growing and eating that McDonald's represents to José is "totalizing" in another way as well. It "de-links" us from the
specifics of who we are—our specific spot of earth, people, climate, culture,
history—that make us different from any other.

But not everyone values that peculiarity of place shaping who we are. Upset
about what some of his far-flung franchises were up to, Ray Kroc, a founder
of McDonald's, once railed, "We cannot trust some people who are noncon-
formists. . . . We will make conformists out of them in a hurry."[1] And he has.
Nearly 800 McDonald's restaurants now pepper José's homeland, and worldwide, you can find 26,000 sets of the telltale golden arches in 119 countries.

Yes, sameness snuffs out cultural differences, and it can be dangerous, too.
Now, for example, the vast majority of potatoes grown in America are of the
same variety, one that needs heavy fungicide protection; so if a single blight
were to hit, we'd be in big trouble. And all those antibiotics fed to animals are
generating antibiotic-resistant strains of salmonella, for example, making us
all more vulnerable.[2] We're losing critical weapons against disease through no
choice of our own.

IN THE GRIP OF MYTH

But sameness—uniformity—is efficient, economists keep telling us, and most of us still believe them.

The night before the festival, at the university, during the question period after José and I spoke, a young man in the audience rose. His lanky frame held an obviously heavy heart. He told us his family's farm had just folded, and he asked what his generation could do to keep the family farm alive.

"We just weren't efficient," he said.

I felt so bad for him. The very fact that family farms are folding is proof that they're inefficient, goes the standard line—and many farmers swallow it. Bearing the loss is hard enough; blaming yourself makes it even worse. But he'd bought the myth, too—the myth that the big, industrial farming model is most efficient, even though studies measuring input against output now prove that the most efficient farms are actually medium-sized family operations.[3]

I can identify with the young man, and with these farmers. I've had difficulty, too, in fighting the myth that survival proves efficiency. In debates with agricultural economists, I've had a hard time not getting pulled onto their turf, where the hidden costs of industrial agriculture are ignored—the costs, for instance, of polluting our environment, of eliminating jobs, of providing dangerous working conditions—all borne by us taxpayers and hidden in the subsidies that the biggest farms get. (By last count, the top 10 percent of U.S. producers received 61 percent of our agricultural subsidies.[4])

But even those who quantify small- and medium-sized farm efficiency often only count how much land, chemicals, fuel, and labor get used up to produce so much. What is difficult to calculate, and challenging to measure, is *life*. It may sound corny, but there is no other way to say it: the life of the farm family sustained by love of the land. The life of the rural community centered around healthy farms. The life of animals living free from misery and disease. The life of the soil itself—the millions of microorganisms that live or die in every handful.

I so wish there had been time that night to say to the young man: "Don't swallow their line. Staying in business doesn't mean you're efficient. It may mean you're willing to eke every bushel from your land, despite the damage it brings. It may just mean you're so big you can cash in on large government subsidies."

Of course, even saying all that, I wouldn't have answered his burning question: "What can we do about it?" Those answers were yet to come.

"Look Mommy, There's Our Farmer!"

It's the middle of a crisp Sunday afternoon, and no one looks up as we enter. All of them—adults and children alike—are too busy. The smell of fresh basil is overpowering. Bunches are scattered on large picnic tables and ready to be tossed into dozens of food processors spotting the room. Bottles of olive oil catch the afternoon sun. This is a farm, not a pesto factory, but it's a farm like none Anna and I have ever experienced.

After a lunch of pesto pasta piled high, we sit in thick grass, our backs to a setting sun. We listen as Barb and David Perkins, both forty-three, tell us how they set out to become farmers and made this pesto party possible.

Five years ago, they sold their house in the city and bought these acres we're sitting on—a long valley nestled between deep green hills.

Two-thirds of Dane County, in which Madison sits, is cropland, and Barb and Dave want to make it healthy farmland like this. They want to protect it against the fast-creeping sprawl of sameness—like the chain stores in the strip malls we drove by on our way here.

From the beginning, Barb and Dave knew they didn't want to farm with chemicals, or to grow food for anonymous customers in a merciless market. So they started their Vermont Valley Community Farm growing food for specific people—farm "members" who pay the Perkinses up front, around $400 a year. By sharing Barb and Dave's risk—paying in the beginning of the season—Vermont Valley members get organic produce all summer and early fall at 80 percent of the retail price, and they get it delivered. And today's pesto party is just one of Barb and Dave's many enticements to get members out to the country.

In this area near Madison, there are several dozen such membership farms—among the greatest concentration anywhere in the country. Called "community supported agriculture" (CSA) here in the U.S., the idea emerged in the mid-'60s in Germany, Switzerland, and Japan. In Japan it is called *teikei,* which carries a meaning close to "food with the farmer's face on it."[5] Fifteen years ago, none existed here, but since 1986, a growing movement of dedicated farmers and consumers has been working to establish CSAs across the country. Today, more than fifty CSAs dot Wisconsin, and from Maine to Washington state there are more than 3,000 CSAs serving more than 30,000 families.[6]

We'd met Barb the night before, her energy undiminished by having delivered to her members 450 boxes of watermelon, basil, tomatoes, cucumbers, leeks, and more. Barb has the spirit and build—even the mud on the knees—of a first-rate soccer player, but it's farmer's dirt beneath her nails.

Barb and Dave have always made sure they're not the only ones getting their hands in the earth. Until last year, all the work at Vermont Valley was done by "worker-shares"—members who paid for their produce by contributing several hours a week of their labor. That is, of course, in addition to the long hours that Barb, Dave, and their two sons and daughter put in. This season, Barb and Dave hired some help, but they still use worker-shares to assist them. When we ask who usually chooses to work, Barb says there is no "usually."

"All kinds of people," Barb says, and counts off with her fingers: "Ministers, teachers, students, a massage therapist, a painter, an insurance adjuster. You name it."

Imagining a lot of good-hearted city folk like myself who don't have a clue as to what a farm needs, I ask, "Isn't it a hassle to get them organized and doing what you need done?"

"Sure," Barb says. "It could be more efficient [there's that word again!] to hire laborers—at least, that's what we're told. But we go to a lot of trouble to give our members a chance instead. We do it because it's a way to get people involved with the farm. It's important for people to have that deep connection.

"After all," she goes on, with a look that says she hopes we already get it, "giving people a connection to the land is why we're doing this. A lot of people come back year after year to work here.

"The vegetables," she says, "are really an aside."

When they bought their farm, Barb, Dave and their children set a five-year goal of 500 members.

"Because beyond that," Barb explains, "we wouldn't remember everyone's names." Anna and I can't help but share in the satisfaction shining across Barb's face when she tells us that this year, their fifth year on the farm, they reached 500 members.

"Every now and then I have a moment that makes all the hard work, all the long hours, all the sweat we've put into this place worth it," Barb says, smiling. "Yesterday, I was at a restaurant in town and I saw this little kid, wide-eyed, grab his mom's arm and point at me.

"He said, 'Mommy, Mommy, look. There's our farmer!'"

THE NEW FAMILY FARM

As we sit together, the sun falls behind the farm's forty-five sloping acres. Four frisky pooches nuzzle up to us, and Barb and Dave apologize; these new additions to the farm's deer-control efforts are still in training. On this organic farm, Dave tells us, deer, not insects, are the biggest intruders.

A worker-share and her friend join us. They've taken advantage of the "U-Pick" tomatoes and carry a piled-high pail of the red treats. The young worker-share tells us that she recently lost her job, so this farm has been a real boon. By working with the Perkinses, she can still afford to eat delicious organic produce.

As the dogs get even friskier, Dave downplays the challenge of growing organic. "It's not that different from conventional farming. Sure, you have more weeds, but we control them by hand and mechanical weeding and by crop rotation. Yeah, insects can be a problem, but if, say, you lose a third of your potatoes, it's not a problem if you have fifty other crops." Dave underscores what farmers have always known: There's security in diversity.

The light is fading fast this balmy evening, but before we head out, Barb and Dave want to be certain we understand the significance of what we're seeing.

"We've been able to make our farm our only source of income since 1998. But in Wisconsin today, earning one hundred percent of your income from the farm is extremely *rare*," says Barb, with a strong emphasis on "rare." Her comment is easier to understand if one keeps in mind that 94 percent of all our farms qualify as "small," with less than $250,000 in gross sales. Sounds like a lot of money, but these are the farms dying out because few families can make ends meet with their average *net* yearly income of $23,000. Contrast their squeeze with the situation of the bigger farms—the top 3 percent of which capture almost 60 percent of the farm sales. These farms are pulling in much more income *and* as much as $460,000 each year in federal farm subsidies.[8]

As we're talking, a tall blond man carrying his toddler walks up to bid Barb and Dave goodbye. He has stayed long after the other members to show his youngest more of the farm. Last year, he tells us, his eleven-year-old visited for the first time. After complaining that there would be "just a bunch of old hippies," his son had come, and then didn't want to leave, he was having such fun picking corn.

Sweeping his daughter back into his arms, he adds, "Most of the old family farms are gone. They were bought out by agribusiness." He nods to Barb and Dave. "These community-supported farmers. They're the new family farm."

Pleasure is Not Merely in Our Tastebuds

The next day, we drive further out of Madison. The green is so green and the farmsteads so picturesque that it takes real effort to keep in mind the heartache of a way of life under threat here. This is the "driftless" area of Wisconsin, called that because the glaciers stopped just north and never had the chance to grind down these hills. I'd heard the term "driftless" before, and it had always evoked romantic images of a place and people not entirely absorbed by the dominant culture.

We're with Jack Kloppenburg, an energetic professor of rural sociology at the University of Wisconsin, who has taken us under his wing to help us make connections and make sense of what we're seeing. I can imagine that at a university heavily involved in biotechnology, Jack, a national leader in sustainable agriculture, may not be the administration's favorite prof.

At a bend in a narrow country road, Jack stops so we can take pictures of a farm—its rows of corn extend in manicured lines as far as we can see, and its towering silos perch like castles on top of a nearby hill. As Anna's camera captures the uncanny perfection, Jack says something I hadn't yet put into words. "Taste is not merely in our tastebuds, but in our knowledge. Knowledge adds to our pleasure in eating."

I immediately think back to Jack's potluck the night before. Maybe the dishes were especially delectable because I had informed tastebuds. They could taste not only the flavors of the just-picked yellow watermelon, squash, basil, and tomatoes, but also the knowledge that the food was grown without chemicals and with the caring hands of the farmers and backyard gardeners— some of whom joined us on the patio that night.

Now I see, too, that knowledge can kill taste—knowledge of what's in our food that's not good for us. Knowledge that it's farms like this one, as Jack explains, that contaminate the earth and water beneath our feet. We'd already learned that one-quarter of U.S. drinking water wells contain nitrates from fertilizer in amounts above safety standards.[8]

"Atrazine, the most widely used herbicide for corn," Jack also reminds us, "has seeped into the ground all around here." As we climb back into the car, he adds, "In some parts of the Midwest, you can't even drink the water."

ACCIDENTAL FARMERS

Just behind José and his host, we pull into the gravel driveway of a handsome 160-acre farmstead, where Matt and Diane Sharp—in jeans and high rubber boots—greet us. One of their sons and a daughter hang back shyly, but close enough so they don't miss a thing.

A large blue-gray barn rises up on the green hill behind them like the inspiration for a Norman Rockwell painting, but Matt's first words after all the how-do-you-do's shatter the serenity.

"Everything changed when our first child was born. At six months, Ian developed a brain tumor. Doctors told us it was caused by exposure to chemicals and that he wasn't likely to survive. It was a really scary time, but he surprised all his doctors. He's sixteen now."

Gesturing to Kathleen, age thirteen, and Gabriel, nine, Matt says, "We decided then that if we were going to have more children, we were going to do everything in our power to help them to be healthy and safe.

"We decided we wanted more control over our family's food," Matt tells us. "We weren't raised on farms, and we didn't get started until four years ago when we bought our first cattle. We're sort of accidental farmers.

"We're registered nurses, and we were seeing higher and higher rates of certain diseases, even some diseases that people never used to get," he says. With his short-cropped hair and wire-rimmed glasses, Matt would fit as well in the E.R. as he does here.

"Asthma, attention-deficit disorder, cancer, depression, obesity, fibromyalgia—an arthritis-like condition—they're all up. That's a scary thing," he says.

For the Sharps, there is no doubt: Americans are getting sicker—even dying—because of what they eat. But, they remind us, it's not just a matter of our food choices. The quality of our food is eroding as well.

"Our big farms have stripped our topsoil by using chemicals and overusing the land. We can't have healthy food without healthy soil," Matt says.

Matt's caution reflects a deterioration in food quality borne out by official surveys which show nutritional values declining in many commonly eaten vegetables.[9] Our drive for production, over all else, has eroded even the nutrition in foods we eat precisely because we think they're going to be good for us!

But it's not just the plants that are affected. "Animals have been affected by the production drive, too," Matt says. "They're pushed to grow faster and bigger, and their lives are spent almost entirely in concrete-floored feedlots. These animals are getting more stressed and more sick.

"Most of the farmers around here," Matt says, bringing home his point, "are spending more on veterinarian bills than I do on my mortgage.

"Older farmers can remember Ol' Bossey living as long as twelve years, but now the average is closer to four. It's common knowledge among farmers that a lot of hamburgers, bologna, and other meat that's ground up is made from culled cows—dairy cows culled from the herd because they're so sick and worn that it's better business to turn them into meat before they die anyway. If I wasn't growing my own animals—if I didn't know where my meat was coming from—I'd be a vegetarian . . . maybe even a vegan."

I know their family's health motivates both Matt and Diane to take the risk they've taken. Their enthusiasm is backed by new studies showing pasture-raised beef like theirs has more "good" omega-3 fatty acids, vitamin E, beta-carotene, and less saturated fat than feedlot fed.[10] Others, though, say beef is beef is beef. It still contains fat and cholesterol—along with carcinogenic substances created when meat is cooked—that scientists link to cancer and heart disease. The only diets that have shown to substantially reduce cholesterol are vegetarian.[11]

BEYOND COMMUNIST AMERICA

Before we climb up the low hill to the pasture, José—his signature pipe in hand—chuckles as he says in a strong French accent, "America is the most communist country ever."

The Sharps look more than a little stunned. If I hadn't heard José talk about totalitarianism at the food festival, I might not have grasped his meaning, either. It's that all of us, every *thing,* is being squeezed into one giant system, in this case a certain way of growing our food and raising our animals. In this system, decisions are far removed from people, and the decision makers are oblivious to the impact. José sees us all becoming the *same*—like the frightening images of gray, uniform communism so familiar to my generation growing up with the Red scare.

The Sharps, however, are doing things differently. As we climb past the barn to the pasture, Diane makes sure José sees that their Highland Hearth Farm is breaking free from the "communist" system. They've chosen to raise their cows—beginning with four in 1996 and now at sixty—on pasture, not on grain.

When I wrote *Diet for a Small Planet,* grain feeding to livestock had just been consecrated as *the* superior way to produce meat. Advertisers told us to love all that marbling. Yumm. Never mind, of course, the tremendous waste in feeding and the cruelty to animals confined in feedlots. And never mind that any nutritionist can tell you marbled meat has more fat of the type linked to disease.

As I pointed out in *Diet,* and as many others have since, livestock give back to us in meat only a tiny portion of the nutrients we feed to them. Yet, worldwide, more and more grain is going to livestock—in many industrial countries as much as 70 percent.[12]

"Ruminants, like cattle," Diane explains, "have always taken solar energy in the form of grasses and turned it into milk and protein that humans can eat.

THE STEAK ON YOUR PLATE

As I was driving home today, one of those pickup trucks that belong more in Wyoming than downtown Boston cut me off. Just before it sped off, I caught a glimpse of its bumper sticker: BEEF, it said, BECAUSE THE WEST WASN'T WON ON SALAD. I chuckled to myself; I'd never seen beef eaters' backlash before. But in a few weeks, I'd see more: a T-shirt that said VEGETARIAN: OLD WEST FOR "LOUSY HUNTER." Maybe it's been inspired by a new president who reigns from a state known as much for its love of steak as its love of two-stepping.

When I see steak, though, I don't picture All-American picnics or the wide-open range. Ever since I was young, when I saw a steak, my mind would conjure up the piles of grain and soy consumed and the gallons of water used to get it to my plate. When I saw steak, I would see the illogic and irrationality of a food system that takes plenty and squanders it. And now, when I see steak, I picture a whole lot more. In my own tally of the price we really pay, I imagine:

- The antibiotics fed to livestock every day that pack on the weight fast and block disease before the animals are even sick;

- The pesticides used on the grain and soy feed, chemicals that become even more concentrated in the meat itself;

We say, let ruminants do what they're designed to do. Plus," she adds, "cattle don't get as sick when they're eating what they're designed to."

The Sharps' approach is in one sense age-old—moving livestock from pasture to pasture so grass cover is maintained, and the animals mimic their movement in the wild. But in another sense, it's brand new. They are part of a movement of farmers—both dairy and beef—reinventing a centuries-old method into managed intensive rotational grazing.

There were some pioneering beef and dairy "graziers"—as they call themselves—starting in the mid-'70s, but this approach really took off in the early 1990s.[13] By the end of the decade, more than one-fifth of Wisconsin's dairy farmers and a growing number of its beef farmers were foregoing grain feeding, at least for the most part, and converting to intensive, rotational grazing.[14]

- The saturated fat and cholesterol, linked to cancer and heart disease; and the possibility of food-borne diseases like those caused by E. coli bacteria;

- The suffering of cattle trapped in crowded feedlots;

- The meatpacking workers, who must get by on some of the lowest wages in the country, even though last year, the world's largest pork-production plant saw its profits double[15];

- Other meatpacking workers whose lives are cut short in a workplace where one out of four workers every year suffers job-related injury or illness, the highest rate of any job in the country.[16] (Our nation's slaughterhouses have been called more dangerous and debilitating now than at any time since Upton Sinclair wrote The Jungle, in 1906.[17]);

- And, next to these faces, the few people who've come to control the meatpacking industry—a concentration so tight that now four corporations control over four-fifths of the beef slaughterhouses in the U.S.[18] Just one, IBP, kills 40 percent of America's feedlot cattle.[19]

So around that small, small steak, I see the chemicals, the fat, and the germs; the drugs and the resources. I see the workers in debilitating jobs, the old-time farmers going out of business, and the corporations making a killing. I have no temptation to eat. My fork never budges.   —Anna

From time to time, they share their knowledge in hyacinth-like get-togethers called "pasture walks."

Matt picks up the end of what looks like a waist-high clothesline wrapped around a long spool. It's actually a solar-powered electric fence—a simple device that allows farmers like Matt and Diane to control their livestock cheaply and effectively. As Matt moves the line, as he does every twenty-four hours, the cows are primed, and they trundle past quickly to a lush new patch.

"You know, this isn't rocket science," Matt says. "Good soil is the key. We've gotten our soil healthy by using clover, alfalfa, grasses, and organic fertilizer. We've doubled our pasture production in just a year by intensively managing the grazing," he adds.

As we talk, Diane rushes ahead and puts out coffee and cookies on the trunk of their car, and I attempt a lame joke about a tailgate party farm-style. As we munch, Diane hands us flyers describing the health benefits of grass-fed meat.

Hearing the Sharps talk about their tasty and healthy beef, I can't quite relate. It's been thirty-plus years since I've had a bite, and the more I've learned about meat, the more convinced I've become that it is not good for us. But here with the Sharps, I do find myself very glad that those who still eat meat can at least now choose to buy from people like them. By that choice, their customers reject the cruelty and pollution of feedlots and factory farms, and they receive in return the security of knowing that the animals were raised without a diet full of hormones, antibiotics, and questionable feed.

When it's time to say goodbye, Matt apologizes that his son Ian couldn't join us. Since his childhood illness, Ian has been severely handicapped and confined to a wheelchair; today's slight breeze would have bothered him too much. As we're leaving, Matt adds, "Ian is the best thing that ever happened to us. He changed our lives. He got us to remember our priorities."

That night in the hotel room, I call a friend back in Boston who grew up on a farm. Yeah, he liked my story of the Sharps, but he pressed me with one question: Will their kids want to farm?

I told him about the Sharps' teenage daughter, Kathleen, with her fresh, freckled face. "Last year I entered the county fair," I overheard her saying to Anna, "and my friend down the road helped me with my entry. It was fun. There aren't many girls who work on farms, but I like it." Pointing to the grassy hill just beyond the house, she told Anna, "That's where I'm going to build my farm."

"It's the Lateness that Bothers Me."

Anna and I are standing under a tall willow tree on John Kinsman's 150-acre farm near the tiny town of LaValle. John, in a blue-and-white-striped shirt and crisp cap, is the lively seventy-four-year-old founder of Family Farm Defenders, a group committed to farming that sustains the earth and gives farmers control over their lives.

I'd crossed paths with John over the years, but we'd never had a chance to really talk. Now, we tour farms near Madison together as John hosts José Bové, whom he'd met twelve years ago in Europe. John, a fifth generation dairyman, immediately took to José because, as he put it, in Europe "farmers have dignity that U.S. farmers have lost. They still believe in themselves." (I'm amused throughout the day as John pronounces José's name "Josie," like the nickname for Josephine.)

John's trim frame and irrepressible grin exude optimism, so his words shock me.

"The problem for farmers is that food has lost its dignity. If you have no dignity, you have no hope. Food has no value. The price dairy farmers get is half the cost of producing it. 'So, aren't they stupid to keep farming?' That must be the attitude of consumers.

"It's getting so late," John continues. "It's the lateness that bothers me." He doesn't mean that evening is falling; he means that only seven-tenths of 1 percent of people in the U.S. are still farmers. With fewer than two million farms remaining in the U.S., we have more people doing time in prison than farming full-time. The number of people considered "farmers" actually dropped so low that as of 1993 the Census Bureau stopped using the category.[20]

"Three or four of my farmer neighbors will be gone in a year," John says, shaking his head. The government reports that in the mid-'90s an average of almost 20,000 family farms folded each year—organizations working with farmers say even that estimate may be low.[21] With farm income down by almost one-fifth this year, John could be losing many more neighbors.[22]

John has survived, he tells us, because he chose to farm differently from his neighbors: organically. But he didn't start out that way.

"I started with the chemical fix like everybody else," John says. "But in a couple of years, I ended up in the University hospital. My legs were numb.

"The doctor asked, 'When did you last use pesticides?' Then he put me in the ward, and I saw we were all farmers. My legs and arms shriveled. The doctor told me my nerve coverings were almost destroyed. Never once did it go in my record, though, what the cause was."

As John describes his ordeal, I have an eerie feeling of recognition. We've now heard a variant of his story from farmers on five continents. They've told of a range of scary symptoms, brought on, they believe, by farm chemicals.

Introduced after World War II, pesticides seemed to hold great promise for high-yield, risk-free farming. So, by the mid-'90s, the U.S. was using roughly a billion pounds of active pesticide ingredients each year—that's about four pounds for every person in the country and 20 percent of the world's pesticide use.[23] We'd also become a major pesticide exporter, even of pesticides deemed too hazardous to allow here. The goal of it all is, obviously, to reduce loss to pests, but we've been losing that fight, too. Despite a tenfold increase in pesticide use, the share of crops lost to pests has nearly doubled since World War II.[24]

"I got treatment and started improving," John continues. "This woke me up. I said, 'No more chemicals.' Today I'm healthier than I was at twenty-one. I eat right, and I have hope.

"The demise of the family farm is not inevitable," John says, standing with his back to his large red barn. It's clear that his passion for saving family farming—actually reinventing it á la the Perkinses and the Sharps—comes out of his own experience.

"When I started in the fifties, this land was so bad it didn't even grow weeds. The topsoil was gone. When we shifted to organic, we just kept adding organic matter. We seeded clover, alfalfa, and grasses. Now in many areas the soil is dark and rich and full of earthworms.

"I can survive with the low prices," John says, referring to his early choice to farm organically. "But most farmers around here can't. They're deep in debt from what they've paid for land, fertilizers, pesticides, and big machinery.

"Just recently, a young man down the road went out, got the mail, found a notice from the bank about his debt, got his gun, and shot himself," John says, somberly. "Another neighbor attempted suicide last Christmas Eve." As John talks, I remember learning that the suicide rate among farmers is three times higher than in the general population.[25]

Lives are being needlessly destroyed, but why? I want to know. "Why aren't your neighbors opting for your lower-cost way, since you're doing so well?" I ask.

"Because they're afraid," is John's emphatic answer. "They don't believe it's possible. They've put so much into a certain way. It's fear of change," he adds, echoing Alice Waters's words.

Change is difficult, but it can be terrifying if we can't see alternatives. John and the other farmers we meet are showing their neighbors it's possible to change and thrive, but most still don't believe it. Part of the problem is that sustainable methods, and their effectiveness, are still largely invisible.

As we were completing our journey, for the first time a worldwide survey of sustainable agriculture initiatives was completed. We held our breath. What would it show? Looking at more than 200 projects in fifty-two countries using about 70 million acres, the university-sponsored research was unequivocal: Sustainable practices can "lead to substantial increases" in production. In fact, some root-crop farmers realized gains as great as 150 percent using more sustainable methods.[26]

Simultaneously, researchers here in the U.S. released in *Nature* magazine one of the first rigorous comparisons of organic and chemical farming, this one focused on apple growing. (This research took on special urgency when Anna and I learned that in a recent study of apples grown in Washington state, 84 percent tested positive for pesticides—and two out of every twenty-five exceeded federal standards. In the case of two types of these apples, a two-year-old eating even half an apple would be exposed to more pesticides than the government deems safe.[27]) The *Nature* study found that the organic orchards produced better soils, superior energy efficiency, and fewer environmental impacts, while achieving comparable yields.[28]

But John's neighbors have heard nothing of these breakthroughs.

Before we say goodbye, John stresses to us that there's a lot more to the farmer's dilemma than what and how he or she grows. They get low prices for a reason. When farmers try to sell their products, they face only a handful of corporate buyers, so they have virtually no bargaining power. Yes, farmers can reduce costs by shifting away from chemicals, but they can also take charge of their predicament, he says, by getting rid of the middleman, marketing directly to consumers. This way, they could get a fair price without consumers having to pay more.

That sounds good, but maybe a little dreamy, too, I think. How can a farmers' marketing cooperative, I wonder, compete with giant agribusiness? There's no time to ask John, but we'll get our answer in a few days—when we least expect it.

GOT MORE MILK?

We arrive at Bob Wills's Cedar Grove cheese factory in the late afternoon, and Bob immediately rushes to the cooler to treat us to fresh juice and get us more ice for Anna's hand, which still throbs days after the sting. Bob, in his wire-rimmed glasses and casual but professional clothes, looks every bit the businessperson who took over the family enterprise. But, with his law degree and a PhD in economics, Bob is not a typical cheese-maker.

"I took my kids—eight and ten years old—to hear you speak the other night," Bob tells us. "They liked how you talked about thinking differently about fear to gain the courage to do what you believe in. I'm also trying to focus on how I can make my world what I want it to be." Like making this one-hundred-year-old factory into a leader in keeping small dairy farms around here in business.

Standing in his airy storefront that's connected to the factory in the back, Bob points to a map with tiny dots scattered across it. "These show where this area's old cheese factories used to be. In 1922 there were almost three thousand," he says. "Today there are closer to a hundred." To get a better sense of the odds Bob is up against, keep in mind the extent of concentration in the cheese industry nationwide. Today, one company, Philip Morris, through its Kraft cheese brand, controls almost half of the entire North American market.[29]

But Bob is not daunted. Though he's watched many of his colleagues go under, he still picks up his 100,000 pounds of milk each morning from forty nearby dairy farms, processes it in his on-location factory, and distributes it across the county and country. Innocuous, no? But actually Bob's little cheese factory sits in the center of hot controversy.

In the late '80s, Monsanto finished developing Posilac, its brand name for the rBGH (recombinant bovine growth hormone) synthetic hormone to stimulate higher production in milk cows. Though, early on, a Food and Drug Administration veterinarian whose job was to evaluate Posilac had found adverse effects on injected cows, the FDA ignored these cautions. It even fired the scientists and approved the product for market in 1994.[30] By the late '90s, Monsanto was claiming that one-third of dairy farms nationally were using the hormone. But, since farmers are not required to tell consumers whether or not they use rBGH, and since most cartons contain milk from different farmers, it's impossible to know what milk comes from rBGH-treated cows.

Not so at Cedar Grove. "I entered the fray when rBGH first came on the market," Bob tells us. "Ours was one of the first dairies in the nation to label milk rBGH-free. We got signed, notarized statements from farmers saying they weren't using rBGH.

"Monsanto tells us there's no difference between rBGH and non-rBGH milk," Bob continues, "and since the FDA agrees, saying rBGH is just a synthesized version of a naturally occurring hormone, they don't require any labeling.

"Immediately, we received warnings from Monsanto that we couldn't advertise our milk as rBGH-free because it implied there was something the matter with their product.

"But I think they're wrong about rBGH. The growth hormone *does* change milk. The more rBGH, the more of an insulin-like growth promoter, called IGF. Milk solids are lower, too, and that means less protein. Plus, producing more takes a terrible toll on the cows' health. There's more disease, more antibiotics, and higher vet bills. When farmers were told rBGH was the answer, no one mentioned these downsides. Now, three out of four of my neighbors have stopped using it."[31]

We've also learned about scientists who've called into question the safety of rBGH, including concerns like Bob's that it increases IGF, a suspected cancer promoter, particularly in the human colon and breast.[32]

Yet, the government still requires no labeling, and people like Bob are threatened for expressing their concerns. Monsanto even sent Bob a letter insinuating they would sue for his labeling practices; they've as yet not made good on their threat.

But Bob is luckier than some. Just after Posilac was released, Monsanto sued two dairies, one in Iowa and one in Texas, for labeling their milk rBGH-free. At the same time, Monsanto sent 2,000 threatening letters to other dairies and natural-foods retail stores across the country.[33] And Monsanto didn't stop at dairies.

In 1996, a Florida television station received threatening letters from Monsanto just days before it was to air a four-part investigative report on rBGH. In response, the news managers and lawyers at Fox-owned WTVT requested that the journalists rewrite the piece. After more than eighty revisions, the station producers cut the report from their programming and fired the journalists. The husband-and-wife team, Jane Akre and Steve Wilson, decided to sue the broadcaster under the Florida state law that protects whistle-blowers from retaliation. After two years of legal fees and lost livelihood, one of them was awarded damages of almost a half-million dollars. Some vindication, yes.

But they've yet to see the money; Monsanto is appealing the verdict. Worse, the public has been kept in the dark; the investigative report never aired.[34]

But in all this turmoil, we come back to the underlying point: We never needed rBGH in the first place. The problem for dairy farmers has long been *too much milk,* not too little. The last thing farmers needed was a drug to produce more milk. (And maybe the last thing consumers needed, too. We've been advised to seriously consider recent studies linking dairy consumption with prostate cancer and insulin-dependent diabetes.)[35] In fact, a milk surplus aggravated by the use of rBGH has helped push milk prices down to their lowest levels in decades. And, as José might say, putting rBGH on the market is totalitarian, making everyone who doesn't conform pay a heavy price.

"Just to keep on doing what we've always done here at Cedar Grove," Bob says, "and reassure customers we're not using rBGH, we have to carry the expense of certifying and labeling. If a dairy uses both rBGH and non-rBGH milk, it costs to keep them separate. The burden falls on us. It's not that the rBGH product is better, but it can insinuate itself into the market anyway, by forcing up the costs of those who don't use it." Bob draws a parallel with organic farmers, who have to carry the costs, for instance, of creating buffer zones between their fields and those using pesticides or genetically modified organisms. Totalitarian indeed.

A VISIT TO THE LITTLE SHOP OF HORRORS

Bob decided to ensure that his factory is a leader not only in discouraging growth hormones, but in encouraging organic farming, too. In the past few years, he's been urging the farmers he buys from to forego chemicals. Now, almost half of the milk he buys is organic.

"Around here," Bob adds, citing lower costs of organic farming and the premium price organic milk commands, "I've never seen an organic farmer go out of business."

Bob's taking his "solve for pattern" approach beyond cheese: He's applying it to his factory's waste, too. Bob had been spending more than $30,000 a year to dispose of his wastewater when he decided to try something different—using nature to clean his water. Risking $150,000 of his own money, plus funds he got from the state, he installed what's called a Living Machine®.

Imagine a greenhouse with big tanks of water instead of soil beds. That's what it looks and smells like—well, an extraordinarily successful greenhouse.

Bob tells us he goes in with a machete, often, because the plants get so tall. This is *The Little Shop of Horrors* with an environmental twist.

"That big one is elephant ear," Bob says, as we make our way past the oversized plants. "There's calla lily; and that one is canna lily. That wooly looking plant with flowers—that's sedge. There's some ginger, too."

These plants are not just ornaments; they *work*. The cheese factory's wastewater flows first into closed aerobic reactors and then into open aerobic reactors—fancy names for tanks, as far as I can tell. Their work is to provide a pleasing environment for communities of bacteria, zooplankton, phytoplankton, snails, and fish, all of which "clean" the water.

"When the water comes out—up to six thousand gallons a day—it's clean enough to flow right into [nearby] Honey Creek," Bob says with satisfaction. He's also happy to report that he'll recoup his investment in just a few years.

"I enjoy having schoolchildren tour, too, to see that technology can work with nature," Bob adds. "I'm on a citizens' advisory committee to the Center for Integrated Agricultural Systems at the university. I want to help redirect research to technology like this that liberates people."

As we leave, Bob tells us about another outcome, one he hadn't expected. "Our employees love this thing. They come over and visit the greenhouse, so they're more aware about waste. There is a lot less wastewater now than there used to be. Everyone's just more careful."

Bob's Living Machine® is exactly the kind of technology we didn't have thirty years ago. No one imagined it. Since then, many people have. They've not only begun to imagine working with nature rather than against it; they're devising technologies that drastically reduce our impact on the earth.

On the edge of this frontier are Amory and Hunter Lovins, creators of the Rocky Mountain Institute in Colorado, whom I've learned from for many years. Their latest book, *Natural Capitalism,* written with Paul Hawken, tells of a myriad of innovations that work with nature like the Living Machine does, including a small firm in Oregon that developed a way to make tomato paste by straining the tomatoes through ultra-fine sieves instead of boiling them. The process improves quality and uses only 5 percent of the energy.[36]

Clearly, Bob's Living Machine® is a similarly brilliant business solution: Reduce your costs, encourage employees to reduce their waste, even create a draw for the local community. Curious, of course, Anna asks how many other cheese factories are using Living Machines®.[37]

"Well," Bob says, "I think there's one in Australia, but I've never seen it."

WHAT I SEE ON TV

I've been working on this chapter all day, and for a break I decide to watch a 20/20 episode I've been meaning to see for months. I pop it in the VCR, and I hear Barbara Walters asking, "Do you think organic food is healthier and safer for you, your family, and the planet? Millions of people do. But can they be wrong?"

Organics, I'm told, do not have higher nutrient levels, and are actually worse for us, than conventional foods. In fact, the report says, many illnesses, even deaths, have been connected to the "nasty bacteria" that can be found in organic foods. Foods grown with chemicals, I'm told, are much less risky for our health. Without a speck of doubt, organic food is simply less good for us and less good for the environment. The show ends with Walters asking, distressed, "But I've been buying organic foods all this time, it isn't dangerous, is it?"

Sounds worrisome, no? Complaints followed, asking the network to re-evaluate. It turns out that their expert, Dennis Avery, is a scholar at a think tank financed in part by chemical giants such as Dow and Novartis. And that study proving that no pesticide residues appeared on conventional foods? Well, actually, it never tested for pesticides. The 20/20 segment reporter did eventually apologize. Millions had watched the original, and few heard the apology.

So the story lives on. The nonprofit PR Watch reports that Avery still gets quoted in articles with titles such as "Organic food—It's Eight Times More Likely to Kill You." How ironic that during this same period, the latest threat of food-borne illness has resulted in the largest meat recalls in history, pulling over 40 million pounds off the shelves and killing at least eight people. I've yet to hear about organic strawberries doing the same.

—Anna

A LIVING CORAL REEF

A few nights before we leave Madison, we're invited to dinner by chef Odessa Piper, Madison's queen of natural, locally grown cuisine. As founder and co-chef of L'Etoile, one of Madison's classiest restaurants, she's been connecting the work of businesspeople like Bob and farmers like the Kinsmans, the Sharps, and the Perkinses with folks in Madison for twenty-five years.

We climb the stairs to L'Etoile's elegant dining room and find Odessa in the kitchen, wearing a wilted white chef's coat, her reddish-brown hair pulled back off her face. Sitting down near the bar—in the calm before the rush— we're immediately captivated by Odessa's story.

"I grew up in the fifties in Portsmouth, New Hampshire, one of fifty nuclear targets of the Cold War. How to select food for the bomb shelter was a big discussion in our house. Packaged, processed foods—that was bomb-shelter cuisine to us, though my parents cooked everything from scratch.

"I moved to Hanover, New Hampshire [home of Dartmouth College] and joined the Wooden Shoe Commune—we used your book," she adds, with a smile. "Though I didn't know it at the time, I got my start as a chef learning how to grow and 'put by' [jar and can] our own food. It was a magical opportunity for a young person. From there I went to Wisconsin and joined a group of back-to-the-landers who were inspired by a visionary named JoAnna Guthrie. JoAnna's mission was to link a restaurant with an organic farm to demonstrate the interdependence between rural and urban life.

"Twenty of us settled to farm near Soldier's Grove [on the western edge of Wisconsin]. Of course, no one knew how to be successful growing organically thirty years ago. That time was the beginning of so much, including our whole approach to farming and cooking as artisans.

"Artisanal products are things we use in our daily lives that nourish both our bodies and our souls," Odessa explains, when she sees my questioning look. "Appreciating the art of farming and cooking is central to what we do. We believe that respect for nature and all that grows is the beginning of the understanding of good food."

Odessa began her path to restaurateur in 1972, when she helped JoAnna open a restaurant. Four years later, at the age of twenty-four, Odessa set out on her own to launch L'Etoile.

"Looking back, I realize I bonded to L'Etoile as a mother to her child. But in the first year we ran up a crippling debt. My partner left, and the stress put me in the hospital. Even the plants froze. That was the turning point. I was at the end of my rope, but I couldn't let L'Etoile die, so I got my family to help me make fresh pastries to sell at the farmers' market to raise money.

"In the early years, L'Etoile was known for our croissants. We sold thousands of them at the farmers' market. One day we got rained out and, of course, all-butter croissants don't keep. So I sent my nephew to the market to give them away to farmers. Several hours later these same farmers came tromping in here to give *me* things—strawberries, bread, apples. That's when I realized L'Etoile's cuisine is one of friendship, of interdependence."

To Odessa, interdependence means choosing organic ingredients when possible and purchasing from small farmers—now roughly one hundred of them—local to the area.

"It's a cuisine of abundance," Odessa emphasizes.

I've sensed over the years that many people assume eating in season, eating plant foods, eating whole foods, eating local foods, all mean denial and self-discipline, not pleasure. To Odessa, it is clearly about pleasure, too.

"We don't have to roll over and play dead in the winter," she adds, "even here in Wisconsin. We have a dozen varieties of apples to choose from in the winter. We serve roasted tomatoes that we've harvested and frozen at the peak of their ripeness and flavor. Local farms root-cellar hundreds of pounds of winter squash for us.

"Our food is not cheap because we are showing the real cost of food. We pay our farmers immediately. We pay our staff as well as we can and offer the benefit every worker should have—a meaningful job. By doing this we are creating what I call deep wealth, and the returns are incredible."

As we talk with Odessa, I realize how rarely I've met a person so completely aligned. Every cell in her body seems attuned to her mission of bringing the full human back into the experience of community, linked through the earth and good food to each other.

"In Madison, we're like a living coral reef, building our cathedral out of little currents into something beautiful. This is a region with a mission, and I'm fortunate, I've been perched here seeing its evolution," Odessa says, with an endearing openness and humility.

We move to the dining room for dinner with two of L'Etoile's farmers, Richard de Wilde and Linda Halley, who started their farm, Harmony Valley, in Viroqua near where Odessa had lived, the same year *Diet for a Small Planet* was released.

"We learned the hard way about farming organically," Richard, with a trim beard and wearing a soft linen shirt, says smiling. "The university laughed at me. They warned me, 'Don't try to make a living doing this.' Now I teach a five-day university course on organic farming—giving away all my hard-earned knowledge! Eleven years ago, maybe forty people would come. Now thirteen-hundred show up," he says, beaming.

After a meal whose flavors will stay with Anna and me for days, we're treated to a blueberry "soup" served, as the dessert menu tells us, with "Ari de Wilde's Charentaise melons." Richard and Linda laugh; Ari is their eleven-year-old son.

Through her menu and other subtle touches, Odessa has made an abstraction like "interdependence" not only palpable but also visible to all who dine here. On the wall near our table is a salmon-colored map of Wisconsin with strings reaching out to the location of all the farmers she depends on—most of them probably older than eleven!

THE ARK OF TASTE

The next day, we encounter another of Odessa's ripples: Tami Lax, about-to-be-chef of the latest whole-foods restaurant in Madison.

"I was the operations manager for a retail music chain," Tami tells us, as we talk in a little café near her almost-restaurant. In her mid-thirties, Tami has a contagious energy and bright eyes behind stylish horn-rimmed glasses. "Even though I grew up on a farm and could remember my grandmother's root cellar, my life was speeding up and I was losing track of what I loved. So I started changing my diet. I remembered my passion for gardening and cooking, and I went to Odessa for advice. She hired me.

"I was Odessa's *chef de cuisine* and 'forager.' Most of L'Etoile's food is locally grown, so part of my job was meeting farmers. I loved it so much that every day off from the restaurant I worked on farms. When one of our suppliers had a stroke, I harvested his apples.

"The more I got to know these farmers, the more I saw how much knowledge we are losing. The number-one dairy farmer where I grew up just went out of business. It's devastating to lose these people. If everyone just did a little bit, we could change it. I know all the farmers I will buy from. If you know people personally, you are not going to treat them as a commodity.

"Through this work, I got interested in the Slow Food Movement."

Slow Food started in 1986, when Carlo Petrini, an Italian outraged over the desecration of a 14th-century piazza and the loss of local culture it symbolized, was inspired to start a movement to save diverse, traditional foods and our personal connection to good eating. Slow Food, self-described as an antidote to the "fast life," now has 60,000 members in more than thirty-five countries.

As the Midwest leader of the Slow Food Movement, Tami plays Noah.

"We have what we call the Ark of Taste," Tami tells us. "Like Noah, we must bring foods onto the Ark if we don't want them to disappear."

Tami's first Ark inductees were three local farmstead cheeses; one is a sheep cheese aged in open-air caves on cedar boughs. These cheeses are made as a craft, produced right on the farm not in factories like Bob's. At the turn of the century, there were a couple thousand farmstead cheeses in Wisconsin—now these are the only three left.

"In Slow Food, we want to stimulate markets for endangered foods," Tami says. "The Ark is one way. Food tastings are another. Our first event in this area was an apple tasting at an orchard with hundred-year-old apple trees and forty-three varieties to taste."

I suppose many Americans would see Tami's efforts as quaint—interesting, but irrelevant—but maybe not if they were aware that, worldwide, 95 percent of our food requirements are now being met from fewer than thirty plant varieties.[38] To appreciate the narrowness of this genetic base, remember our earth is home to literally millions of plant species, many of which have not even been identified.[39] So the Ark of Taste is not just for our pleasure, although certainly it is that, but also for our viability.

Before Tami rushes back to oversee the finishing touches on her restaurant, she tells us, "My father always wanted to be a farmer but was afraid he couldn't support five kids that way. So while he went into paper manufacturing, he kept his hand in the soil.

"We spent summers on the farmstead he'd inherited," Tami continues. "My brothers and sisters and I would make a game of foraging for our evening meal. Sometimes we would make a whole day of it. We'd pick apples, wild greens, walk two miles to the blueberry patch. We'd fish. I can still remember the trout. I've never tasted fish as good."

FROM RAG-TAG TO BIG TIME

When we heard we'd be spending our last day in Madison at the Willy Street Food Co-op, I was dubious. My memory of Willy Street was a tiny storefront. I couldn't imagine enough space for the meetings we're anticipating with more than a dozen people representing other food-community efforts in the area. I shouldn't have worried.

Since I last visited Madison, Willy Street had expanded, big-time, moving into spacious new facilities with a sunny conference room. This co-op, along with others in Madison, is one of more than 300 food cooperatives that have sprouted up across the country since the '70s. (And this in the face of a tightening retail control that may break all records: In the three final years of the last century, the five biggest grocery retailers doubled their share of the market to 42 percent of all sales in the country.[40])

On this, our last day, we want to learn about the farming business, and specifically marketing. All the farmers we've met are inspiring, yes, but are they economically viable? While spending on food in this country since I wrote *Diet for a Small Planet* has jumped from roughly $100 billion to $500 billion a year, the amount going to farmers has only crept up, with virtually no rise since 1980. Today only twenty cents of our food dollar goes to the farmer, down from forty-one cents in 1950—the rest goes to all the other stuff, from advertisers to packagers to distributors.[41]

Earlier, family-farm defender John Kinsman had said that part of the answer was to eliminate the middleman. Great idea, I thought, but how?

Seemingly to answer this exact question, into the co-op walks dairy farmer Jim Miller, fit-looking and fifty-something with graying hair and a square jaw. After a tight-as-a-vise handshake, Jim sits his husky frame down and begins to tell us about Organic Valley, a cooperative of family farms working together to market and distribute organic products. "It used to be called the Coulee Region Organic Produce Pool," he says, "CROPP, for short."

As soon as I hear "CROPP," my heart sinks. I flash back to a small, wooden church in Viroqua, Wisconsin. Over a decade ago, I'd been invited to speak there by the nicest, most earnest people—CROPP's founders. They had just started an organic dairy co-op to cut out the marketing middlemen, and they had big dreams. Mainly, though, I remember sitting on a hard pew thinking how unlikely it was that they would actually make it. Assuming the co-op today couldn't consist of much more than a mélange of well-meaning idealists, I'm afraid that, no matter what Jim tells us, I'll conclude that farmers' marketing efforts are marginal in the big picture.

But Jim is hardly a hippie back-to-the-lander. He was born and raised on the farm, left for what he called the "restaurant business" in the south, but came back to the farm in 1994.

"My father had just died of cancer. He was the one who did all the spraying of the fields. It was a terrible death. We couldn't prove it, but everyone in the family blamed the farm chemicals.

"That's when we decided to go organic, all of us—ten families. We're all related, and we farm together. Neighbors told us, 'You're nuts,' and we did have to suffer through some trying times because it takes three years without chemicals before you can sell as certified organic—and get a premium price.

"I remember the ridicule. As we were shifting to organic, our corn didn't look so good, and one neighbor said, 'Hey, Jim, what are you growing there— pineapples? I've never seen such lousy-looking corn.' Now, farmers who scorned us are asking how they can do it.

"This summer, five fields owned by neighbors of ours are completely dead from the leaf hopper. A neighbor sprayed two or three times to kill the bugs, but it didn't work. The insect damage went right up to the edge of our fields, but our crops are as healthy as they can be. Healthy plants in healthy soil will not be killed by bugs. Bugs scavenge for unhealthy plants."

I shouldn't have worried about that tiny, rag-tag group of founders I met in the church that evening in 1989.

Organic Valley membership has jumped from seven farmers to 300, and last year they sold almost $80 million in organic products from California to Maine—now even Japan. If it continues to grow as fast as it has, Jim tells us, Organic Valley could reach sales over $100 million next year—a far cry from the humble beginning I'd witnessed.[42]

"More farmers want to join us all the time. The market is growing like crazy," Jim says, smiling, and he's right. Nationwide, in each of the last eight years sales of organic food have grown by 20 percent.

"Consumers are smarter now. Once a week there's something in the paper about what's going on—hormones, pesticides, resistance to antibiotics. So the big food chains are responding. They are working with us to get organics into their stores. They are giving deals to companies like Organic Valley because consumers have a vote and they're using it."

I think of what John Kinsman said several days earlier: "With every dollar you spend, you vote. You either vote for big business, or you vote for the family farm." And, I think now, you either vote for big chemical companies or you vote for healthy farmers.

Jim tells us how satisfying it is to learn more each year about better, more sustainable, farming practices—instead of just taking instructions from corporate advertising. I flash to farmer suicides, from India to France to Wisconsin, and am stunned by the tragedy of such wasted life and the contrast with Jim's experience.

As we're saying goodbye, Jim looks at Anna and me. "You know why we're so successful?" he asks with a broad smile. "Because we love what we do."

THE CORAL REEF GROWS

Jim is just the beginning. For the rest of the day we hear more, and our notepads fill. We learn about a soon-to-be-launched food label in the Midwest to help consumers "vote," to use John's and Jim's term, for the changes they want. It builds on the Food Alliance label (described in the last chapter) that's spreading in the Northwest, now in 500 grocery stores. To be certified, farmers can use some chemicals, but must prove to certifiers that their products are safe for consumers and that they provide safe workplaces and fair salaries for their employees.

And we hear much more . . . about Home Grown Wisconsin, a co-op of twenty organic farmers that sells to restaurants in Madison and Chicago. From Rink DaVee, a thirty-five-year-old former Chez Panisse employee and one of Home Grown's founders, we learn how it all started: "It all goes back to Alice Waters," he tells us, grinning. "It just took a while to get to here."

We hear about the blossoming of community gardens, now numbering several dozen in the Madison area alone. Tens of thousands of gardens dot cities around the country.[43] Madison's Troy Gardens has a vision of using its twenty-six surrounding acres in a mix of ways: from a community-supported farm like the Perkinses', to affordable housing, to a farmers' market, to educational activities for kids in the neighborhood.

And we learn about Partner Shares, a program to provide financial support to make it possible for low-income families to join local CSAs.

But it doesn't stop there. For the rest of the day, roughly a dozen people inundate us with stories about everything from the successful community effort to avert Coca-Cola's exclusive "pouring rights" contract with the city's schools to the success of the Willy Street co-op itself. Its spacious new quarters have helped it double its buying and selling of produce in just the last year. Local farmers, we're sure, are applauding.

Through these stories, we understand better what Odessa meant when she described what is growing here as Madison's own "coral reef."

SHOPPING LIKE A CHEF

It's our final morning in Madison, and we're off to see how a "real chef" shops. We're meeting Eric Rupert, Odessa's co-chef, at the local farmers' market. The market started here twenty-six years ago, and increasingly on Wednesdays and

Saturdays it attracts big crowds including, we discover, clusters of white-coat-clad chefs selecting their evenings' ingredients.

On the way to meet Eric, our small side street is partially blocked by an eighteen-wheeler that broadcasts across its long hulk: SYSCO: AMERICA'S LARGEST MARKETER OF QUALITY ASSURED FOODSERVICE PRODUCTS. Turning the corner, we arrive at the market and see before us its colorful array not of *foodservice products,* but of *food.*

The first farmer Eric introduces to us is a robust woman with a silkscreen of a giant tomato across her shirt. Arranged in front of her are heirloom tomatoes—some green, others odd-shaped, some striped with color. A cardboard sign declares, "Bred for taste, not for shipping." As the flavor of one of her samples explodes in my mouth, I wonder how long SYSCO's foodservice products would sell if more Americans could have this experience—not of a product to eat but of a just-picked tomato.

While Eric talks business, Anna and I chat about the organics debate. At the same time organic foods are becoming increasingly popular—the market is growing 20 percent each year and passed $5 billion in sales last year—consumers are getting mixed messages.[44] Critics argue that organics are no better, no different, than conventional foods. Anna and I imagine trying to prove that these heirloom tomatoes have more vitamins and minerals than the hard, flavorless ones we could buy down the street. But is that the only point?

The people we meet remind us what eating organic food is also about. Regardless of quantifiable difference in nutrients, it *is* healthier to eat organic food. It's healthier for the soil and water, for our bodies, and for the farmers and farmworkers who tend crops free from chemicals.

As Anna and I talk, a swarm of kindergartners rush by with their teachers in tow. Eric tells us that many schools take their students to the market to expose them to fresh foods. With farmers' markets nationwide up by more than two-thirds to about 3,000 in just the last six years, more and more kids, like those giddily weaving in between raspberry, pickle, and apple stands, will have this opportunity.[45]

But, we remind ourselves, most Americans still don't have access to organic, locally grown food at local farmers' markets. Many don't even have organic foods in their local grocery stores, and many more can't afford them if they do. We remind ourselves that, in the solve-for-pattern spirit, answers to how to ensure access for all will come only as we weave together many disparate pieces, as the Madisonians are showing us.

If Adriana from Belo Horizonte, Brazil, were here, Anna says, she'd be clear: Answers will come as we realize that if the market isn't working—if it's preventing people from being able to feed themselves, and feed themselves healthy and fresh food—we as a society must step in. There's an economic aspect of citizenship, Adriana would say, calling on society to make sure everyone has income to buy quality food, and making sure this food is readily accessible to all.

Answers will come as we continue to develop and support creative initiatives like the ones Anna and I have learned about, from Madison's Partner Shares to the ex-convicts' garden in San Francisco to other efforts linking farms to homeless shelters and food banks. Or like Just Food in New York City, where low-income community-based groups work *with* community-supported agriculture farms, helping their members access and afford CSA participation.[46]

The answers will come, as René Louail in France suggests, by shifting our taxpayer money, now disproportionately going to large-farm, industrial agriculture, to assist instead our country's smaller farms and to support a transition to organic, sustainable agriculture.

And, at the same time, solutions will arise as those who don't have options like CSAs and who *can* afford to pay the higher price for local, organic food get educated. Some Americans are, after all, finding the extra money to spring for the designer label or the SUV or the latest cell phone. For many, disposable income is not the obstacle. It's that we haven't yet learned to see price accurately. When we walk into a store and there's a choice between organic and locally grown or non-organic food shipped thousands of miles, what do we see? We can learn to see the invisible cost of the apparently cheaper choice. We can grasp what Jean-Yves Griot teaches: the full, but still invisible, cost of today's chemical agriculture.

I'm coming to see that, for many of us, paying for organic and local food isn't a financial decision; it's an emotional one. It's about defining who we are. It's whether buying organic, shopping at places like Willy Street, make us *feel good*—good that we're keeping families on the land, good that we're loving our own families better by avoiding chemicals, good that we're respecting ourselves enough to eat healthfully. And knowledge about the impact of our choices, as Jack Kloppenburg reminded Anna and me, can change what makes us feel good.

COWBOY HATS ARE FLYING

By the time Anna and I get to the airport, we're bursting with images of the ways people's lives here are interweaving, how their efforts are building on one another, how Odessa's coral reef is growing—and it doesn't stop at the airport.

The last boarding call announced, our indefatigable guide—doctoral student and food-citizenship promoter extraordinaire Sharon Lezberg—is still feeding us more.

"But wait, I haven't told you about . . ." she says, handing us still more pamphlets and papers and notes. Our bulging backpacks fill even more, and we think of Odessa's parting words: "This is a region with a mission."

Once on the plane, the farmers'-market tomatoes permanently in our taste buds, Anna and I talk about how the experience in Madison confounded our expectations. How stirring it's been to meet Americans who'd grown up bombarded with the same messages of me-first consumerism that we had, but who are, nonetheless, choosing their own vision of community.

Anna tells me it's a story from Jim Goodman, one of the farmers we met, that captures the essence of this place for her.

"Jim had a neighbor, a guy who thought of himself as a 'real' farmer," Anna says. "When this guy was working the crops near the road, he would always wear his cowboy hat—even in bitter-cold Wisconsin winters. He wanted to seem tough." Anna ducks her head in close and whispers, for dramatic effect, "But when he was back in the fields where he thought no one could see him, he'd take off the cowboy hat and put on a warm, wool one.

"It takes courage to get rid of the cowboy hat," Anna says. "It's the kind of courage we all need—courage to be true to ourselves.

"Just think of the Sharps and the looks they must have gotten. I can imagine the jokes: 'Nurses! Farming?' Think of the Perkinses, who risked it all to try their hand at community-supported agriculture, or Odessa, who almost lost everything building her dream. And think of all the farmers using organic and sustainable methods when the flashy farming magazines and top-dollar advertisements tell them it's backward and old-fashioned.

"Cowboy hats are flying!"

UNITED STATES: AWAKENING OUR SENSES

Fresh Peapod and Rice Salad

CRYSTAL LAKE GARDENS AND GEORGE RIGGIN, FROM THE *Food for Thought Cookbook*, MADISON, WISCONSIN

Serves 4   *Pack this for a picnic supper or a pot-luck get-together. The whole is surprisingly greater than its simple parts. This is a quick and easy recipe—proving that healthy eating can also be convenient.*

¾ cup uncooked wild rice or 6 ounces long-grain and wild rice mix

1½ cups broccoli, chopped

⅓ cup slivered almonds

⅓ cup red onion (1 very small) or scallions (the white and light green parts of about a bunch), sliced

¼ cup of your favorite Italian salad dressing

1 tablespoon lemon juice (1 small lemon)

½ teaspoon lemon pepper

1½ cups edible peapods (snap peas)

Prepare rice. Cool slightly.

Steam broccoli until crunchy-tender. (Feel free to substitute uncooked sweet peppers for the broccoli, or to use half steamed broccoli and half raw peppers to add color.)

Lightly toast slivered almonds on pan in toaster-oven (about 3 to 5 minutes at 350° F). Watch carefully so that they don't burn.

Toss broccoli, rice, and almonds with remaining ingredients and refrigerate 2 to 24 hours.

THE HOMECOMING

TRAVELING
THE EDGE
OF POSSIBILITY

The tree that moves some to tears of joy is in the eyes
Of others only a green thing that stands in the way.

Some see nature all ridicule & deformity . . .
& some scarce see nature at all.

But to the eyes of the man of imagination,
Nature is imagination itself.

As a man is so he sees.

WILLIAM BLAKE, 1799[1]

With our book deadline only a month away, I pull into my dad's place in Vermont for a visit. Climbing out of my little white car, I see his neighbor approaching. "Your dad says you're writing a new book with your daughter. What's it about?" she asks.

I pause barely a second and one word pops out: "Perception."

"Oh," she says, looking confused, "I thought it was something about food and hunger again."

So I try my best to explain. "Actually, it is, but this time we're writing about solutions—the ones emerging all around us. Only we can't see them because they don't fit our expectations, what we're taught to see. We're writing about the unexpected."

Whenever I think about how difficult it is to see the world anew, I'm thrown back to an evening a decade ago. I sat listening to a learned Harvard professor explain to her rapt audience how 18th-century Europeans experienced such a shift in perception—how they finally let go of the notion of the divine right of kings. Pulling out my notebook, I awaited the juicy historical detail. My eyes blinked when she said simply, "They stopped believing in it."

Spunky answer, but I know of course that people didn't "stop believing" overnight. And we won't stop giving our power away to Monsanto, Microsoft, or a mystified market overnight either. We humans, as Erich Fromm reminds us, do seem to fall with ease under the "spell of irrational doctrines."[2] The trait shouldn't surprise us; after all, human beings have a deep need to make sense of our world. We need what Fromm calls a "frame of orientation" or what Anna and I call a "mental map."

But if our mental map blinds us, binds us—telling us, for instance, to bow down to an almighty king—how do we come to believe that something else is possible; to see with new eyes? The people in this book suggest an answer.

On Dissonance and Entry Points

If we're lucky, or if we stretch, or if life simply hits us over the head with the proverbial two-by-four, we can each experience that moment of internal dissonance introduced in *Chapter 1: Maps of the Mind*. It's that feeling that something just doesn't fit right anymore. Something doesn't match up.

A "shift in perception" can sound pretty innocuous. But sometimes the dissonance it takes to jolt us out of a limiting mental map can hurt. Sometimes it's a crisis.

For John Kinsman in Wisconsin, it took lying in a hospital bed with lifeless limbs before he questioned dominant, chemical-drenched industrial farming. For his fellow farmer Jim Miller, it took his father's painful death from cancer. For René Louail in Brittany, it took the seizure of his farm by an agribusiness company. For Negi Singh in India, it took a sinking feeling that his work lacked meaning. For Muhammad Yunus in Bangladesh, it took the shock of walking by starving people and realizing that his teaching did nothing to end the tragedy. For Cathrine Sneed in California, it took a life-threatening kidney disease before she stopped and let the message of *The Grapes of Wrath* sink in.

After such moments—we all have had them, or will—what happens next? Do we grit our teeth, stuff our dis-ease, and go on? And, if we don't . . . if we let ourselves experience the discomfort, what do we do with it?

As we emphasized from the beginning of the book, we need a practical way to *act* on our new sense of possibility. We need a way to "get off the bus," as Wangari would tell us, and climb onto one that's headed in a direction we ourselves have chosen. *We need an entry point.*

In Brazil, the entry point for the landless is, understandably, getting one's own land. From there, formerly voiceless peasants begin together to ask: "What kind of community," and, even, "What kind of Brazil, do we want?" In Wisconsin, the entry point is healthy food and saving the family farm, and from there a multifaceted reweaving of city and countryside begins to emerge. In India, the entry point is the seed, as farmers reclaim indigenous knowledge, and from there they begin to question government and corporate-promoted farming practices.

But the lesson of these stories isn't to *wait* for moments of dissonance to strike. As has been true for so many we met, by simply taking action we create dissonance; we put ourselves in a new place.

Kenyan village women began planting trees with Green Belt; only then did they start to see with new eyes. Suddenly, the forests near their villages became theirs, as public land should be; suddenly, the encroaching desert became something reversible, not inevitable; suddenly, the government became something they could challenge, not a dictatorship to endure; suddenly, hunger became something they could ameliorate by creating their own food security. Each of these realizations, these moments of dissonance, pushed them on.

But what if we haven't experienced such dissonance personally or discovered an entry point? Fortunately, we're social beings, and that means we learn through each other. We can use these stories, these people, as wedges into our consciousness, as ways to create dissonance within ourselves even though we haven't had their experiences directly. We can use others' experience to see entry points that we never knew were there, right before our noses. By telling their stories, we confess, Anna and I are not-so-secretly hoping to trigger vicarious dissonance!

Springing Free from the Thought Traps

But breaking free isn't easy, because we absorb the dominant mental map like invisible ether. Its thought traps tell a powerful story, locking us into certain ways of seeing.

They tell us we face unending scarcity, and if we just keep focused on producing more we'll be able to survive. They tell us our nature is to be selfish and cutthroat, and that's what has made us king of the mountain. They tell us our species' progress lies in ever-more-sophisticated technology and in experts who solve problems by dissecting them into their smallest pieces. Most powerfully, these thought traps tell us we've happily arrived, thank God, at the end of history, settling in globally to a corporate capitalist system that is the best we could design.

The people we met tell a different story.

Amazingly, the *burkah*-cloaked, soft-spoken women of Bangladesh, the kids sharing kale in Berkeley, the guitar-thumping, hand-clapping families in Brazil, the pesto-munching farmers in Wisconsin all have something in common—they all show us the chinks in this mental map.

By revealing the falsity of its thought traps, but more importantly, by giving us something else to believe in, they spring us free. Not with blueprints for an ersatz utopia but through real-world examples of different ways to build economies and organize communities—of transformations we're all capable of experiencing. Thankfully so, as the tragic consequences of the dominant mental map become more evident each day.

Toss out the old thought traps, and the world looks entirely different. After seven months spinning around the globe, we've never found it easier to see the destructiveness of our old mental map and the beauty of new organizing principles emerging. The people we met are, through their lives, communicating what Anna and I have come to perceive as five liberating ideas, powerful antidotes to the five thought traps of the dominant map.

These freeing ideas are arising from parallel experiences of people all over our planet, mostly people who have never met and likely never will. But together they confirm that a new mental map is taking shape, one that thirty years ago seemed about as likely as the Berlin Wall falling, Nelson Mandela becoming South Africa's president, or vegan "hot dogs" selling briskly at Dodger Stadium in Los Angeles.

FIVE LIBERATING IDEAS HELPING US FIND OUR WAY

Unimaginable thirty years ago, the emerging mental map allows each of us to find meaning in our own lives, healing our planet and ourselves.

ONE: SCRAPPING THE SCARCITY SCARE, REALIZING ABUNDANCE

Cutting through the scarcity illusion, we're able to see potential abundance all around us, even in what is now waste. We realize that growing food in ways that sustain the earth and people is not only productive but linked to the changes essential to slowing population growth.

TWO: LAUGHING AT THE CARICATURE, LISTENING TO OURSELVES

Now we can see that the image of ourselves as merely selfish materialists is but a shabby caricature of our true nature. We would never have survived as a species if it wasn't for our need—and our capacity—for effectiveness and connection.

THREE: PUTTING TOOLS IN THEIR PLACE, TAPPING THE SAVVY OF CITIZENS

Now we can turn technologies—even the market itself—into tools, not tyrants. Scientific tools can help us—but only when citizens draw values' boundaries for their application.

FOUR: DISCARDING DISSECTION, SOLVING FOR PATTERN

Now breakthroughs in science and technology allow us to perceive the interrelatedness of diverse problems and their solutions. We have the tools to build on nature's genius and tap the best of ancient wisdom. We can also see more clearly the power in the ripples our own choices make in solving the world's problems.

FIVE: BUSTING FREE FROM "ISMS," CREATING THE PATH AS WE WALK

Now it's clear that global corporate capitalism—economic life cut off from community life—is not inevitable, nor fixed, nor the best we can do. Millions are letting go of all "isms"—ideologies with one unchanging endpoint. They're re-embedding the market in values respecting nature, culture, and themselves.

Liberating Idea One: Scrapping the scarcity scare, realizing abundance. Discovering that we humans create the very scarcity we fear was the irony that launched my life's quest. I saw how human beings, operating from fear, got locked into the narrow view that the only way to solve hunger is to conquer scarcity, and the only way to do that is by endless interventions to boost output. Yet, despite thirty years of myth-shattering evidence, narrowly focused scarcity-fighting continues.

While writing this chapter, we pick up the morning paper to find a long feature on Ingo Potrykus, co-inventor of a bioengineered rice containing Vitamin A. It's dubbed "golden rice" because three new genes, two of them from daffodils, give the rice color. Ingo Potrykus, who experienced hunger himself as a child, is convinced he's found a solution to another scarcity problem. Vitamin A deficiency, he says, causes 3,500 children to die every day.[3]

Ingo sounds like one of the most dedicated and caring people you'd ever meet. But there's one thing wrong with this picture: There is no scarcity of Vitamin A in the world! It is abundant in carrots, spinach, papaya, and leafy green vegetables—leaves of amaranth, coriander, curry, radish, and other foods historically common in, for example, the Indian diet.[4] What's lacking is not a new $100 million intervention to put Vitamin A inside rice.[5] What's lacking is people's access to foods already rich in the nutrient.

To the people we met on our journey, this fact is obvious; they've broken the grip of the scarcity trap to see solutions with fresh eyes. In Bangladesh, Muhammad Yunus told us he rejected an offer from an international aid agency for Vitamin A supplements for Grameen borrowers. "I didn't feel good about it," he said. "If I can encourage people to eat vegetables, that will be a much better solution." Now, one of Grameen's sixteen Decisions—the pledges the borrowers make before receiving a loan—is that they will grow kitchen gardens. In India, Navdanya is promoting the sharing of seeds of foods rich in Vitamin A. And in Kenya, Karangathe and the Green Belt Movement are introducing gunnysack gardens, so leafy greens again grow within arms' reach of villagers' cooking pots.

SEEING ABUNDANCE

Breaking free from the scarcity trap, many are seeing abundance where thirty years ago we saw scarcity; resources where before we saw waste.

Official UN tallies of food that is actually available tell us we have only 2,000 calories a day for every person on the planet—sufficient, but only barely, for us all to survive.[6] Sounds precarious! But more and more people now recognize the abundance such an estimate hides.

It's so low in part because every day, for every man woman and child alive, 1,700 calories in grain are going to livestock, which at best can return only 400 calories to us in meat.[7] Since almost half the world's grain now goes to animals, even modest shifts toward plant-based diets would free up vast resources.

And, happily, research since *Diet for a Small Planet* has confirmed that such a shift is best for our health, reducing risk of disease and lengthening lives, as we outlined in *Chapter 2: The Delicious Revolution*. Investigators have even found a plant-centered diet can help *reverse* the disease process. Heart disease is America's number-one killer, but because a plant-food diet is free of cholesterol and is very low in saturated fat, it can actually undo artery blockage.[8] So, rather than sacrifice, with new eyes we see returning to plant-centered diets as a step toward that which we all desire: better health.

And we can also see more clearly how our fear-fed fixation on producing more blinds us to what is already available if we reduce other losses.

It's estimated that 1,400 calories per person per day are lost during distribution, and in other ways, such as food rotting in storage or being tossed into restaurant dumpsters. That's more than half of our food energy needs—and all of it gone.[9]

And, what is waste and what is potential abundance, anyway? Remember, in Belo Horizonte, Brazil, everyone considered eggshells and manioc leaves nothing but garbage until the city turned this "waste" into fabulously nutritious supplements for flour to feed hungry kids and moms-to-be.

A narrow production focus, it's now clear, also diverts us from realizing the abundance available by tapping existing knowledge of how to avoid losing crops to pests. Today, pests ruin half of our crops worldwide, according to one leading entomologist.[10] Yet knowledge of natural pest control is growing rapidly, and it could make much of the food now munched by critters available for all of us.

Other unseen abundance lies in the uncultivated, wild foods that rural people eat. Across the African continent, for example, rural people consume more than 500 wild plants, but none of these make it into official consumption estimates.[11] In Kenya, it's also unlikely that food like that grown in the gunnysack gardens we saw, providing vital nutrients to villagers' diets, make it into UN statistics.

The scarcity lens also means we don't recognize what should be most obvious: that paying farmers low prices—with real prices for grain sinking by two-thirds since the '50s—itself depresses production. On average, all commodities, save fuel, now fetch for farmers *less than half* as much as they did when I wrote the first *Diet,* and one-third what they did at the beginning of the century.[12] If, as economics Nobel laureate Amartya Sen reminds us, falling prices to farmers put a brake on production, what abundance might we see if farmers received a fair return and were encouraged to use sustainable methods?[13]

Over the years, in debates with those who see humanity facing imminent absolute scarcity, one common argument I've heard goes like this: If we tended the earth with the care we should, some of us would have to starve. If we were to "go organic," the head of the world's largest agribusiness firm, Syngenta, recently warned, we'd face an "enormous food deficit."[14]

In effect, this scarcity mindset is telling us, we have no choice but to continue along the destructive chemical path; if we want to eat now, we can't worry about protecting the earth for future generations. But, as Anna and I learned on our journey, this is a false tradeoff.

What thirty years ago I had hoped was true has since been shown to be. We can grow food, generate healthy soil, and protect biodiversity and water resources, *all at the same time.* I think of Jafri's work with Navdanya farmers in India or of Roland Bunch's breakthroughs in Central America.

"We're just beginning to fathom the full potential," Roland told me from his home in Honduras. "We're learning to imitate the highly productive, millions-of-years-old humid tropical forest to be productive and sustainable here. We should have guessed this all along," he said. Using this approach, farmers whom Roland worked with in Guatemala when I first met him in the 1970s are now achieving yields eleven times greater than they did then.

Roland's discoveries, combining traditional wisdom with the latest science, dovetail what's called "Grow Biointensive" farming, which began in the U.S. about thirty years ago. Horticulturalist Alan Chadwick introduced the approach, based on thousands-of-years-old principles, and since then John Jeavons and his Ecology Center in California have developed it further. Its principles are now being used in more than one hundred countries.[15]

Chemical, mechanized farming in the U.S. uses about three-fourths of an acre to feed one person, but the Jeavons group reports that Grow Biointensive can provide a healthy, diverse plant-food diet without chemicals using as little as one-fifth to one-tenth of an acre. Water use is way down, too; the method requires only one-third to one-eighth as much as industrial-style farming, depending on the crop. Part of the Grow Biointensive genius also lies in carefully linking land use with optimal nutritional output. "Compared to what we thought we could achieve thirty years ago," John tells us, "we've found we can feed a person a healthy plant diet on half as much land."

What Nature Has to Teach

With measly resources devoted to developing sustainable methods—compared to the billions flowing toward chemical agriculture—and in almost no time, we can already document their enormous promise.

Interestingly, one of the biggest "experiments" in sustainable farming began not by design but by a twist of history. With the collapse of the Soviet Union, suddenly Cuba was cut off from its source of pesticides (used by its farmers at twice the intensity of those in the U.S.) and other ingredients of industrial-style farming, including petroleum. It was clear: Go organic or starve. Now, 60 percent of Cuba's non-sugar acres are organic. And urban gardens— with vegetable production doubling or tripling each year since 1994—supply 60 percent of all vegetables consumed in the country.[16]

In the previous chapter, we mentioned the release of the first global survey of the sustainable farming initiatives. Yet while the media bursts this year with stories about the battle over GMOs, not to mention foot-and-mouth disease, we've seen not a single news item reporting the survey's striking findings—findings that suggest the promise of sustainable practices.

In fact, one of the strongest impressions Anna and I share as we end this journey is how *little* we humans yet know about the consequences of the scarcity mindset's focus on extracting every ounce from the earth. How little we know about what it might mean to truly listen to nature. How little we know about the earth we depend on.

We're told, for example, that there's really no nutritional advantage to food grown without chemicals. But what do we really know?

Dick Thompson, a farmer in Boone, Iowa, who had stopped applying chemicals more than thirty years ago, told me that, working with university researchers, he learned that his soil contains twice the organic matter and sixty times the number of earthworms per acre, compared to his neighbor's chemically treated fields. He also compared the roots of his organically grown corn with that of his neighbor's and found his to be more extensive. Do we really know the implications of these differences?

Both he and his wife Sharon laughed as they told me of their surprise when they left both corn plants in the yard, and mice soon devoured the organic corn but rejected that grown with chemicals. It was untouched! "Mice must know something that people don't," they joked.

In the last thirty years, scientists have discovered an entire domain of life, Archaea, one that may hold as much complexity and diversity as that containing all plants, animals, and fungi. This before-unknown domain, like that called bacteria, has no nuclei. It shows up in unique niches, like the hot pools in Yellowstone, but also in great abundance on the roots of plants—that is, on those roots found in organic but not in chemically treated soils. Scientists are still getting to the bottom of what Archaeal microbes on plant roots do, but many suspect that they may mediate the flow of minerals and nutrients and fend off pathogens.[17] As one scientist learning from Archaea said in 1998, "Five years ago, we were very confident and arrogant in our ignorance. Now we are starting to see the true complexity of life."[18]

We mention the Archaea discovery only to underscore how little we know, which should alert all of us to be wary of interventionist strategies, like chemical pesticides and genetic engineering, that disrupt natural systems instead of working with nature's wisdom. But to manifest the potential of this approach, we will have to break free of all five thought traps. Before tackling the remaining four, however, there's a second dimension of rethinking scarcity to consider.

KNOWLEDGE ABUNDANCE

The people we met are discovering that knowledge, if freed from a scarcity mindset—the more for you, the less for me—results in growing abundance, too.

Their on-the-ground discovery of how to generate knowledge abundance is mirrored elsewhere. The experience of the Internet and new thinking in management are nudging this shift along as well. Students of new technology's impact see the logic of the emerging economy, centered in the Internet, as fundamentally different from the old scarcity-grounded one. The old extract-manufacture-dispose economy was driven by secrecy and exclusion—hoarding to enhance value by maintaining scarcity. The new logic, declares *Wired* magazine editor-at-large Kevin Kelly, with almost breathless excitement, turns on its head the notion that scarcity creates value: "In a network economy, value is derived from plenitude," he says.[19] He uses mundane examples, such as fax machines, to suggest that the more that exist, the more value they have to all users. Those we met feel the same way about sharing seeds: Everyone gains as diversity is enhanced.

William Ury, anthropologist and coauthor of *Getting to Yes,* plays the same note in his later book, *The Third Side.* Ury observes a vast culture change, one easy to see in new management styles. Thirty years ago, who could have imagined CEOs spending millions on team-building training seminars? Management is moving from pyramidal structures with top-down control, to networks.[20] Ury views these new management practices as reinventions of what was common in our tribal roots before agriculture. Then, we worked in flexible, self-organizing work teams; today, he notes, we're bringing back that culture.[21]

"Humanity is returning to dependence on a basic resource that is, as in hunter-gatherer times, an expandable pie,"[22] Ury argues. That resource is knowledge. Just as hunter-gatherers relied on the constant exchange of information, so, too, do all of us. Relationships are transforming because we're no longer focused on a fixed pie, but rather on what we create through sharing knowledge. "We are returning to the horizontal relationships that existed among human beings for most of human evolution," Ury writes.[23]

In our paradoxical era, however, this growing energy among executives to "flatten" corporate hierarchies, giving decision-making latitude to managers and even line workers, is matched ironically by a tightening of control over workers in other ways. Corporate leaders fight unions, cut benefits, and link reward ever more directly to output, propelled by both the fear of losing out and by the compulsion for personal accumulation that globalization fuels.

In the same paradoxical vein, while knowledge grows through sharing— as we've seen on our journey—a powerful counter-trend is gaining steam. Increasingly tied to profit-making ventures both inside and outside academia, scientists who previously shared findings freely at scientific gatherings, for example, are now closely guarded—lest a rival get the patent first. An MIT biology professor told me recently of his sadness that the tenor of professional meetings in his field has changed radically in the last decade. Too many scientists are afraid of divulging something that might be patentable. In India it was easy to see the negative potential impact of seed patenting on poor farmers in the tiny villages we visited. Now we're coming to see here in the U.S., too, the knowledge-limiting aspects of patenting plant and animal life.

Simply celebrating the emerging "knowledge society" neglects another obvious fact as well. The market offers no built-in mechanism to draw in the vast majority of the world now excluded from the plenitude Ury exalts. Most of us aren't hopping through phone calls with call waiting or surfing the Web for the latest hot idea. By last count, in fact, less than 3 percent of people living outside of the United States had Internet access, and only a small percentage of people in less-industrial countries even have access to telephones.[24]

Still—despite the counter-trends and technological exclusion of many—Ury and Kelly are onto something that we, too, found: a shift from hierarchy to network in the basic metaphor of relationship, and a spreading appreciation that knowledge and abundance grow by sharing.

In these big shifts, the greatest action is not with technology, though; it's with people, most of whom are low on the technology ladder. Those we met on our journey are just a handful of the millions of people around the world bringing about this transformation—not in boardrooms, but within communities and among them. Remember Hannes Lorenzen's network of economically disadvantaged localities throughout Europe gaining strength by coming together to share knowledge? And, Farida Akhter's group Nayakrishi in Bangladesh, working like the water hyacinth, spreading and expanding by sharing ideas, not hoarding them?

Navdanya in India is more a loose web of people with a common vision than a structured organization. And what Odessa calls the Madison-area "coral reef" is growing not because she or anyone else is orchestrating the next move, but because enough people desire human-scale community life and are sparking each other's courage and creativity to make it real.

These networks are strengthening across borders, too, we were reminded, when we were disappointed in missing José Bové in France because he was in India with thousands of protesting farmers. They are all part of Via Campesina, made up of farmers from almost forty countries, including the Landless Workers' Movement, who share a common vision of sustainable farming.

Liberating Idea Two: Laughing at the caricature, listening to ourselves. Whether this abundance talk sounds pie-in-the-sky, what mental map we carry within us—and ultimately our belief about what's possible for our planet—all depends on one thing: how we size up human nature.

And what if the only definitive thing one can say about human nature is that we love to argue about it? Well, the endlessness of this debate shouldn't make us throw up our hands. If we don't come up with our own best guess, we'll just go on absorbing the culture's caricature of ourselves as selfish materialists—a pretty ugly picture.

Anna and I are coming to see human nature not as fixed, limited to a media-fed caricature, but as full of possibility. So we were glad to see Paul

Ehrlich, author in 1969 of *The Population Bomb,* remind us that we don't have one nature. Rather, as the title of his latest book, *Human Natures,* suggests, we have capacities for a wide range of behavior—from cutthroat to beneficent—depending on what is reinforced all around us.[25]

But we're also convinced a human being is not a tabula rasa, either: Within our multiple "natures" are certain widely shared needs. And one of the things I love most about getting older is that I've seen enough, heard enough, lived enough to have an educated guess as to what they are. It's been rewarding to find that Anna, although with such different experiences and fewer years on the planet, shares the same intuition. For us, they boil down to this: *We need to feel both connected to others and useful toward ends beyond ourselves.*

Everywhere we heard this desire expressed. We heard it in Bengali, Hindi, Portuguese, and Punjabi. We heard it in French, Dutch, and KiSwahili. We heard it in German, English, and KiKuyu. We heard it from the gruff-looking Bangladesh Grameen Bank manager who spoke wistfully about working directly with poor villagers. "It was like a first love," he said. We heard it when Negi in India explained to us why he works with Vandana. "I'm working for what my heart is saying."

So it makes sense to us that scholars drawing on a wide review of anthropological findings uncover the same core needs. In *The Anatomy of Human Destructiveness,* Erich Fromm states that humans need to feel accomplishment, to know they've made a dent. "To be able to effect something," Fromm writes, "is the assertion that one is not impotent, but that one is an alive, functioning human being." In a remake of Descartes's famous maxim, "I think, therefore I am," Fromm sums up our need this way: "I am, because I effect."[26]

Contrast this need for agency with the role we increasingly play within global corporate capitalism. In it, we're diminished to passive consumer, not only in the economic realm but increasingly in the political sphere as well. Even there, we've become mere spectators, with candidates marketed to us alongside Pampers, Prozac, and Pepsi. Little wonder so many people feel that something essential to our happiness is missing in our lives.

Just as strong as this need for agency, Anna and I have come to believe, is our need to connect with others. We're not isolated egoists, social atoms, "utility maximizers," as modern economics posits. We are fundamentally *social* beings. Infants cry at the sound of others crying. Children wither if not nurtured. Isolation makes us go nuts. In fact, banishment has always been one of the harshest punishments human beings inflict on one another—from the parental shout of "Go to your room!" to the sentence of solitary confinement.

Precisely because Adam Smith has been appropriated as the godfather of self-seeking capitalism, I delight in quoting him on our social nature: "How selfish soever man may be supposed," he wrote in 1790, "there are evidently some principles in his nature, which interest him in the fortune of others, and render their happiness necessary to him, though he derives nothing from it except the pleasure of seeing it."[27]

When the guys in the Reagan White House sported Adam Smith neckties to celebrate "me-first" capitalism, you can bet they weren't thinking of this side of Smith.

But we need not rely on Smith—either Reagan's version or ours. We can choose to listen to the voices of the people featured in these pages. We can choose to listen to ourselves.

LEARNING FROM HISTORY, NOT THE MEASLY BIT WE CALL CIVILIZATION

To say anything about our basic makeup, though, shouldn't we also step back, way back, and take in the biggest, longest sweep of human existence?

Toward the end of our journey, on a windless, overcast day, Anna and I stood on gritty sand in Kenya's Rift Valley; in front of us lay dozens of hand axes. I lingered in the thick air, imagining each molecule as a year separating me from my ax-making forbears, *Homo erectus,* who shaped these crudely sharpened stones as many as two million years ago.

This vast expanse of time—the 99 percent of our species' existence during which we lived in small groups, our sustenance coming from gathered plants and hunted animals—is crucial, scientists tell us. Whatever genes shape us today we got long before the advent of agriculture. There just hasn't been enough time since for natural selection to work on us. So what *were* we like during most of our evolution?

Charles Darwin observed that among primeval people actions were no doubt judged "good or bad, solely as they obviously affect the welfare of the tribe—not that of the species, nor that of an individual member of the tribe."[28] And William Ury, after surveying recent anthropological evidence, follows the lead of anthropologist Claude Lévi-Strauss, who with dramatic flair suggests that human beings may have had only one sustainably successful way of life—as hunter-gatherers. "The key to its success lay in our ancestors' highly developed ability to cooperate," concludes Ury. "A more fitting name for our species than the 'killer ape' would be the 'cooperative ape.'"[29]

It's hard for Anna and me to imagine how our species could have survived without these twin needs: for effectiveness—to be active and accomplish something, as Fromm stresses—and for connection expressed in cooperation, as Ury emphasizes. If we're right, then, we must deny our deepest selves when we allow ourselves to be reduced to passive consumers, acquiescing to a world we feel we've never chosen.

The implications are enormous. Just think of the vast untapped human capacity for what we typically call "leadership." Isn't leadership, after all, just the combination of these two dimensions of ourselves—accomplishment through connection?

The face of Landless Workers' Movement member Antonio Capitani immediately comes to our minds, as he explained what it meant to be chosen leader of the family groups, responsible for shaping the development of a whole new community in a settlement of the formerly landless in Brazil.

Or we think of Anthony Travis in the San Francisco garden and recall his obvious pride in his role as manager of brigades planting and nurturing trees throughout the city.

Or we think of Swapna, the former student of Yunus who helped create Grameen. Motivated by a desire to be effective and to connect with women she wanted to help, Swapna didn't allow criticism rooted in cultural mores to stop her. She's the one who carried her *purdah* clothing in her bag when she visited villages, so she could always prove to the women she wanted to help that she was one of them. Over the twenty years since, Swapna has risen to a top leadership post in the Bank.

As Yunus would say, we are all bonsais, our capacities limited only by the size of the pot in which we grow.

Liberating Idea Three: Putting tools in their place, tapping the savvy of citizens. This capacity for accomplishment through connection within each of us, once we let go of the thought traps, brings us to another sweeping shift in perception in the past thirty years. It's a consequence of seeing human existence in the same light with which scientists now see the natural world: from life as divisible and hierarchical to life as an indivisible network in which every node is critical.

Suddenly, every human being has a contribution to make. We revalue the regular citizen—the non-specialist. This shift in perception is happening in so many places, in so many ways, it's hard to perceive what a radical swing it is. Everywhere the notion is under challenge that only the few with specialized knowledge, or official rank, can make decisions guiding our communities and larger societies. (The rapid demystification of experts and officials is also a reaction to feelings of shock and betrayal. Remember, thirty years ago we'd yet to experience Watergate or Three-Mile Island.)

Solutions to our biggest challenges are being found by those closest to the problem, applying their experience, values, and common sense; drawing in the expert or the authority as a partner, not as a superior.

Some see this shift reflected in the growth of civil society—registered in the explosion of nongovernmental citizen organizations worldwide. But it goes far beyond the expanding role for citizen organizations in public life. All across the United States, I've seen this new flowering of appreciation of the contribution of the "non-expert." In the '90s, I traveled from city to city interviewing dozens of "average" Americans for the book *The Quickening of America*. They helped me see how this appreciation is remaking relationships in every arena of American life. In the classroom, kids are being trained to mediate their own conflicts. In the factory, work teams are spreading. In local government, citizen assemblies are making major budget choices. In human-service agencies, patients are being enlisted in their own healing practice. Everywhere, I found the notion of the expert or boss meting out the solution to passive student or client or worker giving way to models of partnership.[30]

Every story in this book reflects this revolution in perception and practice—whether it's the Landless Workers' Movement sitting down with Brazilian government officials to work out details of land distribution, or the Conseil d'Etat in France turning to a panel of citizens to guide state policy concerning genetically modified organisms. Whether it's Indian farmers directing their own seed research, or rural Kenyan women doing what previously it was assumed only foresters could do—creating their own tree nurseries.

Only as we make this shift can we put our "tools"—from technology to economic constructs—in their place, under the watchful guidance of citizens pulling in specialized knowledge as needed.

PUTTING TOOLS IN THEIR PLACE

Humans are consummate toolmakers. We've figured out how to craft everything from shovels to spaceships, from scissors to supertankers. Because we love to make tools and use them, it's understandable that we've jumped at the notion that new tools, like bioengineered food, will save us. Neither is it so surprising that sometimes we forget to put tools in their place. We let tools rule us.

Take the market itself. It *could* be a tool. Instead, the market as rigid ideology has become a tyrant. What financier George Soros calls "market fundamentalism" has spread to virtually every patch of earth. I recall visiting China in 1987, just as communist state-run farms were being dismantled. As we walked to breakfast, loudspeakers mounted on tall poles, which only a few years before were blaring Mao's aphorisms, now were telling us: "The market is a glorious path. It will make us all wealthy!"

Globalization—opening markets, reducing government's role—is the buzzword, and in his book *The Lexus and the Olive Tree*, *New York Times* foreign affairs columnist for Thomas L. Friedman captures its power: Just as each morning the lion must run to catch its prey and the gazelle must run to escape the lion, "so it is with globalization." We all have to keep running, and "not everyone is equipped to run fast."

The message? Get out your Nikes and get in shape, because we're not in control, the market is, and some of us—those Friedman calls "the turtles"— are bound to lose.[31]

No wonder it's hard to see the market as our tool. We're told that we're simply at its mercy. But the people we met on our journey are refusing to be cowed. They're discovering ways to make the market work so it doesn't create exclusion—so it doesn't violate our deepest sensibilities, creating more hunger, slums, crime, child exploitation, prostitution, slavery, and the decimation of the natural world.

Belo Horizonte's leaders certainly didn't toss out the market when they decided that good food is a right of citizenship. Mostly, they began to devise ingenious ways to keep the market honest; to keep good food within reach of all people.

The Wisconsin farmers' cooperative, Organic Valley, is not opposed to the market. It uses the market, and even sells its milk products internationally. But the co-op, by replacing the anonymous global corporation, keeps control in the hands of farmers themselves and allows them to make sure their profits stay at home to build thriving communities.

The fair-trade movement isn't attacking the market, either. It's helping producers and consumers use it. It's reminding us: Each dollar is a vote for the world we want. Now, through green and fair-trade labeling, we can use the market to act on our values. We can, as Paul Rice says, "buycott" to protect the environment and ensure that food producers have decent incomes.

All of these developments remind us what is so easy to forget: Economic life is not about our relationships to things—like land or houses or hair dryers. It's about our relationships with each other; what norms and expectations we hold and honor.

What we see today—economic life as a distinct realm governed by the market—emerged in a blink of historical time. Throughout the sweep of human history, economic life was embedded in a web of family and community relationships, in culture and nature.[32] What we saw on our journey is a "re-embedding," as people create a new vocabulary, a new understanding that leaves behind the tired notion that we have only two choices: Either we hand over control to government or forfeit our future to a corporate-controlled market. The people we met are putting us, citizens, back on the hook! We're responsible. We can become active choosers of the world we want.

And it is happening with remarkable speed. Think of it: Thirty years ago, anyone predicting the developments chronicled here would have been considered a starry-eyed dreamer!

Liberating Idea Four: Discarding dissection, solving for pattern. As we've learned to put tools in their place, so to speak, we've also witnessed astonishing scientific breakthroughs in understanding how the natural world works. With this new knowledge and these technological advances, we can now register and measure the damage done by disconnectedly applying our tools. More than that, we can see interconnections. We can think in systems.

As I like to say, we have the "tools to go beyond tools."

I'd heard about "systems thinking" for decades, but it always struck me as a bit abstract, far removed from what I, as a nonscientist, could grasp. Now Anna and I see it emerging everywhere, from the Living Machine® servicing Bob Will's cheese factory in Wisconsin to Jean-Yves Griot's reconfiguring his farming operation in Brittany after learning that his nitrogen fertilizer was polluting the river and the drinking water.

For the first time in our evolution, we have the capacity consciously to create and function with and within whole systems. Thirty years ago, maybe this wasn't yet practical. We'd long ago lost our predecessors' intuitive, culturally passed-on grasp of natural systems—the interrelatedness of all life—drawn from eons of experience and naked-eye observation. Yet modern chemistry, mathematics, biology, and physics had not advanced far enough for us to figure out how to use science to create *with* nature, as the ancients had done, instead of disrupting and destroying it.

Today, though, something is changing. Signs are popping up everywhere.

A recent news story tells of Peruvian farmers who for centuries used the Pleiades constellation to determine when to plant their crops. But only now, with satellite data on cloud cover and water vapor available, have scientists been able to confirm that this centuries-old technique jibes with their scientific analysis. They've discovered these "star-gazing farmers" are actually accurate long-range weather forecasters.[34] Our technology finally allowed us to catch up with ancient Peruvians!

Satellite imaging is just one example of how, in the last thirty years, stunning breakthroughs in science have allowed us to stop being ruled by our tools and instead to start using our tool-making genius to serve us—to help us see and function within the natural systems of which we are part.

SEEING WHOLE SYSTEMS, "SOLVING FOR PATTERN"

On the five continents of our journey, we met people learning to see connections, to let go of one-dimensional, cause-and-effect thought traps, and to perceive a multifaceted web of causes and consequences. The parallels were striking—whether it is the citizens of Madison grasping the rich interrelationships of their food choices and the quality of community life, or the rural people of Brazil, now for the first time with land of their own, realizing the many interconnected dimensions of creating a better future for their families.

These real-life examples of thinking in whole systems are mirrored in the world of science. On our journey, we had a chance to talk with Fritjof Capra, a physicist, author, and old friend from our years in California whose life work focuses on this shift to whole-system approaches. As a founder of the Center for Ecoliteracy, whose work we highlight in *Chapter 2: The Delicious Revolution,* Fritjof has been striving to bring these abstract ideas to life. Sitting with us in the Mocha Lisa Café near the U.C. Berkeley campus toward the end of our travels, Fritjof explains patiently in a soft Austrian accent: "Yes, we're at a frightening time, witnessing the horror of environmental degradation caused by our belief that we could divide the natural world into parts and manipulate it. But it's also an incredibly exciting time, because science, like quantum physics, is showing us so dramatically that there are no parts.

"Just in the last thirty years, scientists have developed the tools to understand that living systems are self-organizing networks whose parts are interdependent. A mathematical language is even emerging—the mathematics of complexity—allowing a *non*mechanistic understanding of life. It's a mathematics of visual patterns."

As Fritjof talks, I'm struck by the irony that it took technology—high-speed computers able to solve complex nonlinear equations—before we could discover order in patterns beneath nature's seeming chaos.

Scientists have come to see beyond parts to whole systems, allowing lines between distinct disciplines to dissolve. I met a Stanford undergraduate recently whose major weaves together physics, anthropology, economics, biology, and chemistry. It's called "Biosphere"—at his age, I didn't even know the word existed.

Our journey has also reminded us what happens when, even with the best intentions, we cling to the dissection approach and refuse to see the big picture. We focus only on producing more food, and end up as in India, with mountains of grain while children continue to starve. We focus on growing more coffee in Latin America, cutting forest canopies, and end up with farmers sick from pesticides, land degraded, and migratory birds decimated. Similarly, the loss of native fish in Bangladesh or the emergence of pest resistance in the Indian Punjab are symptoms of solving by dissection, not for pattern.

Continuing high birthrates are one of the world's most dramatic examples of failure to solve for pattern. To treat seriously the threat of overpopulation means to address the interwoven roots of population growth—as people described in this book are doing. It means perceiving new connections: Historically, fertility rates have fallen when people, especially women, have access to education, to jobs, and to food to feed their families. When Grameen borrowers began to advance, for example, their family size shrank. In Kenya, the younger women discovering their power through the Green Belt Movement told us how pleased they are to be able to choose to have small families.

Fritjof helped Anna and me see how, in the last thirty years, new concepts and techniques have enabled scientists to shift, as he puts it, "from seeing objects to seeing relationships, from quantity to quality, from substance to pattern."[34] The shift within science is mirrored in the lives of all the people we encountered on our journey. Anna and I can't help but be struck by how similar even Fritjof's choice of words is to those of Hannes, Jean-Yves, the MST farmers. Really, almost everyone we met.

Liberating Idea Five: Busting free from "isms," creating the path as we walk.

Of the five thought traps, Anna and I have come to see the last as perhaps the most paralyzing. It's the notion that what we see today is the grand culmination of human experimentation.

We've tried everything else, and it's all flopped. Thomas Friedman writes: "Communism, socialism, fascism—that promised to take the sting out of capitalism . . . have been discredited." He concludes that we can't really "soften the brutality of capitalism" if we want steadily rising standards of living.[35] It's all we've got if we want the goods.

No, say the people we met this year. Global corporate capitalism is not the best we can do. It is evolving—rapidly, in fact—in two contradictory directions at once.

In one, economic life is being torn farther and farther from the democratic fold. As the pace of corporate mergers quickens, private entities gain more power over our well-being—over jobs, the environment, health care—than elected governments have.

Hearing only of the "magic of the market," as Ronald Reagan loved to call it, we're blinded to the irony that corporate-controlled capitalism actually *undercuts* the market. It destroys the conditions necessary for it to serve us. For the market to work, sellers can't be big enough to influence prices; buying power must be widely spread so our dollar-votes reflect the needs of all of us, not merely the desires of a few; participants must have full information about goods and prices; and sellers must carry the full costs of production, passing them on in prices.[36]

In today's world, with a few corporations dominant within virtually every industry, *none* of these conditions holds. That's what we mean when we say that global corporate capitalism is violating its own rules and thereby destroying the market.

Today, for instance, just ten multinational corporations account for more than half of all food and drink sales in the U.S. That means much of our food fate rests with a handful of people—just 117 men and twenty-one women who serve on the boards of these companies.[37]

And the size of these corporations gives them the capacity to shape the market, making it ever less "free." They can influence government policy, as we saw in the case of the USDA's dietary guidelines. And they can dominate media advertising, for example, to continue to fuel sales of high-fat, high-sugar, processed food—even though overeating a nutrient-poor diet has become a national health crisis. Considering *all* industries—not just food—Coke and McDonald's rank among the world's top ten biggest spenders on advertising.[38]

Since business law evolved hand in hand with narrowing corporate control, most corporate action shaping markets is, *technically*, legal. But with so much power in so few hands, it's not surprising that legal lines get crossed. In 1996, for example, senior executives of Archer Daniels Midland—"supermarket to the world," as ADM describes itself—were charged with price-fixing to rig world markets, costing consumers millions in higher prices. ADM, the world's largest soybean processor and food-additive maker, pleaded guilty, paying one of the largest antitrust fines in American history—$100 million.[39] Today, its almost $19 billion in annual sales suggest that this hand-slap didn't cause ADM to skip a beat. With the market clout that its size alone affords, ADM can profit without breaking the law.

A year before the company's indictment, even ADM's chairman, Dwayne Andreas, acknowledged, "There is not one grain of anything in the world that is sold in the free market. Not one. The only place you see a free market is in the speeches of politicians."[40]

Re-embedding

But in our paradoxical time, powerful forces are pushing the other way, too. These forces are infusing social goods beyond private profit into a system we've long been told would be ruined by such tampering. They're showing how to make the market a tool, not a tyrant, and proving that economic life can be rewoven into the democratic fold. They are evolving capitalism as we know it, with examples arising in many forms.

- Only a few decades ago, redistributing land to the landless was deemed utterly anti-capitalist. Passé at best, "pinko" at worst. "Shouldn't the market decide who gets land?" the thinking went. But Brazil's Landless Workers' Movement (MST) has proven that land redistribution can play a role in making the market work, making it more inclusive—even helping end hunger. In Brazil, babies in MST settlements suffer death rates that are half the national average; their members control their own businesses and farms, earning incomes well above the minimum wage.[41] Even international agencies like the World Bank are starting to acknowledge the effectiveness of land reform in promoting economic and social health.

· Society's understanding of the roles of owner and investor within capitalism is changing, too. At the birth of the corporate form in the 1800s, its responsibility to the public good was clear, but it was lost soon thereafter. Most stock ownership came to have nothing to do with exercising real ownership responsibilities, certainly not responsibility to the wider community.

Now many are seeking to reinstate the corporation's wider accountability. Bangladesh's Grameen mutual fund is a clever way to do just that. The fund not only makes money for its investors but also safeguards the social mission of the companies in which it invests, including the dozen that Grameen itself has created and the thousands of businesses its loans have spawned.

And the practice of taking seriously the responsibility of ownership is beginning to go global—in part through the growing clout of pension funds. In the last few years, pension funds, which have an interest in long-term payoff, not quick profits, have come to own on average more than 15 percent of shares in twenty-five of the world's largest corporations. This share size is more than enough, experts say, to exert significant influence over corporate decisions—to have the kind of power we associate with *real,* not paper, ownership. With this power, some pension funds are starting to push the companies they own to see environmentally- and socially-positive policies as part of sound long-term profit-seeking. The California public employees' retirement fund, for instance, recently began using broad social-responsibility criteria to screen all its investments.[42]

· Another rapidly-changing dimension of ownership could also strengthen corporate accountability: Worker-ownership closes the gap between capital and labor—another "no-no" to those clinging to a fixed notion of how capitalism best functions. Lest we think the idea of borrower-owners, as in Grameen, is way out in left field, note that, in at least six major U.S. industries, worker-owned firms—including United Parcel Service—now rank in the top five. And, in the last thirty years, the number of people owning stock in their own companies, through broad-based employee ownership programs, grew from less than one million to almost 20 million, with worker-owned firms generally outperforming others.[43]

- One fast-growing strategy that individuals are using to influence corporate behavior is to reward responsible companies by selectively investing in them. An acquaintance on Wall Street helping investors direct their money according to their values told me he couldn't even utter the words "social investment" fifteen years ago without being laughed at. Today, nearly one out of every eight investment dollars is placed according to the explicit values criteria of investors—rising from $62 billion in 1985 to $2.16 trillion in 1999.[44] (Interestingly, by 1999, genetic engineering ranked second only to arms manufacturing on the "what to avoid" list among those seeking socially sound places to invest their money.[45])

  The most potent social investing, however, means putting one's money directly into specific efforts that are transforming communities and restoring the environment. Shorebank in Chicago, which collaborated with Muhammad Yunus in creating Grameen, has been using its investors' money directly to vitalize low-income communities, and in the last four years has built a partnership with EcoTrust in the Pacific Northwest to create what they call a "conservation economy."[46]

- Other corporations are redefining themselves—not because their owners are suddenly acting like *real* owners and demanding accountability, but because management is discovering that reducing the company's impact on the environment and treating workers fairly is good business. When I first heard about it six years ago, The Natural Step, an organization helping fold environmental sustainability into corporate decision making, seemed like a pipe dream.[47] Today, more than seventy large corporations use The Natural Step's principles. Its poster child, the world's largest commercial floor-covering company, Interface, Inc., used The Natural Step to redefine itself starting in 1994. That's when Interface founder Ray Anderson experienced his moment of dissonance, suddenly and painfully made aware of the environmental impact of his business— that carpets, for instance, will typically take 20,000 years to decompose in landfills. Dissonance triggered innovation: He started making carpets in sections so just the worn part can be removed— and recycled. Today, Interface even has a solar-powered factory.[48]

Ray underscored the enormity of the challenge and the need for clear measures of success when he explained that, despite his commitment to reduce his company's impact on the environment to zero, so far he's only achieved one-third of his goal of zero environmental impact.

These varied initiatives suggest that, ultimately, the legal structure of the corporate charter will have to be remade, returning the corporation to its original purpose of service to the broad public good. Other emerging trends are working as well to reconnect economic life with community values.

- The Proposed Tobin taxes on currency speculation, for example, which we learned about from Susan George in Paris, could redirect corporate capitalism's wealth toward socially useful ends. Who would have thought that, in only a few years' time, the approach, although not enacted, would be endorsed by several legislative bodies from Canada to Finland to India?

- The growing vigor of civil society organizations worldwide, now increasingly linked through the Internet, is also proving that even global corporations are not immune to old-fashioned citizen pressure.

  Monsanto's grip on 85 percent of all genetically modified germ plasm didn't shield it from stockholder revolt when, in the late nineties, Europeans began to reject the use of GMOs in their food. Monsanto's stock price hit the floor before the company was absorbed into the giant Pharmacia. Following the Starlink debacle—when the nonprofit Friends of the Earth discovered that GMO corn deemed unfit for humans had crossed into our food— the offending company, Aventis, fired key executives and began negotiations to sell its agrochemical business.

  W. R. Grace—remember the attempted co-patenter of neem we heard about in New Delhi?—had to file for bankruptcy in 2001 after spending almost $2 billion against hundreds of personal-injury lawsuits related to asbestos.

  And, in the largest-ever antitrust lawsuit (except perhaps for that against Microsoft), fifteen of the biggest antitrust law firms in the U.S. took action last year against big agrochemical companies on behalf of U.S. and French farmers. They charge Monsanto—and

WHAT YOU CAN'T SEE

How many of us get to spend face-to-face time with ordinary citizens on continents across the globe? Not many. And until this book, neither had I. So, we depend on other people's stories, other people's interpretations. Last year I remember reading Thomas Friedman's *The Lexus and the Olive Tree* ravenously. But when I recently reread his bold claims, I read with new eyes.

This two-time Pulitzer Prize–winner declares that there is no "mass popular opposition to globalization." What little there is, puny and unorganized as it may be, uses crime to express its discontent. A key part of his proof? The Brazilian Sem Teto movement.

Sem Teto, Portuguese for "those without roofs," Friedman reports, is a movement of three and a half million peasants whose members live in encampments by the sides of roads, and who rob banks and steal trucks. They have "no flag, no manifesto." Sem Teto, and, by his extrapolation, all those hurt by globalization, "have only their unmet needs and aspirations." That's why they're "just grabbing what they need . . . and not worrying about the theory or ideology."[49]

You see, Friedman had already concluded that there are only two types of people left: those who "want to go to Disney World" and the few so angry that they can't clamber fast enough "to the barricades." With this frame,

"non-indicted co-conspirators" including Novartis, Dow, and DuPont—with using biotech patents to seize monopoly control of world agricultural markets. Their goal: an injunction barring Monsanto from selling patented genetically engineered seeds.[48]

The media consistently depicts protest against corporate globalization as visionless—as knee-jerk negative, even so parochial and backward as to oppose the exchange of goods, ideas, and practices across cultures. In our experience, nothing could be further from the truth. These initiatives are not simply reactive; they involve heightened interchange across cultures, and they reflect the creative evolution of capitalism taking myriad forms in multiple places.

Friedman literally can't see the millions who want to do neither, and who believe they are building something better than either.

So, Friedman couldn't see what we saw in Brazil: The Landless Workers' Movement with its explicit alternative to corporate globalization—with millions of members turning idle land into small farms and cooperatives. He couldn't see the children I played with who are learning to believe in themselves and find joy outside of consumer culture. He couldn't see Izabel talking about the Movement's philosophy of gender equality, or João Pedro explaining their ideology.

I have to hand it to Friedman, though. He does acknowledge that, like every good journalist, he has a superstory—a lens through which he understands the world. His superstory is that there is no mass popular opposition to corporate globalization. And that's what he found.

When we asked, Friedman told us he hadn't heard of the Landless Workers' Movement when he wrote his book. That this award-winning journalist could be unaware of one of the largest social movements in Latin America and even get basic facts wrong—Sem Teto is actually an urban homeless movement—suggests the power of a superstory. Sadly, Friedman's blinds him, and thus his many readers, to perhaps the most promising developments not just in Brazil, but everywhere on our small planet.

—Anna

The prevailing mental map promises that globalization—the shorthand for giving corporate dominance a free hand, undermining democratic governance and, ironically, the market itself—is the best we've got, and most of us are happy with that map. Here in these pages we've offered another map, one of a different sort. It is woven from insights of people we met all over the world.

Every culture has a map determining what is esteemed and what isn't, what is valued and what is neglected. The question is not whether we have a map, but whether it is life-serving.

When anthropologist Ruth Benedict surveyed her life's work and asked the biggest question—why some societies have been effective and peaceful while others are plagued by conflict—she discovered something we think is pretty telling. Weighing multiple variables, Benedict finally came to see that only one aspect of these cultures consistently distinguished them. In the more conflictive cultures, individuals gained prestige by accumulating goods or acting in other ways benefiting themselves alone, whereas in the better-functioning cultures, the status of individuals rose or fell according to their contribution to the whole.[50]

Many times during our world tour, we thought about Benedict's findings. In the dominant map—now driven by global media—increasingly we lift up for highest esteem and reward the self-seeking, just as did the conflict-ridden, hardscrabble societies that Benedict studied. But from Brazil to Bangladesh we saw new cultures arising in which the individual and the community are reconnected, and in which, therefore, status does indeed come from one's contribution to the whole.

This new mental map emerging doesn't lock us into self-defeating thought traps. It releases us. By drawing lessons from the natural world, and by acknowledging our interdependence, it grounds us without being stifling. It urges us to keep tapping our own intuitions; to trust what motivates us, and to listen, like Negi, to what the heart is saying.

SEEING PAST THE NEXT RIDGE

Walking down the hall at MIT during a break in our travels, I ran into a colleague who'd read our chapter on the MST in Brazil. "You know, many see the MST as a Leninist organization," she told me, "very undemocratic."

Later, speaking at the University of Wisconsin, no sooner had I uttered my last word than a woman in the audience stood to challenge me: "You should do your homework," she said. "Don't you know the Grameen Bank, despite all the hype about loans to women, is really a sexist organization?"

Noticing that I didn't bristle in either of these moments, I realize how much I'd absorbed this fifth liberating idea from everyone we met. It's that we can toss out all "isms," including any notion of a prefab model—something finished, done, delivered. In that spirit, I don't have to, or want to, defend the MST or Grameen, claiming they are models to be mimicked, exemplars to be transplanted wholesale. They're not perfect. Grameen and the MST, and really all the groups whose stories we share, are just examples of the millions of people worldwide, experimenting, struggling, failing, and succeeding in carving new paths and creating a world in line with their deepest values.

The people we met are pushing the edge of possibilities, not asserting that they've reached an endpoint. They are modeling creativity, not modeling models. It's this human capacity for creativity that Anna and I want to celebrate: the notion that by our nature human beings are never finished.

Wangari had it right that night in Nairobi. Our task is to keep walking, not to believe we've arrived. As she would say, there is always another ridge to reach.

The Courage of an Expanding Heart

To gain the courage to climb to the next ridge, to learn to "walk," we can put ourselves in the company of those who by their very being remind us that the dominant culture—the materialism, the brutality, the isolation, the destruction, the polarization—is the great aberration, arising in a mere blink of historical time. We can walk beside people who express those life-affirming qualities of human beings that have endured over eons.

This imprintability of ours is itself a source of hope. I believe we "become" each other in some mysterious way, and it happens without our even knowing. (Why else would we be so concerned about whom our children choose as friends, and how else would we explain the rapidity with which we take on the mannerisms of our mates?) This aspect of our social nature—learning by mimicking, as so many other animals do—opens a clear path of change. As we associate with others who have qualities we want to grow within ourselves, we experience ourselves changing.

Reading what we wrote last winter when we began this book—my view limited to the beige brick wall out my MIT window—I'm struck by how much bigger my view is today. Before we began this journey, I could line up the facts and speak with authority about positive developments emerging, but belief in the real possibility of planet-wide breakthroughs had not permeated my cells. It hadn't sunk from my head to my heart, and into the rest of me.

Now the sense of possibility is palpable: in the sights, the smells, the sounds, and in the hundreds of people we met along the way. I'll carry them with me for the rest of my life.

Anna and I have been to the edge and seen for ourselves what is emerging. Yes, it's spotty, still fragile, but it is everywhere, and it is real. It's not about wishing it to be. It's not about starting the river flowing. It's about jumping in. It's the excitement of knowing that each of us on our fragile planet can do the same.

So why do we hesitate, why aren't we all jumping in?

Partly, it is because to take any risk we have to be motivated, and that means acknowledging how frighteningly *bad* things are.

I realize now that I've always felt torn: I've felt I had to shock people out of resignation by telling them about the horror of needless hunger; yet I also felt compelled to rush in to soften it, to emphasize the positive. I have tended to play the rah-rah role, I confess, fearing that if people knew how awful things *really* are, they'd despair.

Now I know I've been wrong.

Sitting in the Landless Workers' Movement meeting in Paraná, we experienced men and women who in one moment celebrated with wall-shaking song their triumph over landlessness, and whose eyes welled up with tears in the next moment as they turned to an elderly man, still bandaged from an assault by police during a peaceful demonstration. In Wisconsin we met the Sharps, who didn't let one child's devastating illness defeat them, but instead were inspired to secure changes to ensure the healthiest life possible not only for their other children, but for everyone who eats the food they produce. In Africa, we met Karangathe, who lost almost everything in government-fomented ethnic conflict only to discover his real passion: reconnecting Kenyan villagers to their own culture's wisdom.

Anna and I learned a lot about the human heart this year. We learned it can hold more than we thought possible. We learned it can grow.

It can grow big enough to hold the tragedy of children dying while food surpluses rot, the loss of so many species that it will take millions of years for our earth to recover, the needless poisoning of those who labor to feed us, the terror of poor families gunned down by angry landowners. All of it.

This image of an expanding heart suggests a certain kind of courage—and all of us, we believe, long to be courageous; to be heroes to ourselves. But this kind of courage has nothing to do with toughness. It is the courage of a heart that has had horrific experience but has not hardened; that has heard too much bad news but has not been numbed; that has witnessed too much suffering but has not been broken.

Such courage doesn't come by shielding ourselves or in desperately seeking signs of hope, but by opening, opening, opening to experience. It comes if we expand our hearts to let it *all* in, all the messiness, the fear, the sadness, the loss, the longing—as well as the wondrous sense of awakening that this era holds.

LEARNING FROM THE LION

The night that Reverend Timothy Njoya spoke with us in Green Belt's cozy Nairobi guesthouse, Anna and I lay in our bunk beds talking long after the generator shut down and we turned the lights out.

Like Wangari, Njoya had faced condemnation and bloody attacks for daring to question the Kenyan government and support democracy.

Shaken by his ability to tell with laughter and joyful energy his story about almost being murdered, I had to ask, "Dr. Njoya, isn't fear a natural response to threat? Isn't it instinctual? Even people who haven't faced violence experience it, so how have you mastered your own fear?" My heart was pounding.

Sitting deep in the cushioned armchair, his sweet face framed by a stiff white priest's collar, Njoya paused for only a moment. Then he said, "Fear is an endogenous energy—it comes from inside us, not outside. Endogenous energies that form fear are the same ones that form courage. Endogenous energies are neutral. So you can channel them into fear, paranoia, or euphoria—whatever you choose."

He jumped up from his chair, surprisingly agile for his age and all he's suffered. "Imagine a lion," he said, crouching. "When a lion sees prey, or a predator, it senses fear first. But instead of lunging blindly in defense or in attack, it recoils." Njoya moved back too, leaning on his left leg and crouching lower. "The lion pauses a moment, targets his energies. Then he springs."

"We can do the same. We can harness our would-be fears, harmonize our energies, and channel them into courage."

His whole body, his whole life, seemed to tell us, yes, this is possible.

As we lay that night talking, stacked on our bunks, fear now had a different meaning. True, not all of us face jail, death threats, or violent attacks for our out-of-step beliefs. Still, listening to our yearnings and following our own sensibilities will always mean facing fear. Fear of the unknown, fear of being different, fear of failure. If we keep changing, as we must to face this era's life-and-death challenges, we will always meet it.

But I know now I don't have to deny fear, praying that it will—finally, finally—go away. We can instead harness fear and, like the lion taking aim, choose where and what we do with it—like Reverend Njoya; like all of those we met on our journey.

As we do, as we step into the unknown, we help create a new mental map. And as we act from our new insights, we allow more and more people to see with new eyes, to know parts of themselves they have denied and possibilities they could not see before.

So our wish for ourselves and for you is not fearlessness. It is for an expanding heart that can transform our fear energies into courage energies to break us free of the deadly thought traps, these old maps into which our culture is locked. So that you and we don't miss, God forbid, our chance to engage fully—to be fully ourselves—in this extraordinary time of suffering, loss . . . and possibility.

Taking Off

But we have only begun
to love the earth.

We have only begun
to imagine the fullness of life.

How could we tire of hope?
—so much is in bud.

How can desire fail?
—we have only begun

to imagine justice and mercy,
only begun to envision

how it might be
to live as siblings with beast and flower,
not as oppressors.

We have only begun to know
the power that is in us if we would join
our solitudes in the communion of struggle.

So much is unfolding that must
complete its gesture,

so much is in bud.

FROM "BEGINNERS"

IN *SELECTED POEMS*

BY DENISE LEVERTOV

PAUL A. LACEY, EDITOR

(NEW YORK: NEW DIRECTIONS, 2002)

EPILOGUE

Some time after we thought we had put this book to rest—before we remembered that a book is never finished until its publisher yanks it from the writers' hands—we received an e-mail from Wangari Maathai's daughter. Wangari was in jail, again. The arrest was the government's response to an impending Green Belt Movement protest against the sale of public forests.

This wasn't to be our only sobering news from overseas. We also learn about more MST members threatened, injured, and killed in ongoing land disputes in Brazil. Of more farmer suicides in India. Of contamination of vital, ancient strains of corn by Monsanto's genetically modified seeds in Mexico.

News closer to home is troubling, too. We hear of massive, unprecedented recalls of possibly contaminated meat and more deaths from food-borne illnesses. Of the Bush administration's new, toothless rules to stop pollution from feedlots, even as the EPA itself says that 35,000 miles of river were damaged by this waste in the last decade alone.

At the same time, we've gathered courage from other news.

Wangari's jail stay lasted only a few hours. (Maybe the faxes, phone calls, and e-mails from around the world did have an impact.) And a few weeks ago we hear from Wangari's daughter again. Kenya's two-decade-enduring strongman is out. And Wangari has won a seat in parliament. Not only that, Wangari has been appointed deputy prime minister for the environment, her daughter tells us, and women danced in the streets of Nairobi to celebrate!

At about the same time, we hear of another big shakeup—this time in Brazil. The new president, winning by a large margin, made his first presidential pledges, ones we're sure the MST is happy to hear: peaceful land reform and Fome Zero (Zero Hunger). On his third day in office, President Luiz Inázio

Lula da Silva scratched a $760 million order for a dozen new fighter planes, declaring that fighting hunger will make better use of that money.

We take heart in learning that the UN Human Rights Commission deemed intellectual property rules on seed patenting an obstacle to human rights. And after a decade of deliberation—perhaps the most participatory process ever known for an international agreement—thousands of individuals, citizen organizations, and government representatives and groups ratified the Earth Charter, laying out fundamental principles for sustainable development.[1] And, we finish this note, we excitedly anticipate the largest-ever gathering of pro-democracy organizations, with perhaps as many as 100,000 people, at the 2003 World Social Forum, also in Brazil.

Over the last year, we've traveled to more than fifty cities and everywhere heard the same message: that, just as in Belo Horizonte, a citizens' voice is growing, one saying that healthy food *is* a right of citizenship for all.

So, yes, the news has been at times disheartening, at times stirring. But with the voices of the people in this book freshly with us, it's easier to remember that hope does not come from convincing ourselves the good news is winning out over the bad.

Nor does it come from assessing what's possible and going for that. Since it's not possible to know what's possible—we could *never* have predicted the startling turn of events in Kenya and Brazil—we find new energy in this very truth. In the awareness of possibility itself—*always* unknowable—we are free to focus on creating the world we want.

Hope, we're learning, comes from a place deep within. Hope is not what we find in evidence; it is what we become in action. We become hope because we are alive. We become hope because our planet needs us to. And our hope can spur us on—to take our own stand, to choose. The Green Belt slogan rings in our ears: *As for me, I've made a choice.*

Anna Lappé, Brooklyn, New York
Frances Moore Lappé, Cambridge, Massachusetts
February 2003

To support the efforts of those pushing forward hope's edge, consider a contribution to the Small Planet Fund. See page 451 for more information.

ENTRY POINTS

Every choice we make can be
a celebration of the world we want.

As we absorb the lesson of solving for pattern, we begin to see the world in ways that help us grasp the roots of problems and how they interconnect. Suddenly, the entry points are endless. Here are only a few possibilities, among many, to help you on your path.

We wish you Reverend Njoya–type courage as you chart your way.

Here you will find contact information for groups profiled in the book, followed by other resources for bringing the themes of this book to life.

To learn more about any of these groups, find still more resources, see images from our travels, and discover how our story continues to unfold, visit www.hopesedge.com. You can also contribute your own suggestions, stories, and resources on the site.

CHAPTER-BY-CHAPTER ENTRY POINTS

CHAPTER 2: THE DELICIOUS REVOLUTION

THE GARDEN PROJECT
Pier 28, The Embarcadero
San Francisco, CA 94105
Tel: (415) 243 8558 Fax: (415) 243 8221
www.gardenproject.org

THE EDIBLE SCHOOLYARD
Martin Luther King Middle School
1781 Rose Street
Berkeley, CA 94703
Tel: (510) 558 1335 Fax: (510) 558 1334
info@edibleschoolyard.org
www.edibleschoolyard.org

THE CENTER FOR ECOLITERACY
2522 San Pablo Avenue
Berkeley, CA 94702
Tel: (510) 845 4595 Fax: (510) 845 0485
info@ecoliteracy.org
www.ecoliteracy.org

FOOD SYSTEMS PROJECT
A project of the Center for Ecoliteracy
2530 San Pablo Avenue, Suite "C"
Berkeley, CA 94702
Tel: (510) 548 8838 Fax: (510) 548 8849
www.foodsystems.org

CHAPTER 3: THE BATTLE FOR HUMAN NATURE

LANDLESS WORKERS' MOVEMENT /
MOVIMENTO DOS TRABALHADORES
RURAIS SEM TERRA
Secretaria Nacional MST
Rua Alameda Barão de Limeira, nº 1232
Bairro Campos Elíseos
São Paulo, Brazil
semterra@mst.org.br
www.mstbrazil.org

IN THE USA: FRIENDS OF THE MST
c/o Global Exchange
2017 Mission Street, #303
San Francisco, CA 94110
Tel: (415) 255 7296 Fax: (415) 255 7498
dawn@mstbrazil.org
www.mstbrazil.org

CHAPTER 4: BEAUTIFUL HORIZON

For more on "food as a right of citizenship," see *Food First* below.

CHAPTER 5: THE HYACINTH PRINCIPLE

GRAMEEN BANK
Training & International Program
Mirpur Two
Dhaka, 1216, Bangladesh
Tel: 880 11 425 Fax: 880 13 559
www.grameen-info.org
See also www.grameen.org

POLICY RESEARCH FOR DEVELOPMENT
ALTERNATIVES (UBINIG)
Farida Akhter, Executive Director
5/3 Barabo Mahanpur
Ring Road, Shaymoli
Dhaka, 1207, Bangladesh
ubinig@citechco.net

NARIPOKKHO
House 51, Road 9A
Dhanmondi, Dhaka, 1209, Bangladesh
Tel: 880 2 81 9917 Fax: 880 2 81 3310

CHAPTER 6: SEEKING ANNAPOORNA

RESEARCH FOUNDATION FOR TECHNOLOGY,
SCIENCE, AND ECOLOGY / NAVDANYA
Vandana Shiva, Executive Director
A-60 Haus Khas

New Delhi, 110016, India
Fax: 91 11 685 6795
www.vshiva.net

CHAPTER 7: WALKING TO NAIROBI

GREEN BELT MOVEMENT
Wangari Maathai, Founder
P.O. Box 67545
Nairobi, Kenya

Tel: 254 2 571 523 Fax: 254 2 504 264
gbm@iconnect.co.ke
www.geocities.com/gbm0001/

CHAPTER 8: STIRRING THE SLEEPING GIANT

TRANSFAIR USA
Paul Rice, Executive Director
52 Ninth Street
Oakland, CA 94607
Tel: (510) 663 5260 Fax: (510) 663 5264
info@transfairusa.org
www.transfairusa.org

MAX HAVELAAR FOUNDATION
Hans Bolscher, Director
P.O. Box 1252
3500 BG Utrecht, The Netherlands
Tel: 31 30 233 7070
maxhavelaar@maxhavelaar.nl
www.maxhavelaar.nl

GLOBAL EXCHANGE
2017 Mission Street #303
San Francisco, CA 94110
fairtrade@globalexchange.org
www.globalexchange.org/economy/coffee

FORESTRADE
41 Spring Tree Road
Brattleboro, VT 05301
Tel: (802) 257 9157
info@forestrade.com
www.forestrade.com

EQUAL EXCHANGE
251 Revere Street
Canton, MA 02021
Tel: (781) 830 0303
info@equalexchange.com
www.equalexchange.com

FAIRTRADE LABELING ORGANIZATIONS
INTERNATIONAL
FLO - Kaiser Friedrich Strasse 13
53113 Bonn, Germany
coordination@fairtrade.net
www.fairtrade.net

CHAPTER 9: THE LAST TASTE OF PARIS

FORUM-SYNERGIES

Hannes Lorenzen, Director
BEL 3013 Rue Belliard 97-113
B-1047 Brussels, Belgium
Tel: 32 2 284 3362 Fax: 32 2 284 9154
info@forum-synergies.org
www.forum-synergies.org

ATTAC - FRANCE

9bis, Rue de Valence
75005 Paris, France
Tel: 33 01 43 36 26 26
Fax: 33 01 43 36 30 54
attacfr@attac.org
www.attac.org

SUSTAINABLE AGRICULTURE NETWORK

Réseau Agriculture Durable
Jean Yves Griot, Président
14, Boulevard Volclair. BP 56131
35056 Rennes Cedex 2, France
Tel: 02 99 50 77 29 Fax: 02 99 50 94 61
griot@club-internet.fr

CONFEDERATION PAYSANNE IN FRANCE

81, Avenue de la République
93170 Bagnolet, France
Tel: 01 43 62 04 04 Fax: 01 43 62 80 03
contact@confederationpaysanne.fr
www.confederationpaysanne.fr
www.cpefarmers.org (in Europe)

GREENPEACE FRANCE

Bruno Rebelle, Director
22 Rue des Rasselins
75020 Paris, France
Tel: 33 01 44 64 02 02
Fax: 33 01 44 64 02 00
www.greenpeace.fr

GREENPEACE USA

702 H Street NW
Washington, DC 20001
Tel: (800) 326 0959
www.greenpeaceusa.org

CHAPTER 10: TAKING OFF THE COWBOY HAT

WISCONSIN RURAL DEVELOPMENT CENTER

4915 Monona Drive, Suite 304
Monona, WI 53716
Tel: (608) 226 0300 Fax: (608) 226 0301
For information on Madison Area
Community Supported Agriculture
Coalition (MACSAC): *www.macsac.org*

**WISCONSIN FOODSHED RESEARCH
PROJECT**

www.foodshed.wisc.edu

FAMILY FARM DEFENDERS

John Kinsman, Founder
P.O. Box 1772
Madison, Wisconsin 53701
Tel/Fax: (608) 260 0900
ffd@ureach.com
See also: *www.familyfarmer.org*

COMING TO OUR SENSES

CHEFS COLLABORATIVE
441 Stuart Street, #712
Boston, MA 02116
Tel: (617) 236 5200
cc2000@chefnet.com
www.chefnet.com/cc2000

THE ENTRY POINTS CONTINUE

For each one of the following ways we can take action, there are hundreds of
resources with people eager to help you. Here, we have listed just a few, many
of which we discuss in the book's chapters; you'll find more on our website,
www.hopesedge.com.

REALIZING FOOD AS A HUMAN RIGHT

FOOD FIRST/INSTITUTE FOR FOOD AND
DEVELOPMENT POLICY
Co-founded by Frances Moore Lappé in
1975; a great source of knowledge, tools,
networking, and campaigns to make food
a human right.

FOOD FIRST
398 60th Street
Oakland, CA 94618
Tel: (510) 654 4400 Fax: (510) 654 4551
www.foodfirst.org

NURTURING AGRICULTURE THAT SUSTAINS THE LAND AND RURAL COMMUNITIES

We can choose to educate ourselves and to press elected leaders to redirect public subsidies and tax policies to encourage sustainable, family-farm agriculture.

GLOBAL RESOURCE ACTION CENTER FOR
THE ENVIRONMENT (GRACE) AND FACTORY
FARM PROJECT
Tel: (212) 726 9161 Fax: (212) 726 9160
Works for the elimination of the factory
farm as a mode of production, and for its

replacement with a sustainable
food-production system that is healthful,
environmentally sound, economically
viable, and humane.
www.gracelinks.org
www.factoryfarm.org

ACTION GROUP ON EROSION TECHNOLOGY
AND CONCENTRATION (ETC) GROUP
Dedicated to the conservation and
sustainable advancement of cultural and
ecological diversity.
478 River Ave., Suite 200
Winnipeg, Manitoba, R3L 0C8, Canada
Tel: (204) 453 5259 Fax: (204) 284 7871
etc@etcgroup.org
www.etcgroup.org

INSTITUTE FOR AGRICULTURE AND TRADE
POLICY
Promotes resilient family farms, rural
communities, and ecosystems around the
world through research and education,
science and technology, and advocacy.
2105 First Avenue South
Minneapolis, MN 55404
Tel: (612) 870 0453
iatp@iatp.org
www.iatp.org

INTERNATIONAL FORUM ON ORGANIC
AGRICULTURE MOVEMENTS (IFOAM)
A platform for international exchange and
cooperation to further organic farming.
IFOAM Head Office
c/o Ökozentrum Imsbach
D-66636 Tholey-Theley, Germany
Tel: 49 6853 919890 Fax: 49 6853 919899
headoffice@ifoam.org
www.ifoam.org

NATIONAL CAMPAIGN FOR SUSTAINABLE
AGRICULTURE, INC.
Dedicated to educating the public on the
importance of a sustainable food and
agriculture system that is economically
viable, environmentally sound, socially
just, and humane.
P.O. Box 396
Pine Bush, NY 12566
Tel: (845) 744 8448 Fax: (845) 744 8477
campaign@sustainableagriculture.net
www.sustainableagriculture.net

NATIONAL FAMILY FARM COALITION
Thirty-three grassroots farm, resource,
conservation, and rural advocacy groups
from thirty-three states working to
strengthen family farms.
110 Maryland Avenue, NE #307
Washington, DC 20002
Tel: (202) 543 5675
www.nffc.net

VIA CAMPESINA/INTERNATIONAL
FARMERS MOVEMENT
An international movement that coordinates
peasant organizations of small- and
middle-scale producers, agricultural
workers, rural women, and indigenous
communities from Asia, Africa, America,
and Europe.
International Operative Secretariat
Apartado Postal 3628
Tegucigalpa, MDC, Honduras
Tel: 504 239 46 79 Fax: 504 235 99 15
viacam@gbm.hn
www.viacampesina.org

EATING HEALTHFULLY

We can choose a plant-centered, whole-foods, organic diet, lightening our impact on the earth and no longer contributing to cruelty to animals as we improve our own health.

ORGANIC CONSUMERS ASSOCIATION

Promotes food safety, organic agriculture, fair-trade, and sustainable agricultural practices in the U.S. and internationally.
6101 Cliff Estate Rd.
Little Marais, MN 55614
Tel: (218) 226 4164 Fax: (218) 226 4157
www.purefood.org

EarthSave International

Promotes food choices that are healthy for people and the planet.
1509 Seabright Avenue, Suite B1
Santa Cruz, CA 95062
Tel: (800) 362 3648 Fax: (831) 423 1313
www.earthsave.org
www.organicconsumer.org

We can choose to support nourishing school food programs and resist commercialization of our schools.

A GARDEN IN EVERY SCHOOL (CHAPTER 2)

National Gardening Association
1100 Dorset St.,
South Burlington, VT 05403
Tel: (800) LETSGROW
www.kidsgardening.com

COMMERCIAL ALERT

For other information about commercialism in schools and how to get involved in your own community.
4110 SE Hawthorne Blvd. # 23
Portland, OR 97214-5246
www.commercialalert.org

COMMUNITY FOOD SECURITY COALITION

A national coalition working to build equitable, healthful, sustainable, self-reliant and community-based food systems through policy advocacy, education, research, and organizing.
P.O. Box 209
Venice, CA 90294
Tel: (310) 822 5410
www.foodsecurity.org

AWAKENING THE SLEEPING GIANT

We can choose to buy from local, family farms. Two examples of producer-consumer resources on the Internet:

SuperMarket Co-op (chapter 10)

A Project of the Rural Coalition
Rural Coalition
1411 K Street NW, Suite 901
Washington, DC 20005

Tel: (202) 628 7160 Fax: (202) 628 7165
info@supermarketcoop.com
www.supermarketcoop.com

FARMER DIRECT MARKETING (CHAPTER 10)
Wholesale and Alternative Markets
P.O. Box 96456 Room 2642-S
1400 Independence Avenue, SW
Washington, DC 20090-6456

Tel: (202) 720 8317 Fax: (202) 690 0031
To find direct marketing resources by state:
http://www.ams.usda.gov/directmarketing

We can choose to join a community-supported agriculture farm or to shop at farmers' markets. In so doing, we re-embed local economics into communities and support farming that values the people who tend the land and the land itself.

ROBYN VAN EN CENTER (CHAPTER 10)
National CSA Resources
1015 Philadelphia Avenue
Chambersburg, PA 17201
Tel: (717) 261 2880 Fax: (717) 261 2880
info@csacenter.org
www.csacenter.org

LOCAL HARVEST
Resource hub for listings of food coops, farmers markets, CSAs, and family farms.
www.localharvest.org

USDA RESOURCES

FARMERS MARKETS (CHAPTER 10)
www.ams.usda.gov/farmersmarkets/map.htm

ALTERNATIVE FARMING SYSTEMS INFORMATION CENTER
www.nal.usda.gov/afsic/csa/

EVOLVING CAPITALISM

To re-embed economics in life-serving values, we can choose to buy locally made products and buy directly from producers. We can buy products produced in ways that are less damaging to the environment, to animals, and to people. We can buy through fair trade stores like those run by Global Exchange (listed above).

CO-OP AMERICA (PUBLISHER OF NATIONAL GREEN PAGES™)
Connects people with responsible businesses for purchasing and investing.

1612 K Street NW, Suite 600
Washington, DC 20006
Tel: (800) 58 GREEN Fax: (202) 331 8166
www.coopamerica.org

We can take advantage of a growing fair-trade movement to, as Paul Rice tells us, "buycott," and we can choose to support fair-trade practices of local co-ops, supermarkets, cafés, restaurants, and other businesses, and press our local grocers about their purchasing decisions.

FAIR TRADE RESOURCE NETWORK (CHAPTER 8)
P.O. Box 33772
Washington, DC 20033
www.fairtraderesource.org

OXFAM INTERNATIONAL MAKE TRADE FAIR CAMPAIGN
www.maketradefair.com

We can choose to turn businesses we control or influence toward environmentally sound business practices.

THE NATURAL STEP, US (CHAPTER 11)
A nonprofit environmental education organization working to build an ecologically and economically sustainable society.
116 New Montgomery St., Suite 800
San Francisco, CA 94105
Tel: (415) 318 8170 Fax: (415) 974 0474
www.naturalstep.org

LIVING MACHINES, INC. (CHAPTER 10)
Inspired by ecosystems, Living Machines® are a revolutionary natural wastewater treatment system that accelerate nature's own water-purification process.
125 La Posta Road
8018 NDCBU
Taos, NM 87571
Tel: (505) 751 4448 Fax: (505) 751 9483
www.livingmachines.com

We can choose union and sustainable-farming labels and choose to support companies we know and companies we respect.

UNION LABEL
Lists union-made products and union-provided services and includes a "do buy" and "boycott" list.
www.unionlabel.org

THE FOOD ALLIANCE (CHAPTER 8)
1829 NE Alberta, # 5
Portland, OR 97211

Tel: (503) 493 1066 Fax: (503) 493 1069
info@thefoodalliance.org
www.thefoodalliance.org

IDEALSWORK
Idealswork gives information to consumers about what companies do, enabling us to be more conscious consumers.
www.idealswork.org

ECO-LABELS

The Consumers Union guide to
environmental labels.

www.eco-labels.org

In addition to the buying and investing choices we make, we can choose to
support fairer taxation, including new initiatives like the Tobin Tax, as well as
policies that encourage fairer wages and working conditions.

INTERNATIONAL INNOVATIVE REVENUE
PROJECT / CENTER FOR ENVIRONMENTAL
ECONOMIC DEVELOPMENT (CHAPTER 9)
Spearheads campaign for Tobin Tax on
currency speculation in U.S.
P.O. Box 4167
Arcata, CA, 95518-4167
Tel: (707) 822 8347 Fax: (707) 822 4457
www.ceedweb.org

UNITED FOR A FAIR ECONOMY
A "movement support" organization to
help address the widening income and
access gap in the U.S.
37 Temple Place, 2nd Floor
Boston, MA 02111
Tel: (617) 423 2148 Fax: (617) 423 0191
www.ufenet.org

We can choose to support micro-credit enterprises that work to fight poverty,
and we can get involved with poverty-fighting in our own communities.

GRAMEEN FOUNDATION USA (CHAPTER 5)
Works in partnership with the Grameen
Bank to fight poverty all over the world.
1029 Vermont Avenue NW, Suite 400
Washington, DC 20005
Tel: (202) 628 3560 Fax: (202) 628 3880
www.gfusa.org

RESULTS USA
A nonprofit, grassroots citizens' lobby
working to create the political will to end
hunger and poverty.
440 First Street NW, Suite 450
Washington, DC 20001
Tel: (202) 783 7100 Fax: (202) 783 2818
results@resultsusa.org
www.resultsusa.org

We can choose to place investment dollars in businesses aligned with our values, to support the evolution of capitalism from a single-minded profit motive
to a multiple bottom line.

SOCIAL ACCOUNTABILITY INTERNATIONAL (CHAPTER 11)

(formerly Council on Economic Priorities) Dedicated to improving workplaces and communities by developing and implementing socially responsible standards.

220 E 23rd Street, Suite 605
New York, NY 10010
Tel: (212) 684 1515
www.sa-intl.org

SHOREBANK BANKING CENTER (CHAPTER 11)

The country's oldest and largest community development bank, Shorebank works to improve the economic health of the neighborhoods they serve and uses investors' dollars for community building.

7054 S. Jeffery Boulevard
Chicago, IL 60649
Tel: (773) 288 1000
info@shorebankcorp.com
www.shorebankcorp.com

We can join in efforts to challenge and remake the corporate structure itself, so that democracy governs our economic life.

PROGRAM ON CORPORATIONS, LAW AND DEMOCRACY (CHAPTER 11)

Instigates democratic conversation and actions to contest the authority of corporations to govern and to establish citizen sovereignty through the democratic process.

P.O. Box 246
S. Yarmouth, MA 02664-0246
Tel: (508) 398 1145
www.poclad.org

ECONOMIC DEMOCRACY PROJECT

Working to make corporations more responsible.

P.O. Box 8439
Minneapolis, MN 55408
Tel: (612) 879 0695
www.DivineRightofCapital.com

DEMOCRATIZING GLOBALIZATION

We can choose to support initiatives to make international bodies, such as the World Trade Organization and World Bank, representative and accountable to citizens' concerns.

PUBLIC CITIZEN (AND GLOBAL TRADE WATCH) (CHAPTERS 6 AND 9)

Public Citizen is the "consumer's eyes and ears in Washington," fighting for safer drugs and medical devices, cleaner and safer energy sources, a cleaner

environment, fair trade, and a more open and democratic government.

1600 20th Street NW
Washington, DC 20009
Tel: (202) 588 1000
www.citizen.org/trade

INTERNATIONAL FORUM ON
GLOBALIZATION
Representing more than sixty organizations
in twenty-five countries, IFG researches
the impact of corporate globalization and
helps galvanize a constructive response.

1009 General Kennedy Avenue #2
San Francisco, CA 94129
Tel: (415) 561 7650 Fax: (415) 561 7651
www.ifg.org

We can choose to support international debt relief as well as rules governing trade, aid, and gene-and-seed patenting that protect workers, consumers' health, local culture, and the environment.

JUBILEE USA NETWORK
(CHAPTERS 3 AND 8)
Dedicated to working for a world free of
debt for billions of people.
222 East Capitol Street NE
Washington, DC 20003
Tel: (203) 783 3566 Fax: (202) 546 4468
www.jubileeusa.org

THE TREATY INITIATIVE TO SHARE THE
GENETIC COMMONS (CHAPTER 6)
Nearly 200 citizen groups and tribal bodies
seeking a formal international treaty
prohibiting the patenting of life forms.
Foundation on Economic Trends
1660 L Street NW, Suite 216
Washington, DC 20036
Tel: (202) 466 2823 Fax: (202) 429 9602
treaty@foet.org

SEEING WITH NEW EYES, EXPERIENCING OTHER CULTURES

We can put ourselves in new places and cultures to meet people who are choosing to listen to the land, and tap nature's wisdom and the earth's abundance.

EUROPEAN CENTER FOR ECOLOGICAL
AGRICULTURE AND TOURISM/POLAND
(CHAPTER 9)
Promotes small-scale organic farming
together with eco-tourism.
Jadwiga Lopata, Director
34-146 Stryszow 156
Poland

Tel/Fax: 48 33 879 7114
jadwiga@eceat-pl.most.org.pl
www.eceat-poland.w.pl

GLOBAL EXCHANGE REALITY TOURS (CHAPTER 9)

The tours educate people about how we, individually and collectively, contribute to global problems and suggest ways in which we can contribute to positive change. The tours offer a variety of educational programs that address contemporary political, economic, environmental, and cultural issues around the world.

2017 Mission Street, #303
San Francisco, CA 94110
Tel: (800) 497 1994
www.globalexchange.org/tours
realitytours@globalexchange.org

HOW TO LIVE YOUR DREAM OF VOLUNTEERING OVERSEAS

We also suggest reading this book, which is full of great resources for anyone in the United States interested in doing volunteer work abroad.

www.volunteeroverseas.org
info@volunteeroverseas.org

SOKONI PROJECT (CHAPTER 7)

Sokoni organizes educational and solidarity "safaris" to the Green Belt Movement in Kenya and is exploring a new approach to intercultural relations that is creative, sustainable, and mutually enriching.

P.O. Box 194
Cross River, NY 10518
Tel: (914) 763 5790
www.sokoniproject.org

THE FIVE THOUGHT TRAPS & THE FIVE LIBERATING IDEAS

FIVE THOUGHT TRAPS BLOCKING OUR PATH

From Chapter 1:
Maps of the Mind

The mental map that limits our imagination, helping to create the hunger, poverty, and environmental devastation all around us.

ONE: THE ENEMY IS SCARCITY, PRODUCTION IS OUR SAVIOR.

With the word's population potentially doubling in fifty years, there aren't enough food, jobs, land—or just about anything—to go around. We must keep single-mindedly focused on producing ever more, just to survive.

TWO: THANK OUR SELFISH GENES.

We are selfish by nature. To survive as a species, we had to be self-centered and competitive. While these traits aren't always pretty, they drive the entrepreneurial spirit and the creativity that have gotten us this far. Who can argue with survival of the fittest?

FIVE LIBERATING IDEAS HELPING US FIND OUR WAY

From Chapter 11:
Traveling the Edge of Possibility

Unimaginable thirty years ago, the emerging mental map allows each of us to find meaning in our own lives, healing our planet and ourselves.

ONE: SCRAPPING THE SCARCITY SCARE, REALIZING ABUNDANCE

Cutting through the scarcity illusion, we're able to see potential abundance all around us, even in what is now waste. We realize that growing food in ways that sustain the earth and people is not only more productive, but linked to the changes essential to slowing population growth.

TWO: LAUGHING AT THE CARICATURE, LISTENING TO OURSELVES

Now we can see the image of ourselves as merely selfish materialists is but a shabby caricature of our true nature. We would never have survived as a species if it wasn't for our need—and our capacity—for effectiveness and connection.

THREE: LET THE MARKET DECIDE, EXPERTS PRESIDE.

Since we humans are so self-seeking, thank goodness we can turn to the impersonal law of the market. What the market can't decide, we had best leave to the experts—the people who know what they're doing—because only our technological genius keeps us one step ahead of scarcity.

FOUR: SOLVE BY DISSECTION.

The world's problems are so huge that our only fighting chance to solve them is by dissection. We must break down our mammoth global challenges and tackle them piece by piece, one by one.

FIVE: WELCOME TO THE END OF HISTORY.

Communism, socialism, and fascism have failed. Human evolution has finally triumphed in the best system we can create: global corporate capitalism, in which everyone stands to benefit from the creativity and wealth it unleashes.

THREE: PUTTING TOOLS IN THEIR PLACE, TAPPING THE SAVVY OF CITIZENS

Now we can turn technologies—even the market itself—into tools, not tyrants. Scientific tools can help us—but only when citizens draw values boundaries for their application.

FOUR: DISCARDING DISSECTION, SOLVING FOR PATTERN

Now breakthroughs in science and technology allow us to perceive the interrelatedness of diverse problems and their solutions. We have the tools to build on nature's genius and tap the best of ancient wisdom. We can also see more clearly the power in the ripples our own choices make in solving the world's problems.

FIVE: BUSTING FREE FROM "ISMS," CREATING THE PATH AS WE WALK

Now it's clear that global corporate capitalism—economic life cut off from community life—is not inevitable, nor fixed, nor the best we can do. Millions are letting go of all "isms"—ideologies with one unchanging endpoint. They're re-embedding the market in values respecting nature, culture, and themselves.

COMING TO OUR SENSES

Thirty years ago, I began what would become my lifelong work—extolling the virtues of plant-centered, whole-foods diets. For someone raised in the '50s in Fort Worth, Texas, this was a mighty leap. Remember, back then, no house-wife would dare call it "dinner" without meat. When I was growing up, soy was what you fed to livestock, pesticides were an unalloyed blessing, and "or-ganic" was nothing but a college course chemistry students dreaded. It was then—as my world turned upside down upon discovering that a grain-fed, meat-centered diet was an unhealthy symptom of a destructive farming sys-tem—that I became convinced of the power of our everyday food choices.

Because eating is such a personal choice, and one we make many times every single day, I believe that consciously choosing what we put into our bod-ies, based on the knowledge of what is good for us and for the earth, has tremendous power. It strengthens us in every sense of the word. What delight I took as a young woman experimenting in the kitchen with new recipes with ingredients I'd never even heard of before—much less seen, smelled, or tasted. What delight in feeling healthier as well as clearer about my place on the planet.

Then I was winging it! As your palates will discover in the recipes in this book, a whole new cuisine has sprouted since I wrote *Diet for a Small Planet*. The chefs and restaurateurs who generously share their recipes here represent some of the pioneers in this redirection of our diet.

Inspired by Anna Thomas's 1972 *Vegetarian Epicure*, Mollie Katzen's

1974 *Moosewood Cookbook,* and Laurel Robertson and coauthors' 1981 *Laurel's Kitchen,* millions across the country began enjoying sumptuous meals centered in plant foods, organic whole foods, foods grown in season by nearby farmers.

Over this period visionary restaurateurs—Alice Water of Chez Panisse in Berkeley, Judy Wicks of the White Dog Cafe in Philadelphia, Nora Poullion of Restaurant Nora in Washington, D.C., and many more—also began to show Americans that fine dining can be enhanced, not compromised, by attending to the well-being of the earth and farmers.

In 1993 many such forward-thinking chefs created the membership organization called Chefs Collaborative to promote sustainable cuisine by teaching children, supporting local farmers, and inspiring their customers to choose healthy foods. Among the group's principles—one they share with our friends in Belo Horizonte, Brazil—is that good, safe, wholesome food is a basic human right. Many of the recipes in our book come from Chefs Collaborative members.

We believe humans learn through all our senses, so we hope these recipes—along with those throughout our book—will not only please our palates but open our minds, too, helping us make new choices and sense more fully that each choice we make can be a celebration of the world we want.

THE CONFESSIONS OF A FORMER KITCHEN-PHOBE—ANNA

I'll admit it. I used to be the kind of person who didn't really understand the idea of cooking. It always seemed like too much work; it always seemed to take too much time. I am known for this. When I told friends I was writing a book with recipes in it, I could sense the not-so-suppressed shock—*You,* cooking?!

I have one friend who is famous for hosting amazing multiple-course meals; but if you received an invitation for dinner from me, you knew what to expect: hummus; and what to bring: the pita. In my former life, a bagel for breakfast, lunch, and dinner, with the added tofu or vegetables or cream cheese, seemed to do just fine. Granted, I had grown up with a mother who constantly explained the cancer-fighting qualities of broccoli, who made sure I ate enough beans and rice to get my daily recommended dose of protein. I had been raised around the dining-room table. Still, as my friends will attest, when I set out on my own, cooking never became a priority. And though I knew how important a good diet is, I never felt I had the time or money to eat any differently.

But when I sat down with the dozens of recipes we've included here, I asked myself just what I was going to do when that first person said: *I just love those parsnip patties!* Nod knowingly? I didn't think so.

So I took a deep breath and said: It's time to start cooking. We'd hired a wonderful tester who was more versed in pots and pans and teaspoon measurements than I, but I decided to find out for myself what lay behind these recipes' words. It began, I confess, as work. But I soon started discovering the mystery of the kitchen, the magic of bringing food to life, the satisfaction of serving delicious, unexpected food. And what had always seemed time-consuming and burdensome—cooking meals—became a source of pleasure. In fact, I felt these meals were giving me time rather than taking it away. I was always more relaxed and at the same time more energized after each meal. I even started to understand how different it feels to eat in season and eat food from people you know. So this is my honest admission and my heartfelt thank you: Before I met these chefs through their recipes, I never knew I had it in me to—gulp—cook.

There's an open-air produce market around the corner from where I live now in Paris, and when I go there in the mornings, I talk with the vendors about how I'm using the fruits and vegetables. You should have seen their eyes pop when I told them I had just made watermelon soup for dinner!

Especially for those of you with skeptical, die-hard meat-eating friends, or for those of you who *are* die-hard meat-eaters, I have one more story to tell. The other night I invited several French friends over to try some dishes. One came reluctantly, explaining, "You know, I've always liked the *idea* of being a vegetarian, but I'm just never *full* after a meal without meat." At the end of dinner, she put down her fork, grinning. Her plate was empty. She smiled and gave me a look that said, *I get it.* I suppose the Grilled Vegetable Haystack on Polenta with Summer Gazpacho on page 384 showed her what being a vegetarian can really be about.

You know we're onto something if we can turn *foie gras* fanatics into fennel lovers.

Bon appétit!

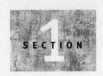
RECIPES FROM PIONEER VEGETARIAN AND WHOLE-FOODS COOKBOOK AUTHORS

ANNIE SOMERVILLE, author of *Fields of Greens: New Vegetarian Recipes from the Celebrated Greens Restaurant*

🍴 *Corn and Bulgur Salad with Cilantro and Lime*

🍴 *Butternut Squash Soup with Apple Confit*

🍴 *Linguine with Golden and Green Zucchini, Cherry Tomatoes, Pine Nuts, and Gremolata*

ANNA THOMAS, author of *The Vegetarian Epicure*

🍴 *Watercress and Radicchio Salad*

🍴 *White Bean and Garlic Soup with Chard*

🍴 *Kabocha Squash Stuffed with Savory Rice Pilaf*

🍴 *Caramelized Apple Pudding with Aged Cheddar Cheese*

MOLLIE KATZEN

Author of *The Moosewood Cookbook*

- 🍴 *Tunisian Eggplant Appetizer*
- 🍴 *Indian Summer Casserole*
- 🍴 *Watercress Salad with Currants and Walnuts*
- 🍴 *Chocolate Eclipse*

With close to four million books in print, writer/illustrator/chef Mollie Katzen is listed as one of *The New York Times*'s best-selling cookbook authors. She is a charter member of both the Natural Health Hall of Fame and the Harvard School of Public Health Nutrition Roundtable. Mollie is credited with helping to move healthful cooking from the fringes of American society onto mainstream dinner tables. Her books include *The Moosewood Cookbook, The Enchanted Broccoli Forest, Still Life with Menu, Vegetable Heaven,* and two cookbooks for children, *Pretend Soup* and *Honest Pretzels.* Since 1995, Mollie has hosted her own cooking show on public television, and she remains a lasting influence on several generations of Americans.

Tunisian Eggplant Appetizer

Serves 6   *Here is a South Mediterranean version of caponata (the famous Italian eggplant salad) featuring two outstanding guest stars: green olives and marinated artichoke hearts. It is so good it must be served as a course unto itself, accompanied by wedges of pita bread. (If you serve it with anything else, the other dish, no matter how good, might go unnoticed.) It keeps beautifully, so go ahead and make it three or four days ahead of time, if that is the most convenient for you.—Mollie*

¼ cup olive oil (or more, as needed)

1 medium-size onion, finely chopped

2 to 3 medium-size cloves garlic, minced

½ teaspoon salt (or more to taste)

1 large eggplant (peeling optional), cut into
    1-inch cubes

3 tablespoons tomato paste

¼ cup red wine vinegar

1 cup small pitted green olives

1 small jar (6 ounces) marinated artichoke
    hearts (drained, each piece cut into 2 or
    3 smaller pieces)

pinches of dried tarragon, basil, and/or
    oregano (optional)

Heat the olive oil in a large skillet. Add the onion, garlic, and salt, and sauté over medium heat until the onion is soft and translucent (5 to 8 minutes).

Add the eggplant cubes, stir, and cover. Cook until the eggplant is very well done (15 to 20 minutes), stirring occasionally. Add small amounts of additional oil, 1 tablespoon at a time, if needed to prevent sticking.

Stir in tomato paste and vinegar, and heat to the boiling point. Add the olives and remove from heat.

Stir in the artichoke hearts, then cool to room temperature. Taste to adjust the seasonings, adding the optional herbs if desired.

Cover tightly and chill. Serve cold or at room temperature.

Indian Summer Casserole

Serves 4 · *Highly seasoned vegetables are combined with olives, chilies, and cheese, and baked in custard. This recipe is named in honor of that time of year when corn, peppers, and fresh basil are peaking, and late crops of tomatoes are barely ripe. If you can't get green tomatoes, use the firmest and least-ripe red ones available. (The recipe below can be made in advance to the point where you spread the mixture in the pan. Then it can be stored, tightly covered, in the refrigerator for up to several days. Bring to room temperature and add the custard just before baking.)—Mollie*

2 cups corn (fresh or frozen)

3 large bell peppers (combined red, yellow, and green, if possible), chopped

2 medium-size green tomatoes, diced

2 to 3 large cloves garlic, minced

1 cup scallions (whites and greens), chopped

1 tablespoon olive oil

1 teaspoon salt

1 to 2 teaspoons ground cumin, to taste

½ to 1 teaspoon dried oregano, to taste

several leaves fresh basil, minced (or 2 teaspoons dried basil)

¼ cup fresh parsley, minced

lots of freshly ground black pepper

cayenne pepper to taste

½ cup chopped olives (black and/or green)

1 small Anaheim or poblaño chili, minced, or 1 4-ounce can diced green chilies

½ cup (packed) grated mild white cheese

4 eggs (okay to delete up to 2 yolks)

½ cup plain yogurt or buttermilk

paprika for the top

Preheat the oven to 375° F. Butter or grease the equivalent of a 6 x 9–inch baking pan.

In a large skillet, sauté the corn, peppers, tomatoes, garlic, and scallions in olive oil with salt, cumin, and oregano. Sauté quickly over medium-high heat, stirring. After about 8 minutes, remove from heat.

Stir in basil, parsley, black pepper, cayenne, olives, and chilies. Stir in the cheese until it melts. Spread mixture into the prepared pan.

Beat the eggs together with the yogurt or buttermilk. Gently pour the custard over the top. Dust modestly with paprika.

Bake uncovered 30 to 35 minutes.

Watercress Salad with Currants and Walnuts

Serves
3 to 4

This is a subtle and elegant salad, lightly dressed, and with small touches of scallions, walnuts, and currants. Balsamic vinegar is the first choice to use here, but champagne vinegar or any fruity variety will be just as effective. Red wine vinegar will also work. If you clean and dry the greens ahead of time, the salad will take just minutes to prepare. Store the cleaned greens in a bunting of paper towels, sealed in a plastic bag in the refrigerator.—Mollie

1 medium-sized head butter (Boston)
    lettuce, or similar soft lettuce
1 small bunch fresh watercress
1 to 2 perfect scallions
1 handful currants
2 handfuls walnuts, lightly toasted (use a
    toaster oven or a cast-iron skillet on the
    stove top)

2 to 3 tablespoons walnut oil
1 scant tablespoon balsamic vinegar
a small amount of salt
a generous amount of freshly ground black
    pepper

Clean the greens and dry them thoroughly. (For best results, use several vigorous whirls in a salad spinner, followed by some firm patting with paper towels.) Put them in a salad bowl.

Finely mince the scallions. Add them to the greens along with the currants and walnuts.

Drizzle in the oil; toss well, then sprinkle in the vinegar and some salt and pepper. Toss again and serve immediately.

Chocolate Eclipse

Serves
8 to 10

*This dessert is fashioned after one of my mother's specialties that she would make about once a year (usually when a grade-school teacher came over for lunch). It is a soft, moist chocolate cake with a built-in pudding-like fudge sauce that ends up underneath. Even though Chocolate Eclipse tastes very rich, it is actually less so than a regular chocolate cake. It has a similar amount of chocolate and sugar, but contains only 2 tablespoons of butter and no eggs. Chocolate Eclipse tastes best about an hour or two after it has emerged from the oven.
—Mollie*

2 tablespoons butter

2 ounces (2 squares) unsweetened
  chocolate

2 cups buttermilk or sour milk (2 cups milk
  plus 2 teaspoons vinegar)

1 teaspoon vanilla extract

2½ cups unbleached white flour

2¼ cups (packed) brown sugar

3 teaspoons baking powder

1 teaspoon baking soda

½ teaspoon salt

1 cup semisweet chocolate chips
  (optional)

½ cup plus 2 tablespoons unsweetened
  cocoa

2½ cups boiling water

Preheat the oven to 350° F. Grease a 9 x 13–inch baking pan.

Melt the butter and chocolate together.

In a separate saucepan, heat buttermilk or sour milk gently until just a little warmer than body temperature (don't boil or cook it). Remove from heat and combine with chocolate mixture and vanilla.

In a large mixing bowl, combine flour, 1 cup of the brown sugar, baking powder, baking soda, and salt. Mix well (use your hands, if necessary) to break up any little lumps of brown sugar, making as uniform a mixture as possible. Stir in chocolate chips, if desired.

Pour in the wet ingredients and stir until well combined. Spread into the prepared pan.

Combine the remaining 1¼ cups brown sugar with the unsweetened cocoa in a small bowl. Sprinkle this mixture as evenly as possible over the top of the batter.

Pour on the boiling water. It will look terrible, and you will not believe you are actually doing this, but try to persevere.

Place immediately into the preheated oven. Bake for 30 to 40 minutes, or until the center is firm to the touch.

Cool for at least 15 minutes before serving. Invert each serving on a plate so that the fudge sauce on the bottom becomes a topping. Serve hot or at room temperature.

LAUREL ROBERTSON

Author of *The New Laurel's Kitchen: A Handbook for Vegetarian Cookery and Nutrition*

🍴 *Tomato Soup and Gingery Tomato Soup*

🍴 *Chinese Asparagus*

🍴 *Parsnip Patties*

The best-selling coauthor of the popular vegetarian classic *Laurel's Kitchen*, Laurel has written other well-loved cookbooks, most recently, *Laurel's Kitchen Caring: Recipes for Everyday Home Caregiving*. With its compassion and wholesome vegetarian recipes, this latest book has been called the perfect aide for any caregiver.

Tomato Soup

Makes about 8 cups

A fine basic tomato soup, spectacularly good when the tomatoes are garden-fresh and ripe. Delicious as is, or as a good base for any kind of red-brothed soup.—Laurel

1 medium onion, chopped

1 tablespoon oil

2 stalks celery, chopped

1 carrot, chopped

¾ teaspoon oregano

1½ teaspoons dried basil

4 cups cut-up tomatoes, fresh
   or canned

2 to 3 cups hot vegetable stock

salt and pepper to taste

In a big soup pot, sauté the chopped onions in oil, adding the celery and carrot when the onion is partly cooked. Cook together until the onion is soft.

Add oregano, basil, and tomatoes to the pot and simmer gently until the tomatoes are very soft. If you want a smooth, creamy texture, purée the soup. (Using a food mill for puréeing will remove the tomato seeds and skins, making a velvety soup. You can also peel and seed the tomatoes before adding to the pot, if you want that texture and don't have a food mill.)

Add the hot vegetable stock, adjusting the amount to get the quantity and thickness you want. Bring to a boil and simmer on low heat for 5 minutes. Season with salt and pepper to taste.

Gingery Tomato Soup

Makes
about
5 cups

Tangy, fruity, light, and refreshing. Wonderful steaming from a big mug any time, but especially when you have a cold. Ginger aficionados will make it a heaping tablespoon.—Laurel

2 teaspoons oil	3 cups chopped tomatoes, fresh or canned
2 cloves garlic	2 cups vegetable stock
3 shallots (or 1 onion), chopped	1 tablespoon shoyu
1 tablespoon ginger, minced	fresh black pepper to taste

Heat oil in a heavy saucepan and add whole garlic cloves, then onion. Sauté. Add ginger, and stir; add tomatoes, and simmer until tomatoes are soft. Put through a sieve or food mill. Add stock, shoyu, and black pepper to taste.

Chinese Asparagus

Serves 4

A classic dish that fits in anywhere. Have you ever tasted fresh water chestnuts? They are as much better than the canned ones as fresh asparagus is better than canned. Chinese groceries often have them even if others don't, and they are worth looking for. Choose firm nuts that haven't shriveled at all. Peel and rinse, then use as you would the canned ones.—Laurel

Suggestion: Depending on the season, you can also use snow peas or snap peas instead of asparagus.

1 tablespoon shoyu or tamari	1 tablespoon ginger, minced
½ teaspoon honey	2 cloves garlic, minced
2 teaspoons cornstarch	8 water chestnuts
1 tablespoon water	½ cup flavorful broth
1 pound asparagus	2 teaspoons toasted sesame seeds
2 teaspoons oil	(optional)
1 medium leek, sliced thin	

Combine the shoyu, honey, cornstarch, and water, and set aside.

Trim the asparagus and cut diagonally into 1-inch slices. Prepare the remaining ingredients. Heat a wok or big, heavy skillet; when hot, add the oil and then the leek. Cook just a minute, then add ginger and garlic, stirring for only a few seconds. Add water chestnuts and asparagus, stir once more, and add the broth. Reduce heat, cover, and simmer gently until the asparagus is tender.

Stir the sauce to dissolve the cornstarch completely. Uncover vegetables, turn heat on high, and pour the sauce over them. Bring to a boil, stirring constantly for about a minute or until the sauce is thick. Serve sprinkled with sesame seeds if you like.

Parsnip Patties

Makes 12 patties. Serves 6

Parsnips are an old-fashioned vegetable being newly rediscovered. Use young, tender parsnips for steaming; older ones will get rubbery, so stir-frying is better for them. These Parsnip Patties are truly outstanding. Don't leave out the walnuts. Alongside broccoli, green beans, or kale, with a dollop of applesauce, they are very fine eating.—Laurel

4 cups raw parsnips, peeled and cut into chunks

1 onion, minced

1 tablespoon vegetable oil

1 teaspoon dried tarragon

2 eggs, beaten briefly

1 teaspoon salt

½ cup finely chopped walnuts

2 cups whole-grain bread crumbs

Preheat oven to 350° F. Steam parsnips until tender (10 to 15 minutes). While parsnips are cooking, sauté onion in oil. Add tarragon.

Mash parsnips with potato masher, a few lumps are okay. Stir onion into mashed parsnips, then eggs, salt, and walnuts.

Form parsnip mixture into patties, using about ½ cup for each. Spread half the bread crumbs on a greased baking sheet and place patties on crumbs. Press remaining crumbs on top of patties. Bake for 20 minutes.

ANNIE SOMERVILLE

Greens Restaurant, San Francisco, California

Author of *Fields of Greens: New Vegetarian Recipes from the Celebrated Greens Restaurant*

🍴 *Corn and Bulgur Salad with Cilantro and Lime*

🍴 *Butternut Squash Soup with Apple Confit*

🍴 *Linguine with Golden and Green Zucchini, Cherry Tomatoes, Pine Nuts, and Gremolata*

Under Annie Somerville's guidance as executive chef, Greens Restaurant has become a culinary landmark, known since its opening in 1979 for a mix of casual elegance, fine vegetarian food, and its message of health and harmony. Annie's *Fields of Greens: New Vegetarian Recipes from the Celebrated Greens Restaurant* showcases many of the restaurant's delicious recipes and includes a wealth of information on farmers' markets, sources for seeds, plants, and other resources, as well as hands-on tips for gardeners and farmers' market aficionados.

Corn and Bulgur Salad with Cilantro and Lime

Serves
4 to 6

A zesty summer salad with a fresh, hearty taste that's quick and easy to put together. The bulgur has a nutty flavor and texture that mixes deliciously with the sweet kernels of corn.—Annie

½ cup boiling water

½ cup bulgur

1 tablespoon light olive oil

3 cups corn kernels (approximately 3 ears of fresh corn)

¾ teaspoon salt

½ cup (1 small) red onion, diced into ¼-inch cubes

1 jalapeno chili, seeded and thinly sliced

1 tablespoon fresh lemon juice

1 tablespoon fresh lime juice (1 small lime)

pinch of cayenne pepper

1 tablespoon cilantro, coarsely chopped

1 tablespoon fresh sage (about 5 large leaves), coarsely chopped

Place the bulgur in a medium-size bowl and pour the boiling water over it. Cover and let sit for 20 minutes.

Meanwhile, heat the oil in a skillet. Add the corn and ¼ teaspoon of salt and sauté over medium heat for 5 minutes. Add the onions and sauté for about 3 minutes, until the corn is tender. Allow to cool, then toss with the bulgur, chili, lemon and lime juice, ½ teaspoon of salt, and a few pinches of cayenne, to taste. Add more salt if necessary. Toss in the cilantro and sage just before serving.

Butternut Squash Soup with Apple Confit

Makes
8 to 9 cups

This is a delicious, satisfying soup for fall and winter. The squash purée is the smooth background flavor, with bits of apple throughout. Calvados (distilled from French cider) is the unusual ingredient here. The tart confit adds a lively touch, you can even serve it as a relish alongside a potato or winter squash gratin.—Annie

3 cups vegetable stock

1 tablespoon light olive oil

2 cups (1 medium) yellow onion, thinly sliced

1½ teaspoon salt

five-pepper mix or white pepper

2 tablespoons Calvados (or hard cider)

6 cups (about 4 pounds) butternut squash, peeled, seeded, and cut into large cubes

APPLE CONFIT

1 tablespoon unsalted butter

2 McIntosh or other flavorful, not-too-tart apples, peeled, cored, and sliced

1 tablespoon Calvados (or hard cider)

½ cup apple juice

½ cup crème fraiche (optional)

Warm the stock over low heat. Heat the olive oil in a soup pot and add the onions, ½ teaspoon of salt, and a pinch of pepper. Sauté over medium heat until the onions are lightly caramelized (about 15 minutes) adding a little stock and using a wooden spoon to scrape them as they stick to the pan. Add 2 tablespoons of the Calvados and cook for 1 or 2 minutes, until the pan is almost dry.

Add the squash and 1 teaspoon of salt to the onions. Add just enough stock to barely cover the squash (about 2 cups); the squash breaks down quickly and releases its own liquid as it cooks. Cover the pot and cook over medium heat for 20 to 30 minutes, until the squash is very soft. Purée the soup in a blender or food processor and thin it with stock to reach the desired consistency. Return the puréed soup to the pot, cover, and cook over low heat for 30 minutes.

While the soup is cooking, make the Apple Confit. Melt the butter in a medium-size skillet and add the apples. Sauté over medium-high heat, stirring to coat the apples with the butter. When they're heated through, add 1 tablespoon Calvados and cook for 1 or 2 minutes, until the pan is almost dry. Add the apple juice, cover the pan, and cook over medium heat for 15 to 20 minutes to reduce the liquid. Mash the apples with a fork or a masher, making sure the confit retains some texture.

Stir half the confit into the soup, saving the rest to stir into each serving. Season the soup with salt and pepper to taste. Add a spoonful of apple confit and a swirl of crème fraiche (if desired) to each serving right before serving.

Linguine with Golden and Green Zucchini, Cherry Tomatoes, Pine Nuts, and Gremolata

Serves
2 to 4

This easy summer pasta is a great way to show off brightly colored squash and a variety of cherry tomatoes. The fresh taste of gremolata—garlic, lemon zest, and Italian parsley—brings out all the flavors.—Annie

½ pound summer squash (use ¼ pound each of any combination of zucchini, yellow summer squash, sunburst, or pattypan squash)

1½ cups cherry tomatoes. (Recommended: Sweet 100, Sungold, Red or Yellow Pear)

3 cloves garlic, finely chopped

2 teaspoons lemon zest (the yellow skin of the lemon), finely chopped

2 tablespoons Italian parsley, chopped

3 tablespoons extra-virgin olive oil

1½ teaspoons salt

⅛ teaspoon ground pepper

½ pound fresh or dried linguine

1 tablespoon lemon juice

2 tablespoons pine nuts, toasted

grated Parmesan cheese to taste

Set a large pot of water on the stove to boil.

If you're using zucchini or summer squash, cut them in half lengthwise and slice them diagonally into ¼-inch-thick pieces. If you're using sunburst or pattypan squash, cut them in half through the stem end and slice into ½-inch-thick wedges. Cut the cherry tomatoes in half if they are large. Set aside 1 teaspoon garlic to sauté with the summer squash.

Make the gremolata by combining the remaining garlic with the lemon zest and Italian parsley in a small bowl. Set aside.

Heat 2 tablespoons of olive oil in a large skillet and add the squash, the reserved teaspoon of garlic, ¼ teaspoon of salt, and pepper. Sauté over medium-high heat for 2 to 3 minutes, just long enough to heat the squash through.

When the water is boiling, add 1 teaspoon of salt. Add the linguine and cook until just tender (about 45 seconds for fresh, and approximately 6 minutes for dry). Before you drain the pasta, add ½ cup of the cooking water to the sauté pan, along with the cherry tomatoes and remaining olive oil. Immediately drain the pasta, then add it to the pan. Toss in the gremolata, lemon juice, pine nuts, ¼ teaspoon of salt, and a few grinds more of pepper. Reduce the heat and toss well. Sprinkle with Parmesan and serve immediately.

ANNA THOMAS

Author of *The Vegetarian Epicure*

(♨) *Watercress and Radicchio Salad*

(♨) *White Bean and Garlic Soup with Chard*

(♨) *Kabocha Squash Stuffed with Savory Rice Pilaf*

(♨) *Caramelized Apple Pudding with Aged Cheddar Cheese*

In the 1970s, while a graduate student in film, Anna Thomas wrote the now-classic *The Vegetarian Epicure*, bringing a gourmet vision to vegetarian cooking and setting the table for a counterculture ready to feast with both earnestness and pleasure. Her latest cookbook, *The New Vegetarian Epicure: Menus for Family and Friends,* is inspired by her time spent in France, Italy, Mexico, and in her current home, southern California, as well as by her Polish roots. Organized around seasonal menus for both simple and lavish meals, the book exudes Anna's love for good food, her joy in preparing it, and her delight in sharing it with all of us.

Watercress and Radicchio Salad

Serves 8
as a side
salad

The peppery watercress salad is a perfect foil for the squash's natural sweetness and the pilaf's slightly exotic flavor. The salad can be served alongside the squash or as a separate course. This recipe calls for pumpkinseed oil, which has a rich, nutty flavor, and apple balsamic vinegar, the most subtle and gentle of vinegars. Both are marvelous, but not a stock item in many cupboards, so feel free to substitute a good, virgin olive oil and the wine vinegar of your choice. But go easy on the vinegar.—Anna

3 cups torn fresh watercress

1 large head red radicchio

3 medium Belgian endives

1½ tablespoons pumpkinseed oil

3 to 4 teaspoons apple balsamic vinegar

salt and pepper to taste

3 tablespoons toasted, salted pumpkin
   seeds

Wash the watercress thoroughly, as it tends to be muddy, and remove any thick stems, then tear it into pieces. Wash and tear the radicchio, and slice the endive crosswise into thin half-moons. Spin all the salad greens to remove excess water, or dry them by rolling them up in a kitchen towel.

Toss the salad with the pumpkinseed oil until all leaves are glistening. Add the vinegar, salt, and pepper, and toss again, then sprinkle on the pumpkin seeds.

White Bean and Garlic Soup with Chard

Serves
8 to 10

The white bean soup is an old favorite, and very simple to make; you do have to let the beans simmer for hours with garlic and sage, but that just perfumes your house as no potpourri could. This soup works well with chard, but would also be wonderful with kale, or with beet greens; whichever you use, be sure your greens are firm and glossy. Additional olive oil can be passed at the table to drizzle on top, or Parmesan cheese. I like to serve plain bruschetta with this—slices of baguette brushed with olive oil and rubbed lightly with garlic, then toasted or grilled.—Anna

1 pound small white beans (dried)	2 medium onions, chopped
1 head garlic, separated and peeled	1 large bunch Swiss chard (about 12 ounces)
2 teaspoons crumbled dried sage leaves	4 to 6 cups light vegetable broth
2 to 3 tablespoons olive oil	fresh ground black pepper to taste
1 teaspoon salt	1 teaspoon fresh lemon juice

Put the beans into a large, heavy-bottomed pot, and add about two quarts water, the garlic cloves (reserving one), the sage, and 2 or 3 teaspoons of olive oil.

Bring the beans to a boil, turn down the heat, and simmer them gently until they are tender. This could take anywhere from 2 to 5 hours, depending on the age of the beans. During this time, check the beans occasionally, and add water as needed to keep the beans well covered. When the beans are almost tender, add a teaspoon of salt.

Cook the chopped onions gently in a tablespoon of olive oil, stirring often, until they are evenly light brown, soft, and sweet.

Wash the chard thoroughly, cut off tough stems, and coarsely chop the greens or cut them into 1-inch strips. Chop the reserved clove of garlic, heat it in 2 teaspoons olive oil, and add the chard, tossing it in the hot oil until wilted.

When the beans are perfectly tender, scoop out about a cup and a half of them and reserve them. Add the caramelized onions to the remaining beans and bean broth, along with about 2 cups of the vegetable broth. Purée this mixture in a blender, in batches, until it is smooth and creamy.

Pour the purée back into the pot and add the reserved white beans, the sautéed chard, and 2 to 4 cups more of the vegetable broth—enough to get the consistency you like in the soup.

Season the soup with fresh ground black pepper, more salt if needed, and fresh lemon juice.

Kabocha Squash Stuffed with Savory Rice Pilaf

Serves
8 to 10

The stuffed kabocha squash is tasty, festive, and fun to serve. I bring the whole steaming squash to the table on a platter, lift its "lid," and cut it into fat wedges as I would a cake. The fragrant, colorful rice pilaf spills out over each wedge of squash as it's served, and more pilaf can be added to the plate around it. Don't be put off by the long list of ingredients. Many of them are the spices that give this pilaf its intriguing, slightly exotic flavor.—Anna

1 large kabocha squash (4 pounds or 2 medium)

1 large eggplant (1 pound)

salt to taste

2 tablespoons olive oil

1 large onion, chopped

2 cloves garlic, minced

1½ tablespoons fresh ginger, minced

1 teaspoon ground coriander

½ teaspoon cinnamon

1 teaspoon turmeric

pinch of crushed red pepper

1¾ cups uncooked basmati rice (or other long grain rice)

2 cups vegetable broth

2 cups water

12 ounces tomatillos, peeled, cut into ½-inch dice

½ cup green onions (bulb and light green sections), thin-sliced

½ cup dried cranberries or sour cherries

½ cup raisins

1 cup fresh cilantro leaves, packed

½ cup toasted pine nuts

1 tablespoon butter

fresh cilantro sprigs for garnish

Preheat the oven to 375° F. With a very sharp knife, cut an even circle, about 4 inches across, from the top of the kabocha squash. Lift the top off, and scoop out all the seeds and strings, scraping the inside of the squash until it is clean. Replace the lid, put the squash on a baking sheet, and roast it in the oven for about 45 minutes; it will be partly cooked.

Dice the eggplant into 1-inch cubes, salt it, and drain it in a colander for about half an hour, then gently squeeze out any excess moisture.

Meanwhile, heat a tablespoon of olive oil in a large, non-stick pan and sauté the onion and garlic in it for about 5 minutes. Add a dash of salt, the ginger, coriander, cinnamon, turmeric, crushed red pepper, and rice, and stir over medium heat for another 2 to 3 minutes.

Add the vegetable broth and water, then stir in the tomatillos, green onions, dried fruit, and half the cilantro. As soon as the liquid simmers, lower the heat, cover the pan, and cook the rice gently for 20 minutes. Turn off the heat and leave the pan covered for another 5 minutes. In another non-stick pan or wok, heat the remaining tablespoon of oil until a drop of water sizzles in it. Sauté the eggplant in it, stirring constantly, until it is tender and beginning to color. Taste, and add salt only if needed.

Fluff up the pilaf, and stir in the remaining cilantro, pine nuts, and eggplant. (The pilaf should be on the moist side, to balance the dense texture of the kabocha squash. If you want to make this recipe with another juicier type of squash, slightly reduce the liquid.)

Rub the butter over the inside of the squash, and sprinkle lightly with salt. Fill the squash with rice pilaf, nudging it in under the sides and tapping it down. If the pilaf seems dry, sprinkle it with a bit of broth or water. Replace the lid of the squash, fitting it snugly into its place.

Bake the squash at 350° F for another 45 minutes. Put the remaining pilaf into a buttered casserole, cover it, and put it in the oven with the squash for the last 15 minutes.

Bring the hot roasted squash to the table on an ample platter. Cut it into wedges, slicing right through the skin, which is now very soft. This is the fun part—the wedges fall out from the center, and the squash blossoms out like a flower, with pilaf spilling from the center. Lay a wedge of squash on each plate, and spoon on more pilaf from the casserole as you like.

Garnish plates with fresh cilantro sprigs.

Caramelized Apple Pudding with Aged Cheddar

Serves 8

This apple pudding is caramelized to a glazed golden-brown, like an old-fashioned upside-down cake with less cake to it. I love the sharp taste of a well-aged, crumbly piece of cheddar cheese with the sweetness of the apples. The apples are the most important thing here—they must be firm, juicy, sweet, and tart, and hold their shape through cooking. Fuji apples are my choice, but you could also use Granny Smiths or Golden Delicious.—Anna

7 slices home-style white bread	3 pounds Fuji or other firm apples
1½ cups milk	2 tablespoons butter
2 large eggs	½ teaspoon cinnamon
1 teaspoon vanilla	dash of nutmeg
pinch of salt	sharp, crumbly, aged cheddar
1 cup sugar	

Preheat the oven to 350° F. If the bread has thick crusts, trim them off (soft crusts are fine), then tear or cube the slices. Beat together the milk, eggs, vanilla, salt, and ¼ cup of the sugar. Add the bread to the custard, pushing it down into the liquid, and let it soak for at least 30 minutes. There should be very little liquid left.

Quarter, peel, and core the apples, and cut the quarters lengthwise into thick wedges, about ½ inch at the outside. Melt the butter in a nonstick pan and cook the apples in it for about 5 minutes. Add the remaining sugar, the cinnamon, and the nutmeg, and continue cooking, stirring gently, for about 10 more minutes. The apples should be tender but not falling apart, and should have released their juice. Remove apples with a slotted spoon, reserving the juices in the pan.

Butter a 9- or 10-inch nonstick springform cake pan. Arrange the cooked apples in the bottom of the pan, either making a pattern or pressing them in free-form, but cover the bottom of the pan completely. Stir up the bread and custard mixture and spoon it over the apples, distributing it evenly and pouring any remaining custard over the top.

Bake the pudding in the preheated oven for 35 minutes. The bread pudding on top should be puffed and golden brown.

Allow the pudding to cool on a rack for about 10 minutes, then slide a knife around the edge to loosen it, and remove the springform sides. Place a platter upside down on the pudding and invert the pudding onto the platter. Remove the pan bottom carefully, again sliding a thin knife between pan and pudding to loosen it if necessary. (It sometimes happens that apple slices fall out of place— just fit those escapees back where they belong and everything will be fine.)

Heat the reserved apple juices and boil them down to a thick syrup, then drizzle evenly over the apple pudding. Serve the pudding warm or cold, with a sharp, crumbly cheddar cheese.

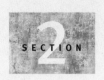

RECIPES FROM PIONEER CHEFS AND RESTAURANTS

BRINGING US ORGANIC AND WHOLE FOODS, AND CELEBRATING LOCALLY GROWN CUISINE

Á LA CARTE

SALADS

CANDLE CAFÉ, New York, New York
Chef Jonathan Grumbles

Aztec Salad

L'ETOILE, Madison, Wisconsin
Chef/Proprietor Odessa Piper

Warm Salad of Roast Wild Mushrooms and Sprouted Nuts

OLEANA, Cambridge, Massachusetts
Chef/Owner Ana Sortun

Carrot Salad with Hot Goat Cheese Crotin

Soup

MILLENNIUM RESTAURANT, San Francisco, California
Head Chef Eric Tucker

🍽 *Yellow Doll Watermelon Ginger Soup with Cardamom Cream*

Entrées

ANGELICA KITCHEN, New York, New York
Chef Pete Cervoni

🍽 *Marinated Tofu over a Roasted Yukon Gold Potato Caponata with Sun-Dried Tomato and Basil Coulis*

CHEZ PANISSE, Berkeley, California
Chef/Owner Alice Waters

🍽 *Pizza with Red and Yellow Peppers with Homemade Pizza Dough*

FRONTERA GRILL AND TOPOLOBAMPO, Chicago, Illinois
Chef Rick Bayless

🍽 *Simple Chipotle Chilaquiles (Tortilla "Casserole")*

HIGGINS RESTAURANT & BAR, Portland, Oregon
Chef/Owner Greg Higgins

🍽 *Fennel and Hazelnut Potato Cakes with Fall Vegetable Slaw and Two Chutneys*

MENUS

FLEA ST. CAFÉ, Menlo Park, California
Owner Jesse Cool

🍽 *Sweet Potato Hash with Barley*

🍽 *Beet Soup with Dill Cream*

(¶) *Swiss Cheese Broccoli Timbales*

(¶) *Tempeh, Spinach, and Ricotta Parmesana*

(¶) *Silken Tofu Mocha Pudding with Crystallized Ginger*

THE ROSS SCHOOL, East Hampton, New York
Executive Chef Ann Cooper

(¶) *Grilled Summer Vegetable Haystack on Polenta*

(¶) *Summer Gazpacho*

ST. MARTIN'S TABLE, Minneapolis, Minnesota
Chef/Restaurant Manager Karen Franzmeier

(¶) *Thai Tofu Spread*

(¶) *Curried Potato, Leek, and Kale Soup*

(¶) *Lemon Ginger Snaps*

REAL FOOD DAILY, Los Angeles, California
Founder Ann Gentry

(¶) *Skillet Corn Bread with Scallion "Butter"*

(¶) *Red Bean, Squash, and Okra Stew*

(¶) *Garlicky Greens*

CAFÉ FLORA, Seattle, Washington
Executive Chef Cathy Geier/Co-owner Scott Glascock

(¶) *Oaxaco Tacos*

(¶) *Black Bean Stew*

(¶) *Pico de Gallo*

(¶) *Lemon Garlic Vinaigrette with Chard*

(¶) *Crème Fraiche and Lime Crème Fraiche*

WHITE DOG CAFE, Philadelphia, Pennsylvania
Executive Chef/Partner Kevin Von Klause

- Spinach and Fennel Salad with Curried Pears and Hazelnuts
- Orange-Rosemary Vinaigrette
- Chilled Cucumber Soup with Tomato-Tarragon Relish
- Wild Mushroom–Barley Risotto
- Harvest Fruit Crisp

RESTAURANT NORA, Washington, DC
Chef/Owner Nora Pouillon

- Arugula and Melon Salad with Lime Dressing
- Grilled Eggplant Steak with Roasted Red Peppers, Feta Cheese, Black Olives, and Pita Bread
- Russian Blueberry and Raspberry Pudding

SALADS

CANDLE CAFÉ
New York, New York
Chef Jonathan Grumbles

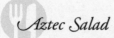

Aztec Salad

Serves 4

You can vary the vegetables in this salad depending on what is in season and what is locally available. This version is best in summer when these vegetables are at their peak.—Jonathan

1½ cups uncooked quinoa	1 tablespoon olive oil
2¾ cups water	½ teaspoon chili powder
1 tablespoon salt	2 cups cooked black beans (or 1 can drained)
2 ears sweet corn	
1 cup pumpkin seeds, toasted	1 red onion, diced

1 bunch cilantro, chopped

1 red pepper, diced

1 lime

lettuce of your choice

DRESSING FOR SALAD

4 Roma tomatoes, roasted

1¼ cups extra virgin olive oil

½ cup red wine vinegar

1 tablespoon plus 1 teaspoon salt

1 teaspoon black pepper

1 teaspoon crushed red pepper

2 cloves garlic, minced

2 tablespoons fresh cilantro, coarsely
   chopped (optional)

Add the quinoa to boiling, salted water and bring to a simmer. Reduce heat, cover, and cook for 20 to 25 minutes. Fluff and then remove quinoa from pot. Put in a large bowl (to avoid stickiness) and allow to cool.

Pre-heat the oven to 375° F. While the quinoa is cooking, cook the corn in salted water. Remove the kernels by scraping them off. Toss the pumpkin seeds with 1 tablespoon of olive oil, 1 teaspoon of salt, and ½ teaspoon of chili powder. Spread the seeds on a baking sheet and cook at 375° F for 5 to 7 minutes. Seeds will start to pop. Toss all ingredients together (except pumpkin seeds and lettuce) and add the juice of 1 lime. Mix in the cooled quinoa.

To Make Dressing:

Cut the Roma tomatoes in half. Toss with 1 tablespoon of olive oil, and ½ teaspoon of salt and black pepper. Place the tomatoes on a sheet pan (cut side down) and roast them at 400° F for 20 to 25 minutes. The skin will blister. Remove and let cool. Combine all ingredients in a blender and blend until smooth.

To Assemble Salad:

Place a handful of your favorite lettuce or salad mix in a bowl. (Watercress or young lettuces from a local farmers' market are recommended.) Lightly dress the lettuce. Place the quinoa mixture in a bowl and toss it with the desired amount of dressing. Place about 1 cup of dressed quinoa mixture on top of lettuce. Sprinkle with pumpkin seeds and drizzle with small amount of dressing.

L'ETOILE

Madison, Wisconsin

Chef/Proprietor Odessa Piper

Odessa Piper moved to Madison in 1969 where she helped her mentor, JoAnna Guthrie, open a restaurant that featured organic produce grown on JoAnna's farm. Odessa's excitement with the exceptional quality and diversity of the region's foods inspired her to create menus reliant on season and locality. This was the impetus to open her own restaurant in 1976, L'Etoile, referring both to nature's edible stars and the French culinary mother tongue of her Midwest interpretations.

Warm Salad of Roast Wild Mushrooms and Sprouted Nuts

Makes
4 to 6
servings

This perennially popular dish at L'Etoile accommodates every season and most diets; its nutty, rich flavors are as nutritious as they are tasty. Since we never know when our wild mushroom gatherers will find a cache of mushrooms, we combine wild with cultivated varieties to sustain a good mix. If you are lucky enough to have access to wild mushrooms, try mixing some in; the ones we use range from morel, chicken of the wood, chanterelle, blue foot, hen o' the woods, lobster, and puff balls.—Odessa

6 cups assorted exotic, cultivated or wild
    mushrooms such as:
        2 cups (½ pound) portabello, cut into
            wedges
        2 cups (¼ pound) shiitake, stems
            removed
        1 cup (⅛ pound) crimini
        1½ cups (¼ pound) oyster
        ½ cup (¹⁄₁₆ pound) enoki
4 teaspoons vegetable oil
2 teaspoons kosher salt flakes or sea salt

1 teaspoon freshly ground pepper
1 cup sprouted nuts and legumes (a mix of
    lentils and sunflower seeds, etc.)
½ cup unsalted peanuts
½ cup almonds
1 tablespoon Dijon or other prepared
    mustard
2 tablespoons champagne vinegar
¾ cup light vegetable oil
8 cups mild salad greens
salt and pepper to taste

Preheat the oven to 350° F. Wipe dirt off mushrooms with a towel or mushroom brush. (Do not wash; that makes them soggy!) Remove stems from tough varieties such as shiitake. Cut mushrooms into pieces large enough to show off their variety and colors. Toss them in vegetable oil, salt, and pepper. Spread the wild or thicker mushrooms (morel, shiitake, gold chanterelles, chicken o' the woods, lobster, portabello) one layer thick on a baking sheet. Roast in the oven for 20 to 30 minutes.

While the mushrooms are roasting, coarsely chop peanuts and almonds, and lightly toast in oven for 3 to 5 minutes. Watch carefully so they don't burn. Whisk mustard, vinegar, and oil to make a vinaigrette. Set aside. Wash and dry salad greens.

Just before serving, add the more delicate mushrooms, the sprouted legumes, and the nuts to the baking sheet. Roast again at 350° F for 5 more minutes, until warmed through. Toss the greens with a small amount of vinaigrette to moisten them, then toss through the warm mushrooms, legumes, and nuts to slightly wilt them.

Center portions of salad on plates, pulling the mushrooms up to the top and spooning the nuts that have fallen to the bottom of the bowl around the plate rims. Drizzle remaining vinaigrette over the nuts. Serve with salt and freshly ground pepper.

OLEANA

Cambridge, Massachusetts

Chef/Owner Ana Sortun

Chef Ana Sortun is committed to cooking responsibly and healthfully. She works closely with local farmers to get fresh, organic products. How food looks is the last thing Ana concentrates on; "in between, there's how it *feels*." This salad, however, scores on both fronts.

Carrot Salad with Hot Goat Cheese Crotin

Serves 4   *Fresh herbs are essential in this recipe. The parsley, mint, and dill spark up the Jerusalem-style shredded carrot salad; the warm coated goat cheese coins contrast in temperature and texture. When topped with the toasted pine nuts, the salad sings with flavor.—Ana*

3 teaspoons garlic (2 cloves), finely minced

¼ cup lemon juice (about 3 small lemons)

¼ teaspoon salt

⅛ teaspoon sugar

¼ teaspoon freshly ground black pepper

1 tablespoon white wine vinegar

1 tablespoon plain yogurt

4 tablespoons extra virgin olive oil

3 carrots

½ cup parsley leaves (about 8 sprigs), loosely packed

½ cup mint leaves (about 8 sprigs), loosely packed

2 tablespoons dill (about 4 sprigs)

4 tablespoons pine nuts

2 4-ounce logs of goat cheese

2 eggs

1 tablespoon water

pinch of salt

½ cup flour

1 tablespoon extra virgin olive oil

In a small stainless steel mixing bowl, let the garlic sit with the lemon juice, salt, and sugar for 5 minutes. Whisk in the pepper, vinegar, yogurt, and olive oil, and taste for seasoning.

Peel and grate the carrots. Wash and dry the herbs, and finely chop them. Toast the pine nuts in a toaster oven set at 400° F or in a dry cast-iron skillet until lightly browned, watching carefully so that they don't burn.

Toss the carrots with the dressing, herbs, and pine nuts. Taste for seasoning.

Cut each goat cheese log into four thick coins. Beat the eggs with the water and salt in a small bowl. Put flour on a plate. Coat each side of the cheese coin in flour, then egg mixture, then flour again.

Heat the oil in a small frying pan and brown the goat cheese coins on both sides. Serve hot on top of the carrot salad. You can make the salad a couple of hours ahead of time and refrigerate. Let it come to room temperature before serving, and reheat cheese for 4 minutes in a 400° F oven or toaster oven.

SOUP

MILLENNIUM RESTAURANT

San Francisco, California

Head Chef Eric Tucker

Eric Tucker has been the Executive Chef of Millennium since it opened in 1994. Millennium is an avid supporter of local organic farmers and vendors. His vegan cooking blends cuisines from different ethnic backgrounds and has been praised for its innovative combinations and unexpectedly rich flavors. A coauthor of *Millennium Cookbook: Extraordinary Vegetarian Cuisine,* which is filled with vegan recipes for the artistic cook, Eric says: "My mission is to show the public that you don't have to compromise flavor and texture as you cut out fat and animal products. At Millennium we dispel the stereotypes and misconceptions held by many about low-fat foods and vegan cuisine."

Yellow Doll Watermelon Ginger Soup with Cardamom Cream

Serves 6   *A perfect way to start a meal in the August heat. Really refreshing and palate-invigorating—and absolutely beautiful, whether you use the yellow doll watermelon or substitute the familiar red.—Eric*

4 cups either yellow doll or regular
    watermelon flesh, seeds removed

1 tablespoon minced ginger

2 cups water

3 tablespoons fresh lime juice (2 small limes)

1 teaspoon sugar (optional, to taste)

¼ teaspoon cayenne

¼ teaspoon salt (or to taste)

Cardamom Cream (recipe follows)

2 tablespoons small peppermint leaves

In a blender, blend the melon, ginger, water, lime juice, sugar, and cayenne until smooth. Add salt to taste and refrigerate until well chilled. Serve with two teaspoons of Cardamom Cream, and scatter peppermint leaves over the soup. The Cardamom Cream will form lovely little droplets on top of the soup.

Cardamom Cream

¼ cup cashews, lightly toasted

1 teaspoon white (shiro) miso

½ teaspoon ground cardamom

¼ teaspoon salt

½ cup water

Place all ingredients in a blender and blend until smooth.

ENTRÉES

ANGELICA KITCHEN

New York, New York

Chef Pete Cervoni

Pete Cervoni, former chef of Angelica Kitchen, confessed to us that years ago in one of his Political Science courses he skipped the required reading—*Food First* and *Diet for a Small Planet*. After studies in political science and law, he graduated from the Culinary Institute of America.

"I had been armed with a great deal of knowledge, not the least of which was the ability to take just about any once-living animal and make it dinner." One day, in the middle of roasting 200 pounds of veal bones for the demi-glace he made weekly for one of New York's finest restaurants, he stopped and looked around. He didn't like what he saw. He began regretting his skipped reading. "About a year later," Pete says, "I found a better way—vegan. I realized I didn't need to rely on animals for nourishment. I could make food taste good without animal products."

Marinated Tofu over a Roasted Yukon Gold Potato Caponata with Sun-Dried Tomato and Basil Coulis

Serves 4   *This dish may appear complicated at first glance, but it really is not. Simply view the dish in three phases: Tofu, Potatoes, and Sauce. It is a rustic, hearty dish with simple, uncomplicated flavors. The caponata is not a traditional one. Actually, it is a hybrid, a cross between a caponata and a ratatouille and, in this application, serves as starch and vegetable together.—Pete*

MARINATED TOFU	2 teaspoons freshly ground pepper
1 pound extra firm tofu	1 cup apple cider
2 teaspoons anise seed	¼ cup apple cider vinegar
2 teaspoons fennel seed	⅓ cup extra virgin olive oil
½ teaspoon salt	

ROASTED YUKON GOLD POTATO CAPONATA

2 cups eggplant, diced into ¼-inch cubes

⅔ cup onion (1 small), diced into ¼-inch cubes

2 cups zucchini, diced into ¼-inch cubes

1 cup yellow summer squash, diced into ¼-inch cubes

½ cup red pepper, diced into ¼-inch cubes

1 tablespoon garlic (2 cloves), minced

2½ tablespoons extra virgin olive oil

2 cups (2 small) Yukon Gold potatoes, diced into ¼-inch cubes

2 teaspoons fresh rosemary, minced, or 1½ teaspoons dried

1 teaspoon salt

½ teaspoon freshly ground pepper

1 tablespoon capers, minced

⅓ cup kalamata olives, minced

SUN-DRIED TOMATO AND BASIL COULIS

⅓ cup onion, diced to ¼-inch cubes

1½ teaspoon garlic (1 small clove), minced

pinch of red pepper flakes

¼ teaspoon salt

¼ teaspoon freshly ground pepper

1½ teaspoons extra virgin olive oil

1½ teaspoons balsamic vinegar

½ cup sun-dried tomatoes, dry

2 cups water

⅓ cup fresh basil, cut into fine strips

4 cups tightly packed washed and stemmed spinach leaves

MARINATED TOFU

Begin by marinating the tofu, which you can do up to a day ahead of time. Press excess liquid from the tofu by placing beneath a weighted plate. Alternatively you can boil the tofu for 10 minutes, then drain. Slice the tofu into 8 equal pieces.

Grind the anise and fennel seeds in a coffee grinder or blender. Mix the ground seeds, salt, pepper, apple cider, and apple cider vinegar, then whisk in the olive oil as if you were making a dressing. In a shallow baking dish just big enough to fit the 8 pieces of tofu without the pieces touching, place the tofu and cover with the marinade. Allow to marinate for at least 1 hour or as long as overnight.

Just before you are ready to bake the tofu, preheat the oven to 350° F. Bake the tofu for about ½ hour to 40 minutes, or until most of the marinade has been absorbed and the edges of each piece are beginning to brown. Reserve warm.

(This is when it's useful to have two ovens, because to make the caponata, you need about 45 minutes and a 400° F oven. If you don't have two ovens, do the tofu first, then cover it with foil. To reheat, place uncovered in the oven for the last five minutes that the vegetables are roasting. Alternately, you could make the caponata a day ahead, cover and refrigerate, and warm in the oven the last 10 minutes the tofu is baking.)

ROASTED YUKON GOLD POTATO CAPONATA

For the caponata, preheat the oven to 400° F. Toss the diced eggplant and onion with a teaspoon of oil and place in a large baking dish (it will eventually house all of the vegetables except the potatoes, and you want the vegetables spread fairly thin so they can roast, not steam). Roast the eggplant and onion for 10 minutes. Meanwhile, toss the diced zucchini, squash, red pepper, garlic, and pepper in 1 tablespoon oil. In a separate bowl, mix the diced potatoes with 1 tablespoon of oil, the rosemary, salt, and pepper.

After 10 minutes, add the zucchini vegetable mix to the eggplant and onion, stir, and roast in the oven for 30 to 35 more minutes. At the same time, put the potatoes in an oiled baking dish and roast until done, about 30 to 35 minutes.

SUN-DRIED TOMATO COULIS

While the vegetables are roasting, make the Sun-Dried Tomato Coulis. In a small saucepan, sauté the onions, garlic, red-pepper flakes, salt, and pepper in the olive oil over medium heat for about 2 minutes. Add the balsamic vinegar and stir, then add the sun-dried tomatoes and the water. Bring to a boil, and reduce heat. Simmer for 10 minutes. Turn off the heat. Cover the pan and let the mixture steep for another 10 minutes.

Carefully purée the mixture in a blender until smooth, and return to the sauce pan, keeping warm until needed. Just before serving, add the basil and stir. (The coulis can be made a day ahead of time and refrigerated, just keep out the basil until just before serving. Reheat slowly on the stove, adding basil and stirring until smooth.)

While the coulis is cooking and the vegetables are roasting, wash, stem, and spin dry the spinach leaves. Set aside.

To serve, on each plate place a bed of spinach, then a fourth of the potato caponata, and on top of that, 2 tofu pieces. Top it all with the coulis—and you have a dish of contrasting colors and flavors. Start with a soup and serve this as an entrée, or serve it by itself for a special lunch.

CHEZ PANISSE

Berkeley, California

Chef/Owner Alice Waters

Alice Waters opened Chez Panisse in 1971, serving a five-course, fixed price menu that changes daily. To this day, the set menu format remains the heart of Alice's philosophy of serving the highest quality products according to season. Alice is author and coauthor of several books, including *The Chez Panisse Menu Cookbook, Fanny at Chez Panisse,* a storybook and cookbook for children, and, most recently, the encyclopedic *Chez Panisse Vegetables.*

Pizza with Red and Yellow Peppers with Homemade Pizza Dough

Makes 1 12-inch pizza

When garnishing a pizza, anticipate flavor and balance. A light hand with weighty ingredients such as cheese, tomatoes, and so on, and bold amounts of fresh herbs, garlic, anchovies, flavored oils, and the like, works best. It is better to err on the side of flavor.—Alice

3 bell peppers—1 red, 1 orange, 1 yellow

½ small red onion

¼ cup parsley leaves

¼ cup basil leaves

3 tablespoons olive oil

1 teaspoon red wine vinegar

salt and pepper to taste

2 ounces mozzarella cheese

1 clove garlic

homemade pizza dough for 1 pizza (recipe
    follows)

Preheat the oven—with a pizza stone in it—to 450° to 500° F. Slice thin the peppers and onion, and roughly chop the parsley and basil. Toss in a bowl with 2 tablespoons of the olive oil and the vinegar, and season to taste with salt and pepper.

Coarsely grate the cheese. Chop the garlic fine and mix it with the remaining tablespoon of olive oil.

Roll out a disk of pizza dough 12 to 14 inches in diameter and place it on the back of a lightly floured sheet pan or a pizza peel. Using a pastry brush or your fingers, brush the garlic and oil mixture onto the dough, leaving a ½-inch border. Sprinkle the grated cheese on top of the oiled dough. Spread the pepper mixture on top of the cheese. Slide the pizza directly onto the pizza brick and bake for 4 to 6 minutes or until the dough is crispy and thoroughly cooked. Slice and serve immediately.

Note: For another version of pepper pizza, season the pepper mixture with chopped marjoram or oregano, and thyme, and sprinkle the crust with a large pinch of hot pepper flakes. Garnish with chopped parsley before serving.

Another variation is to season a pepper pizza with chopped cilantro and a julienned jalapeno pepper (seeded or not, as your taste dictates), and to garnish it with cilantro leaves and a squeeze of lemon juice.

For the most volcanic pepper pizza of all, use only jalapenos: Slice about 10 jalapenos into wagon-wheel rounds and macerate them in rice wine vinegar, salt, chopped cilantro, and a little olive oil; bake on a pizza crust, as above, and serve, garnished with cilantro leaves.

Homemade Pizza Dough

Makes 1 12-inch to 14-inch pizza, or several small ones

¼ cup lukewarm water	1 tablespoon milk
2 teaspoons active dry yeast	2 tablespoons olive oil
¼ cup rye flour	½ teaspoon salt
½ cup lukewarm water	1¼ cups unbleached all-purpose flour

Make a sponge by mixing together the ¼ cup warm water, yeast, and rye flour. Let it rise 20 to 30 minutes, then add the rest of the ingredients.

Mix the dough with a wooden spoon, then knead on a floured board. It will be soft and a little sticky. Use quick light motions with your hands so the dough won't stick. Add more flour to the board as you knead, but no more than is absolutely necessary. A soft, moist dough makes a light and very crispy crust. Knead for 10 to 15 minutes to develop strength and elasticity in the dough. Put in a bowl rubbed with olive oil, and oil the surface of the dough to prevent a crust from forming. Cover the bowl with a towel and put it in a warm place, approximately 90° to 110° F. An oven heated just by its pilot light is a good spot. Let the dough rise to double its size (for about 2 hours), then punch it down. Let it rise about 40 minutes more, then shape and bake it.

One of the very best ways to bake a pizza is directly on the floor of a wood-fired brick or stone oven. Not too many households have one, but the effect can be approximated by putting a layer of unglazed ceramic tiles on a rack in your oven. Preheat the oven to 450° to 500° F. Use a wood paddle or the back of a baking sheet to put the pizza in and remove it from the oven.

Flatten the dough on a heavily floured board. Use a rolling pin to roll the dough to roughly 12 to 14 inches in diameter. (When you roll and shape the dough, feel free to make it any shape you wish. Large flat pizzas with uneven bubbly edges have a rustic appeal. Small individual-sized pizzas, served as a savory accompaniment to a meal instead of bread, are very satisfying.) The dough should be ⅛- to ¼-inch thick. Transfer the dough to a paddle or baking sheet, also heavily floured.

Have your toppings ready, at room temperature, and work quickly putting them on the pizza, because after a minute or so the dough will begin to stick and will be impossible to slide off the paddle. To prevent a soggy bottom, tomatoes and other wet foods should be drained of excess liquid. Whatever is on the top must be able to cook in 15 minutes, or should have had some partial cooking beforehand.

Beware of spilling anything wet or oily between the dough and paddle, as that too will prevent it from sliding. Give the paddle a few shakes back and forth to make sure the dough is loose. Slide the pizza from the paddle onto the hot tiles in the oven with abrupt jerking motions of your wrist. This takes a certain knack, but comes easily after a few tries. The pizza will be browned and cooked in 12 to 15 minutes.

If your oven cannot maintain an intense heat of 450° to 500° F, then the dough will perform better if rolled a little on the thick side, ¼ inch or more. When you are deciding whether the pizza is cooked, check the bottom to make sure it is quite crisp. The crust always softens a bit when it cools down.

FRONTERA GRILL AND TOPOLOBAMPO

Chicago, Illinois

Chef Rick Bayless

Simple Chipotle Chilaquiles (Tortilla "Casserole")

Serves 4
as a casual
main dish

One of my nineteenth-century Mexican cookbooks defines chilaquiles as a soup made with day-old tortillas. But in modern-day Mexico's version, the tortillas are fried first, like chips, giving them a more toothsome texture in the brothy sauce. That is, if you eat the chilaquiles right away and if you use crisp-fried tortillas, those with some heft to them—not the thin melt-in-your-mouth kind we Americans nosh; they'll only make soft chilaquiles hash. My simple, traditional Chipotle Chilaquiles begin with a simmering pot of tomato broth flecked with the smoky sizzle of chipotle chilies (you can substitute jalapenos or serranos, if you want). Add the thickish chips, then set a lid in place and turn off the heat. Over the next few minutes, the chips soften perfectly, infusing themselves with Mexican flavor. Spoon the chilaquiles into a deep plate like you would saucy pasta. Then add a sprinkling of full-flavored dry grating cheese like the Mexican queso añejo *or a drizzling of cream, and sliced raw onion, which gives the perfect counterpoint of fresh crunch.—Rick*

12 (10 ounces total) corn tortillas, cut into sixths and fried or baked to make chips, or 8 ounces (8 to 12 loosely packed cups, depending on thickness) thick homemade-style tortilla chips (such as ones you buy at a Mexican grocery)

1 28-ounce can good-quality whole tomatoes in juice, drained, or 1½ lbs (about 3 medium-large round or 9 to 12 plum) ripe tomatoes

2 to 3 canned chipotle chilies en adobo or 2 to 3 dried chipotle chilies, stemmed

1½ tablespoons vegetable or olive oil

1 large white onion, sliced ¼-inch thick

3 garlic cloves, peeled and finely chopped

2½ cups vegetable broth or water, plus a little extra if needed

salt to taste

about ⅓ cup homemade cream, crème fraiche, or store-bought sour cream thinned with a little milk

1½ cups finely crumbled Mexican *queso anejo* or other dry grating cheese such as Romano or Parmesan

2 cups sliced red chard leaves or lamb's quarters (quelites) (optional)

3 tablespoons fresh epazote, roughly chopped, or ½ cup fresh cilantro, chopped (optional)

The brothy sauce can be completed up to 3 or 4 days ahead of time and stored in the refrigerator, covered. Homemade chips for chilaquiles are also fine made a day or two in advance. Chilaquiles lose texture once they're made, so I complete the simple tasks of cooking and serving them when everyone's ready to eat.

Note: If you're using dried chipotles, first toast them in a dry skillet over medium heat for about a minute, turning frequently, until very aromatic. Then place in a small bowl, cover with hot tap water, and let rehydrate for 30 minutes. While they're rehydrating you can prepare these other ingredients.

The Chips

Measure out store-bought chips or make the chips by cutting corn tortillas into sixths and baking or frying until crispy.

The Brothy Sauce

If using drained canned tomatoes, place them in a blender jar. If using fresh tomatoes, spread them onto a baking sheet and place them 4 inches below a very hot broiler. When they're darkly roasted after about 6 minutes (they'll be blackened in spots), flip them over and roast the other side. Five or 6 minutes more will give you splotchy-black and blistered tomatoes that are soft and cooked through. Cool. Working over your baking sheet, pull off and discard the blackened skins and, for round tomatoes, cut out the hard "cores" where the stems were attached. Transfer to a blender, along with all the juices on the baking sheet. If using canned chipotles, add them to the blender, seeds and all. If using dried chipotles, take the chilies that you've rehydrated, drain, and add to the blender. Blend the tomatoes and chilies to a purée, but one that still retains a little texture. You should have 2¼ cups of purée.

Over medium heat, set a medium-large (4- to 5-quart) pot or Dutch oven, or a deep, large (12-inch) skillet (you'll need a lid for whatever vessel you choose). Measure in the oil, add half of the onion, and cook, stirring regularly, until golden (about 7 minutes). Add the garlic and stir for another minute, then raise the heat to medium-high. Add the tomato purée and stir nearly constantly for 4 or 5 minutes, until the mixture thickens somewhat. Stir in the broth or water and season with salt, usually about 2 teaspoons if you are using salted chips. Cover the pot if not cooking and serve the chilaquiles right away. You should have about 4½ cups of broth mixture.

Cooking and Serving the Chilaquiles

Set out the remaining onion, cream, and cheese. Put the pot over medium-high heat until the broth sauce boils. Stir in chard or lamb's quarters and the tortilla chips, coating all the chips well. Let return to a rolling boil, cover, and turn off the heat. Let stand 5 minutes (no longer). Immediately uncover and carefully stir to coat the chips evenly with the sauce and to check that the chips have softened nicely—they should be a little chewy, not mushy. (If they're too chewy, stir in a few tablespoons more broth, cover, and set over medium heat for a couple minutes more.) Sprinkle with the epazote or cilantro, if using.

Either spoon onto warm individual plates in the kitchen or serve directly from the vessel it was made in. Drizzle the chilaquiles with the cream (or one of its stand-ins), strew with the remaining sliced onion, and dust generously with the finely crumbled cheese.

HIGGINS RESTAURANT & BAR

Portland, Oregon

Chef/Owner Greg Higgins

Fennel and Hazelnut Potato Cakes with Fall Vegetable Slaw and Two Chutneys

Serves 6

2½ pounds Yukon Gold potatoes, peeled and cut into ¾-inch cubes

1 pound fresh fennel bulb, sliced thin and blanched

4 tablespoons fresh ginger, minced

½ teaspoon asafetida

½ teaspoon ground black pepper

1 tablespoon toasted cumin seeds, lightly ground

1 teaspoon garam masala

1 teaspoon sesame oil

¼ cup grape seed oil

6 ounces toasted chopped hazelnuts

salt and pepper to taste

Fall Vegetable Slaw (recipe follows)

Carrot-Habanero and Cilantro-Hazelnut Chutneys (recipes follow)

Boil the potatoes in lightly salted water until tender. Drain well and rice the cooked potatoes in a food mill. Combine the potatoes and all ingredients except hazelnuts in a large bowl. Mix well and adjust the seasoning to taste with salt and pepper. Portion the mix into 12 balls and roll these in the toasted hazelnuts. Using a spatula, flatten them into patties on a lightly oiled baking sheet. Bake in a pre-heated 400° F oven until lightly browned (20 to 25 minutes). Serve with Fall Vegetable Slaw, Carrot-Habanero, and Cilantro-Hazelnut Chutneys. Try serving over basmati rice.

Fall Vegetable Slaw

1 carrot, peeled

1 chioggia beet, peeled

1 golden beet, peeled

1 parsnip, peeled

1 turnip, peeled

2 tablespoons rice wine vinegar

1 tablespoon toasted cumin seeds

salt and pepper to taste

Finely julienne the peeled root vegetables on a mandolin or other shredding utensil. Dress with the rice wine vinegar and cumin seeds. Season to taste with salt and pepper.

Cilantro-Hazelnut Chutney

1 bunch cilantro, coarsely chopped

3 jalapeños, roasted, peeled and de-seeded

2 tablespoons garlic, minced

2 ounces toasted, chopped hazelnuts

3 limes, juiced

salt and pepper to taste

Purée all ingredients in a blender until smooth and season to taste with salt and pepper.

Carrot-Habanero Chutney

3 carrots, peeled and sliced ½-inch thick

1 habanero pepper, stem removed

1 cup white wine vinegar

salt and pepper to taste

water as needed

Bring the carrots, vinegar, and habanero to a simmer over medium heat. Cook until carrots are tender, adding water as needed to keep them covered in a liquid. Purée the cooked carrots and pepper in a blender until smooth, seasoning to taste with salt.

MENUS

FLEA ST. CAFÉ
Menlo Park, California
Restaurant Owner Jesse Cool

- *Sweet Potato Hash with Barley*
- *Beet Soup With Dill Cream*
- *Swiss Cheese Broccoli Timbales*
- *Tempeh, Spinach, and Ricotta Parmesana*
- *Silken Tofu Mocha Pudding with Crystallized Ginger*

Jesse Cool is the owner of Flea St. Café, jZcool Eating and Catering, and the Cool Café at the Cantor Arts Center at Stanford University—what she calls "a tiny organic restaurant empire attempting to be sustainable in as many ways as possible." For twenty-six years she has been committed to organic products and celebrating the sensuous aspects of wholesome food. Jesse's *Your Organic Kitchen: The Essential Guide to Selecting and Cooking Organic Foods* is an organic feast for the senses, giving readers all the information they need to create their own organic kitchen at home.

Sweet Potato Hash with Barley

Serves 6
as a side
dish

Next to my organic raised beds is a coop with four chickens, who give me the best eggs in the world! I make this hash and top it with a couple of those fresh eggs poached or fried over easy. The yolks seep into the hash and the only thing left to reach for is the bottle of hot sauce.—Jesse

2 tablespoons vegetable or light olive oil

½ cup uncooked barley

1 small yellow onion, chopped coarsely

1 medium sweet potato or yam, peeled and
    cut into ¼-inch pieces

1 cup water or vegetable stock

salt and freshly ground pepper to taste

In a heavy-bottom, medium-size sauce pan with a lid, heat the olive oil over medium heat and toast the barley for a few minutes until it is nutty brown. Add the onions and potatoes. Stirring occasionally, brown both slightly.

Add the barley and the water or stock. Reduce the heat to medium-low. Simmer for about 15 minutes, or until barley is softened and all the liquid is gone. Stir often. Season generously with salt and pepper.

Suggestion: Add smoked or grilled tofu to make this a complete and very healthy dish.

Beet Soup with Dill Cream

Serves
6 to 8

My Jewish background is filled with old-world food combinations, including beets, potatoes, sour cream, and dill. As with any good soup, neither the ingredients nor the technique need be complicated.—Jesse

6 cups water or vegetable broth

1½ pounds beets (red or golden)

3 tablespoons red wine vinegar

1 medium yellow onion, sliced thin

1 bay leaf

5 whole peppercorns

3 whole cloves

¼ to ½ cup sugar to taste (depending on
   the sweetness of the beets)

½ pound boiling potatoes (not russets)

½ cup buttermilk or sour cream

1 green onion, white and light green parts,
   sliced thin

2 tablespoons fresh dill, chopped

salt and pepper to taste, for both soup and
   potato cream

Scrub the beets, and cut off the greens and tips. In a large soup pot, put the water, vinegar, beets, onion, bay leaf, peppercorns, and cloves. Simmer over medium heat for about 30 minutes or until the beets are tender when you stick a fork in them. When done, pour everything into a colander, catching all the strained juices in a large bowl. Return the juices to the pan and keep simmering over low heat.

Run cold water over the beets and remove them. Using your hands, slip the skins off of the beets. Cut them into ½-inch cubes and return them to the beet juice. Add sugar to taste (the beets may be sweet enough on their own), and season with salt and pepper.

While the beets are cooking, bring a small pot of salted water to a boil. Peel the potatoes and cut into ½-inch cubes. Cook the potatoes until very soft. Strain the potatoes. In a medium bowl, mash them with a fork or potato masher along with the sour cream or buttermilk, green onion, and dill (save a little dill for garnish). Season the potato cream with salt and pepper.

Ladle the beets and broth into bowls. Spoon a generous dollop of the potato cream on top. Garnish with extra chopped dill.

Swiss Cheese Broccoli Timbales

Serves 4 as a
main course,
8 as an appetizer

These little broccoli "cupcakes" are delicious as an appetizer or entrée. Serve them warm or even at room temperature. If you want a really luscious treat, top them with a classic béchamel or white sauce.—Jesse

1 cup vegetable stock

½ cup yellow onion, finely chopped

2 cups broccoli florets, finely chopped

2 tablespoons butter

3 tablespoons unbleached white flour

1 cup milk

1 teaspoon nutmeg

1 large egg

1 cup grated Swiss cheese, divided

salt and freshly ground pepper to taste

oil for the timbale molds, cupcake tins, or glass ramekins

Preheat the oven to 375° F. In a medium saucepan, over medium heat, simmer the yellow onion and broccoli in the stock until very soft. Drain off excess stock (you don't have to save it) and transfer the broccoli and onions to another bowl.

Return the same saucepan to the stove and melt the butter. Cook the flour in the butter for 3 minutes or until bubbly. Using a whisk, gradually add the milk, stirring constantly. Cook for about 5 minutes or until the sauce thickens. Add the nutmeg. Stir in the cooked broccoli and onions.

Whisk the egg and quickly add to the mixture. Add ½ cup of the Swiss cheese, and season with salt and freshly ground pepper.

Spoon the mixture into 8 lightly oiled timbale molds, cupcake tins, or glass ramekins; each should be about ⅔ full. Sprinkle the remaining ½ cup of cheese over the top of the cups. Place them on a rack in a baking pan and fill the pan with hot (not boiling) water to the level of the filling. Bake for about 30 minutes or until the timbales puff slightly and are brown on top. (If a sharp knife inserted in the center comes out clean, the timbales are done.) Remove from the oven and cool for 15 minutes. Run a knife around the outer edge, and unmold onto individual plates or a platter.

Tempeh, Spinach, and Ricotta Parmesana

Serves 4

Moist and saucy, this dish can convert just about anyone to the virtue and versatility of tempeh. I like to serve it with a side dish of tiny orzo pasta that has been tossed with a little olive oil, garlic, and fresh chopped parsley.—Jesse

1 pound tempeh (1 4-ounce cutlet per person)

2 teaspoons extra virgin olive oil

½ cup red onion, finely chopped

1 cup drained cooked spinach (frozen works)

1 to 2 cloves garlic, minced

1 cup low-fat ricotta cheese

salt and freshly ground pepper to taste

2 cups prepared tomato sauce of your choice

1 tablespoon oregano, finely chopped

6 ounces low-fat mozzarella

2 tablespoons grated Parmesan cheese (or more, to taste)

2 tablespoons fresh parsley, chopped

Preheat the oven to 375° F. Place the tempeh in a large shallow baking dish with plenty of room around each cutlet. Bake in the oven for 10 minutes.

Meanwhile, in a medium-size sauté pan, heat the olive oil and cook the onion until soft. Add the spinach and garlic, and cook for a couple of minutes. Set aside to cool slightly and then add the ricotta cheese. Season with salt and pepper to taste.

Mix the oregano into the prepared tomato sauce.

When the tempeh is done, remove pan from the oven. Leaving the tempeh in the pan, mound ¼ of the spinach and ricotta mixture onto each cutlet. Spoon ¼ of the tomato sauce over each, and then sprinkle first with ¼ of the mozzarella and then ¼ of the Parmesan. Bake for 20 to 30 minutes or until hot throughout. Remove from the oven, place a cutlet on each of four plates, sprinkle with parsley and extra Parmesan if you choose, and serve.

Silken Tofu Mocha Pudding with Crystallized Ginger

Serves 6   *Look for crystallized ginger in the baking section or candy section of your grocery store. It is the ginger that is candied and has sugar crystals on the outside. This pudding is creamy and light.—Jesse*

2 cups silken tofu

½ cup semi-sweet chocolate, melted

1 tablespoon dehydrated coffee or espresso

1 teaspoon boiling water

½ cup sour cream

3 tablespoons sugar

1 teaspoon vanilla

½ teaspoon ground cinnamon

2 tablespoons crystallized ginger, chopped

Drain the tofu and whisk until smooth. Whisk the melted chocolate into the tofu.

Reconstitute the coffee in 1 teaspoon of boiling water and add it along with the sour cream, sugar, vanilla, and cinnamon to the tofu. Mix or blend until creamy.

Transfer to individual serving cups and sprinkle the ginger on top. Chill thoroughly.

THE ROSS SCHOOL

East Hampton, New York

Executive Chef Ann Cooper

   🍴 *Grilled Vegetable Haystack on Polenta*

   🍴 *Summer Gazpacho*

Chef Ann Cooper of The Ross School has been a chef all of her adult life. By the time Ann became the Executive Chef of The Putney Inn in Putney, Vermont, she had fallen in love with local products and decided to create menus around them. "It struck me that as a chef it is my responsibility to teach the next generation about our food supplies, sustainability, and seasonality," she writes in the introduction to her book, *Bitter Harvest: A Chef's Perspective on the Hidden Danger in the Foods We Eat and What You Can Do About It.*

Grilled Vegetable Haystack on Polenta with Summer Gazpacho

Serves 4

Marinated Grilled Summer Vegetable   Creamy Polenta (recipe follows)

Haystack (recipe follows)   Summer Gazpacho (recipe follows)

> Grill all of the vegetables. Place polenta in middle of large bowl or plate. Spoon the gazpacho around the polenta. Place the "haystack" of vegetables on top of the polenta.

Marinated Grilled Summer Vegetable Haystack

Serves 4

bayonet-cut (in thin strips) summer   Japanese eggplant, 4 pieces each

   vegetables, such as: (1 small eggplant)

      summer squash, 4 pieces each   leeks, 4 pieces each (1 small leek)

         (1 small squash)   ½ cup Shallot and Maple Syrup Marinade

      zucchini, 4 pieces each   (recipe follows)

         (1 small squash)

      sweet peppers, 4 pieces each

         (1 small pepper)

Cut all vegetables. Place in deep dish large enough to hold them all. Drizzle with Shallot and Maple Syrup Marinade and marinate for at least two hours. Grill on a charbroiler. Reserve warm until ready to serve.

Shallot and Maple Syrup Marinade

Approximately 2 cups

⅓ cup shallots, finely diced

1 cup extra virgin olive oil

5 tablespoons balsamic vinegar

2 tablespoons maple sugar or maple syrup

1 teaspoon fresh thyme, finely chopped

½ teaspoon fresh rosemary, finely chopped

1 teaspoon sea salt

½ teaspoon black pepper, freshly ground

Whisk all ingredients together and taste for seasoning.

Creamy Polenta

Serves 4

The roasted corn of this rich polenta adds a pungent undertone, but frozen or canned corn also serves well when fresh corn is not in season. If possible, use fresh rather than dried tarragon.—Ann

½ cup corn, 1 small ear (unshucked), or canned or frozen

¾ cup milk

¾ cup water

⅓ cup polenta (coarse yellow cornmeal)

8 tablespoons (1 stick) butter

4 ounces goat cheese, cut into pieces

1 teaspoon salt

1 teaspoon black pepper, freshly ground

1 teaspoon tarragon, freshly chopped, or ½ teaspoon dried

1 teaspoon chives or scallion tops, freshly chopped

If using fresh corn, wet the outside of the unshucked corn and then place in a 450° F oven for about 10 minutes. Remove ear from the oven, cool slightly, shuck, and cut kernels off cob. If using canned corn, drain well. If using frozen corn, thaw and drain.

Bring milk and water to a simmer and whisk in polenta. It will look as if there is not enough cornmeal to make it work, but within about 10 minutes of cooking over low heat (stirring occasionally), all the liquid will be absorbed. At this point, add butter, cheese, salt, pepper, and corn.

Add tarragon and sprinkle with chopped chives.

Summer Gazpacho

Approximately 1 quart

3 large tomatoes

1 medium red pepper, seeded

2 stalks celery

1 small onion

1 clove garlic

1 small fennel

2 cobs of corn, unshucked

4 tablespoons olive oil

1 medium cucumber, peeled and
   seeded

1½ cups V-8 or tomato juice

6 tablespoons balsamic vinegar

6 tablespoons extra virgin olive oil

½ teaspoon kosher salt

⅛ teaspoon black pepper, freshly ground

½ teaspoon Tabasco sauce

½ teaspoon Worcestershire sauce

1 teaspoon flat parsley, chopped

2 teaspoons cilantro, freshly chopped

1½ tablespoon chives, preferably fresh

Rub the tomatoes, peppers, celery, onions, garlic, and fennel with olive oil and roast in a 350° F oven until al dente (about 15 minutes). Place corn, unshucked, in oven for 20 minutes. Let corn cool slightly, shuck, and cut from cob. Small-dice half of all the vegetables except for the corn and garlic. Purée the other half of the vegetables and the garlic. Mix all of the ingredients together and add seasonings to taste. Serve immediately or keep chilled in the refrigerator until ready to serve.

ST. MARTIN'S TABLE

Minneapolis, Minnesota

Chef/Restaurant Manager Karen Franzmeier

🍴 *Thai Tofu Spread*

🍴 *Curried Potato, Leek, and Kale Soup*

🍴 *Lemon Ginger Snaps*

Karen Franzmeier is the Restaurant Manager of St. Martin's Table, a nonprofit restaurant and bookstore supported by The Community of St. Martin, an ecumenical, faith-based community.

"St. Martin's Table embodies the values of peace, social justice, and respect for the earth through the food we serve, the growers we support, the books we sell, and the space we provide," Karen says. "The restaurant has a simple menu, serves vegetarian and vegan food, uses primarily organically and locally grown food as much as possible, has volunteers serve the food and give away their tips to hunger-related organizations, and minimizes the amount of waste generated in the kitchen."

Since opening in 1984, St. Martin's Table volunteers have donated more than $434,000 to hunger-alleviation organizations.

Thai Tofu Spread

Makes 2 cups

Everyone at St. Martin's Table raves about this spread. If you're leery of tofu, this spread will convert you!—Karen

8 ounces firm tofu

¼ cup carrot, grated

½ teaspoon garlic, minced

2 tablespoons red onion, minced

2 tablespoons cilantro, chopped fine

¼ cup smooth peanut butter

¼ teaspoon lime zest

¼ teaspoon cayenne pepper

2 tablespoons fresh lime juice (1 lime)

3 tablespoons tamari

Squeeze extra water from tofu, then mash tofu with a pastry cutter or fork. Combine tofu, carrot, garlic, onion, and cilantro in a mixing bowl.

In a separate bowl, blend together until smooth peanut butter, lime zest, cayenne pepper, lime juice, and tamari. Fold into tofu mixture. Adjust seasonings to taste. Enjoy on your favorite crackers, pita, or other bread. Store refrigerated.

Curried Potato, Leek, and Kale Soup

Serves 8   *On a cold winter night, this soup will warm body and soul. Although it is made with vegetable stock, it is creamy and thick.—Karen*

2 tablespoons olive oil

3 cups leeks (about 3 medium, white part only), chopped

¾ cup onions, chopped

1 tablespoon garlic (2 cloves), peeled and minced

1 tablespoon curry powder

1½ teaspoon salt

1 cup carrots (4 ounces), sliced

2 cups russet potatoes (1 large or 2 small), peeled and diced into 1-inch cubes

¾ teaspoon fresh black pepper

1 quart vegetable stock

1 cup tomatoes, diced, peeled, and seeded (or canned)

½ bunch kale, thinly sliced just before serving (or substitute spinach)

Sauté leeks, onions, garlic, curry powder, and salt in oil in a stock pot until tender (about 5 minutes). Add carrots, potatoes, and pepper. Add vegetable stock and tomatoes, bring to a boil, then turn down heat and simmer until potatoes and carrots are tender (about 15 minutes). Just before serving, thinly slice ½ to 1 bunch of kale (or spinach) and add to the soup.

Lemon Ginger Snaps

Makes 30 to 36 large cookies, about 70 small ones   *These tasty cookies really do snap your tongue to attention with their ginger and lemon. They're also delightfully easy to make. —Karen*

2 cups brown sugar

1 cup butter

2 teaspoons lemon extract

2 large eggs

3 cups unbleached all-purpose flour

2 teaspoons powdered ginger

1½ teaspoons baking powder

½ teaspoon salt

½ cup granulated white sugar

Preheat the oven to 350° F. Using an electric mixer, cream together the brown sugar and the butter. Add lemon extract and eggs. In a separate bowl, mix flour, ginger, baking powder, and salt. Add dry ingredients to wet ones and mix.

Put sugar on a small plate. Form cookie dough into ice-cream-scoop-size balls for large cookies or inch-wide balls for small ones, roll in sugar, place on ungreased cookie sheet, and flatten with a fork or cookie stamp.

Bake at 350° F for 10 to 12 minutes or until done.

REAL FOOD DAILY
Los Angeles, California
Founder Ann Gentry

- Skillet Corn Bread with Scallion "Butter"
- Red Bean, Squash, and Okra Stew
- Garlicky Greens

Chef Ann Gentry brings eighteen years of food experience to Real Food Daily, one of the only restaurants in Los Angeles that serves a vegetarian menu using exclusively organic foods. Ann embarked on her self-taught culinary education in the early 1980s, combining the essential elements of the Eastern macrobiotic teachings with her distinctly American culinary style to create what she terms "gourmet whole-food cuisine."

Skillet Corn Bread with Scallion "Butter"

Serves 8 — *Easy to make and fun to serve in the pan, this corn bread is dense and delicious. Use real maple syrup if at all possible. If you want a Southwest feel, add any or all of the optional ingredients: corn, scallions, and jalapeños. If made with soymilk, this, along with its accompanying "butter," is a vegan recipe.—Ann*

2 cups corn meal

1 cup whole wheat pastry flour or unbleached all-purpose white flour

1 cup unbleached white flour

2 teaspoons baking powder

2 cups soy milk or regular milk

Optional: ½ cup corn, 2 tablespoons each minced scallions and jalapeños

½ cup vegetable oil (preferably canola oil)

½ teaspoon salt

⅓ cup maple syrup

2 tablespoons olive oil

Scallion "Butter" (recipe follows)

Preheat the oven to 400° F. Sift corn meal, flours, and baking powder into a large bowl and mix well. In a separate bowl combine milk, oil, salt, and maple syrup. Blend well. Combine wet and dry ingredients and mix only until blended.

If you'd like, add the optional corn, scallions, and jalapeños and mix well.

Heat the olive oil in an 11-inch round cast-iron skillet until it starts to smoke. Add the batter and place the skillet in the oven for approximately 40 minutes, or until lightly browned and a toothpick inserted in the center emerges clean.

Scallion "Butter"

Makes
1 cup

You can serve this recipe with the corn bread, or use its unusual flavors to turn crackers into an appetizer. It also makes an excellent, unique spread for sandwiches.—Ann

6 scallions (cut off 2 inches from top and discard, roughly chop the rest)

6 tablespoons toasted sesame butter or tahini

2 tablespoons umeboshi paste (available at health food stores or Asian markets)

3 tablespoons fresh lemon juice (1 large lemon)

6 tablespoons parsley, chopped

1 teaspoon fresh ginger, minced

Place all ingredients in a food processor and purée. Refrigerate two or three hours before serving.

Red Bean, Squash, and Okra Stew

Serves
6 to 8

This recipe makes a flavorful stew you can make ahead of time and serve to a crowd. If you'd like it milder, adjust the heat by cutting down on the chili flakes and the chili powder. Alternatively, this stew can be made with zucchini. Just substitute the okra for the same amount of zucchini.—Ann

3 cans red beans

3 bay leaves

3 tablespoons olive oil

3 cups onion (1 large onion, ¾ pound), cut into ½-inch dice

1 cup carrots (2 large carrots), cut into ½-inch dice

1 cup celery (3 stalks), cut into ½-inch dice

3 cups butternut squash (2 pounds), cut into ¾-inch dice

1 cup red pepper (1 small pepper), cut into ½-inch dice

1 cup green pepper (1 small pepper), cut into ½-inch dice

¼ cup garlic, minced (divided)

1 tablespoon chili powder

2 tablespoons dried sage

1 teaspoon red chili flakes

4 cups okra (1 pound), cut into ½-inch cubes

1 tablespoon salt

1 3-ounce can tomato paste

2 cups (15-ounce can) whole tomatoes and juice

¼ cup tamari

1 cup cilantro, minced

In a small pot, place beans and bay leaves. Cover, and simmer for 15 minutes.

In a large stock pot, heat oil, onions, and carrots. Sauté for 5 minutes. Add celery, squash, red and green peppers, garlic, and spices. Sauté for five minutes. Add okra, salt, and tomato paste, and cook over low heat. In a food processor, blend whole tomatoes with their juice.

Add to the pot. Add beans and bean liquid. Cover, and simmer for 20 minutes. Right before serving, add tamari and cilantro. Serve hot.

Garlicky Greens

Serves
4 to 6

Quick, assertive, and rich in color and flavor, these greens convince even those who don't think they like leafy food that it's easy being green. Feel free to use pre-chopped garlic and other greens if you wish; spinach and Swiss chard work especially well. Experiment with combinations of the freshest greens you can find to enjoy this 10-minute miracle.—Ann

10 cups uncooked kale (2 bunches)

10 cups uncooked collard greens (1 big bunch)

2 tablespoons olive oil

2 cups onion (1 large onion), cut into half moons

½ cup garlic (about 1 head), minced

1 teaspoon salt

1 tablespoon tamari

Wash the kale and collard greens. Remove and discard tough stems. Cut the leaves into ½-inch strips.

In a large skillet, heat the oil. Add the onions and salt. Sauté for 5 minutes or until the onions are well cooked.

Add greens and garlic and a splash of water if greens are not still wet from washing. Cover to steam for 2 minutes. Uncover, add tamari, and sauté for 3 minutes.

Serve hot.

Café Flora

Seattle, Washington

Scott Glascock, Co-owner

Cathy Geier, Executive Chef

🍴 *Oaxaco Tacos*

🍴 *Black Bean Stew*

🍴 *Pico de Gallo*

🍴 *Lemon Garlic Vinaigrette with Chard*

🍴 *Crème Fraiche and Lime Crème Fraiche*

"We want to showcase that tasty, eye-catching, and satisfying dishes can be made without the sacrifice of animal life," Scott says about his Café Flora in Seattle. "We are especially interested in reaching people who don't identify as vegetarians but who see the benefits of moving toward a more plant-based diet. We also wanted to model what a restaurant can do environmentally, both in terms of how we designed the Café and how we run it. We wanted to create a humane, respectful workplace, with decent benefits—a place where people would feel good about getting up in the morning and going to work.

We like to think that we add something of real value to our immediate community and to the city as a whole.—Scott

We've included these recipes as Café Flora shared them with us. You can, of course, choose to prepare any one of these dishes on its own or in any combination with the others. We suggest starting with the black bean stew and, while the beans are cooking, prepare the Crème Fraiche, Pico de Gallo, and Lemon Garlic Vinaigrette with Chard. Then, put all the ingredients together in the Oaxaca Tacos.—Anna and Frances

Oaxaca Tacos

Serves 4
generously

By far one of our most popular dishes, Oaxaca Tacos have been on our menu practically since we opened. Our first chef, Jim Watkins, created a dish that demonstrates what's appealing about Café Flora: hearty food beautifully presented with bold flavors and varied textures. Much of our menu consists of "composed plates," and here we have provided recipes for all the individual elements of this dish. We serve the spicy mashed potato tacos with crumbled feta and Lime Crème Fraiche alongside Black Bean Stew, Pico de Gallo, and steamed Swiss chard dressed with Lemon Garlic Vinaigrette. Although you can serve Oaxaca Tacos with your favorite beans or salsa, the many guests who have requested this recipe want to serve the dish just as we do at Café Flora.—Cathy

3 large russet potatoes (2 pounds) peeled, cut into 2-inch chunks

2 tablespoons butter

½ teaspoon salt

1 cup (1 small) red or green bell pepper

½ cup smoked mozzarella cheese

½ cup cheddar cheese

⅛ teaspoon crushed red pepper flakes

8 thin corn tortillas

3 tablespoons vegetable oil

wooden toothpicks

¼ cup crumbled feta cheese for topping

4 sprigs cilantro for garnish

Black Bean Stew (recipe follows)

Pico de Gallo (recipe follows)

Lemon Garlic Vinaigrette with Chard (recipe follows)

Lime Crème Fraiche (recipe follows)

Preheat the oven to 400° F. Boil the potatoes until soft (about 10 minutes) and mash with the butter and salt; cool completely.

While potatoes are boiling, dice the pepper into ¼-inch chunks. Shred the cheeses. Mix the mozzarella with the cheddar and the red pepper flakes and set aside.

Brush the tortillas with oil, making sure that they are completely coated. Once oiled, put them in a warm skillet or in a pan on top of a hot oven. The warmth (and the oil) will keep them pliable and prevent cracking.

Place each oiled tortilla on a flat surface. Place a scoop of mashed potatoes in the middle of each tortilla (use an ice-cream scoop or a ⅓-cup measure). Pat the scoop with your hand to flatten it a little.

Sprinkle with 1 tablespoon of the diced green peppers and 2 table-spoons of the cheese mixture. Roll the tortilla so both edges overlap (into a tube) and fasten by inserting a toothpick at an angle between each edge and into the filling. (You may have to use 2 toothpicks.)

Place the filled tortillas on a sheet pan or cookie sheet (with at least ¼ inch in between them) and bake in a 400° F oven for 15 to 20 minutes until the cheese has melted and the tortillas start to brown and crisp on the edges.

To serve Oaxaca Tacos: Remove the toothpicks from the tacos. Place ½-cup of Black Bean Stew on one half of a plate. Place one taco in the middle of the beans, then place the other taco on top at an op-posing angle. Drizzle one or two tablespoons of Lime Crème Fraiche over the tacos and then top with a tablespoon of crumbled feta and a cilantro sprig. Place ½-cup Pico de Gallo and ¼ of the Lemon Garlic Vinaigrette with Chard next to each other on the other half of the plate, opposite the tacos and beans.

Black Bean Stew

Makes
4 cups

Subtle spices that pack a punch combine with black beans and corn to create a stew that satisfies the tongue and warms the soul.—Cathy

1 cup dry black beans or 2 cans black beans	½ teaspoon crushed red pepper flakes
5 cups water (if using dried beans)	½ teaspoon ground cumin
1 cup frozen or canned corn	½ teaspoon chili powder
2 cloves garlic, minced	½ teaspoon dry oregano
¼ cup cilantro, chopped	¾ teaspoon salt
½ tablespoon brown sugar (optional)	vegetable stock (optional)

If you are making your own black beans, pick through and rinse dry beans. Put in a 3- or 4-quart pot or Dutch oven. Add water and bring to a boil. Reduce to a simmer, partially covered, for 1½ to 2 hours or until beans are tender. You may need to add more water as the beans cook to keep liquid above the beans until they are finished cooking. If using canned beans, place in pot and heat. When beans are tender, add all remaining ingredients and simmer 15 minutes until corn is cooked, adding water or vegetable stock to get a looser consistency if necessary.

Pico de Gallo

Makes
3 cups

Determining the heat of pico de gallo can sometimes be difficult. Cathy's advice: If I called the following recipe "hot" half the people that made it would say it has the perfect amount of heat, and the other half would say it is too hot. If you are at all sensitive to chilies, cut the amount of jalapenos by half. We make this salsa year round at the restaurant, so much of the time we use Roma tomatoes. Of course, take advantage of the season's ripest when they are available.—Cathy

8 Roma tomatoes, cored, coarsely chopped

½ red onion, finely diced

4 teaspoons garlic (about 3 cloves), minced

1 jalapeno pepper, split, with seeds
   removed, minced

2 tablespoons lime juice (about
   2 limes)

1 teaspoon salt

2 tablespoons (around 12 big sprigs)
   cilantro, leaves removed and chopped

Combine tomatoes, onion, garlic, jalapeño, lime juice, and salt in a bowl. Add cilantro just before serving.

Lemon Garlic Vinaigrette with Chard

Serves 4

This vinaigrette has been a staple in our kitchen for years. You will want to keep a jar of this in your own fridge for drizzling on steamed vegetables and greens, making quick cold pasta salads, and for spreading on sandwiches.—Cathy

10 cloves garlic

10 black peppercorns

½ teaspoon salt

¼ cup lemon juice (3 small lemons)

1 cup olive oil

10 cups red or green Swiss chard, washed
   and most of the stem removed (1 big
   bunch, around 10 ounces)

To make the Lemon Garlic Vinaigrette, combine garlic cloves, peppercorns, salt, and lemon juice in a blender and blend until smooth. With the motor running, slowly add the olive oil until emulsified. Taste for salt. You can make it ahead of time and store in the refrigerator for up to 2 weeks.

For Chard Vinaigrette, bring vinaigrette to room temperature. Just before serving, steam chard until tender (about 5 minutes). Drain excess water and toss with ¼ cup Lemon Garlic Vinaigrette.

Crème Fraiche and Lime Crème Fraiche

Makes
2 cups

Crème fraiche is very easy to make and quite versatile. Unlike sour cream, it does not curdle when cooked, so it is great for adding a creamy tang to soups and pasta. You can flavor crème fraiche with citrus juice or zest, chili purées, or toasted and ground spices like cumin and fennel. We drizzle flavored crème fraiche on Oaxaco Tacos, sweet or savory pancakes, and quesadillas. Crème fraiche will keep for several weeks in your refrigerator.—Cathy

2 cups heavy cream

1 tablespoon buttermilk

½ teaspoon lime zest, minced

2 tablespoons fresh lime juice

Pour the cream into a container, add the buttermilk, and stir the mixture together. Put a lid on the container, but leave it ajar. Place the container in a warm part of the kitchen and let sit for 24 to 48 hours. Cover the container and refrigerate.

For Lime Crème Fraiche, mix ½-cup Crème Fraiche (or sour cream) with ½ teaspoon minced lime zest and 2 tablespoons fresh lime juice.

WHITE DOG CAFE

Philadelphia, Pennsylvania

Executive Chef/Partner Kevin Von Klause

- *Spinach and Fennel Salad with Curried Pears and Hazelnuts*
- *Orange-Rosemary Vinaigrette*
- *Chilled Cucumber Soup with Tomato-Tarragon Relish*
- *Wild Mushroom–Barley Risotto*
- *Harvest Fruit Crisp*

Executive Chef/Partner Kevin von Klause has been a partner of proprietress Judy Wicks at the White Dog Cafe in Philadelphia for fourteen years. The use of organic and humanely raised foods from local farmers are both Kevin's trademark and passion, just as social responsibility is the trademark and passion of the White Dog. Kevin is on the National Board of Overseers for the Chefs Collaborative and is also a member and lecturer for the Pennsylvania

Association for Sustainable Agriculture. His first book, *White Dog Cafe Cookbook: Multicultural Recipes and Tales of Adventure from Philadelphia's Revolutionary Restaurant,* cowritten with Judy Wicks, is dedicated to the organic family farmers of America.

Spinach and Fennel Salad with Curried Pears and Hazelnuts

Serves 4   *Believe it or not, you can have a fresh seasonal salad in the dead of winter. This composed salad takes advantage of ingredients found at the peak of ripeness and availability during the colder months. Young tender fennel, warm spiced pears, juicy navel oranges, and ever-green spinach are combined with toasted hazelnuts for a festive first course.—Kevin*

CURRIED PEARS

¼ cup fresh orange juice

1 tablespoon good-quality Madras curry powder

½ teaspoon ground ginger

1 tablespoon plus 1 teaspoon packed light brown sugar

¼ teaspoon salt

¼ teaspoon freshly ground black pepper

¼ cup olive oil

2 ripe (not too ripe) Bosc pears, halved and cored

SPINACH AND FENNEL SALAD

4 cups spinach leaves (10 ounces), tightly packed, washed, and stemmed

1 small fennel bulb (stalks removed), cored and thinly sliced to make 1 cup

½ cup red onion (1 small onion), sliced into thin rings

¾ cup Orange-Rosemary Vinaigrette (recipe follows)

¼ cup hazelnuts, skinned and toasted

Prepare the pears: Whisk together the orange juice, curry powder, ginger, brown sugar, salt, and pepper in a small bowl. Slowly whisk in the olive oil. Add the pears and toss to coat with the marinade. Let marinate at room temperature for at least 2 hours, or cover and refrigerate for up to 2 days.

About 30 minutes before you plan to bake the pears, preheat the oven to 400° F.

Place the pears, cut sides down, in a baking dish; pour the remaining marinade over them. Bake until tender, about 20 minutes.

To prepare the salad: Toss together the spinach, fennel, onion, and vinaigrette in a large bowl. (Put vinaigrette on at the last minute.) Divide the salad among 4 chilled plates. Top each salad with a warm pear half and ¼ each of the toasted hazelnuts.

Orange-Rosemary Vinaigrette

1 cup fresh orange juice (it's important that it be fresh)
½ teaspoon minced orange zest
1 teaspoon fresh rosemary leaves, chopped, or ½ teaspoon dried

1 teaspoon minced shallot
2 teaspoons apple cider vinegar
3 teaspoons olive oil
pinch of salt and fresh black pepper

Whisk together all ingredients in a small bowl. Set aside at room temperature for at least 30 minutes to allow the flavors to meld.

Chilled Cucumber Soup with Tomato-Tarragon Relish

Serves 6

Pastel green and garden-fresh, this soup typifies the kind of food we like to make in the summer at the White Dog Cafe. It can be prepared in a few minutes (without turning on the stove), and is invigoratingly icy—perfect for lunch on a blazing summer day.—Kevin

SOUP

6 cups cucumbers (4 large, about 3 pounds), peeled, seeded, and cut into large chunks
1½ cups buttermilk
½ cup plain yogurt

½ cup scallions (2 whole, green and white parts), thinly sliced
1 teaspoon salt
¼ teaspoon freshly ground pepper

RELISH

¾ cup ripe tomato (1 medium), peeled, diced, seeded
2 tablespoons fresh tarragon leaves, chopped

2 tablespoons extra-virgin olive oil
pinch of salt
½ teaspoon garlic, minced (optional)

To prepare the soup, place the cucumbers in a food processor or blender and process until liquefied (about 1 minute). Remove the purée to a bowl and whisk in the buttermilk, yogurt, scallions, salt, and pepper. Cover and refrigerate until well chilled (at least 1 hour). (The soup may be made 1 day in advance and will keep refrigerated for up to 3 days; however, the relish should be made just before serving.)

While the soup is chilling, prepare the relish: Combine the tomatoes, tarragon, oil, salt, and optional garlic in a small bowl and toss to combine.

To serve, whisk soup to make smooth. Divide the soup among 6 chilled bowls or plates. Top each serving with a spoonful of the relish.

Wild Mushroom–Barley Risotto

Serves 4 to 6

Risotto is a classic Italian specialty in which onions and Arborio rice are sautéed in butter or olive oil and the rice is stirred constantly as hot broth is gradually added to the pot. The friction from stirring softens the outer hull of the rice grains, creating an inimitable creaminess. In this dish we substitute barley for the rice, so technically it's not a risotto, but the results are surprisingly similar. The stirred barley retains its nubby texture while exuding a luxurious creaminess; its nutty flavor perfectly complements the woodsy porcini.—Kevin

½ ounce dried porcini or other dried wild mushroom

6 cups water

2 tablespoons extra-virgin olive oil

⅓ cup shallots (about 3), minced

1 tablespoon garlic (2 cloves), minced

3 cups portobello or button mushrooms, chopped

2 cups raw barley, pearl or whole (1 pound)

½ cup dry Marsala wine or dry sherry

1 cup freshly grated Parmesan cheese

1½ teaspoons salt

½ teaspoon freshly ground black pepper

1 tablespoon fresh thyme leaves or 1 teaspoon dried thyme

Combine the dried mushrooms and the water in a saucepan, bring to a boil over high heat. Remove from the heat and set aside to steep for 15 minutes. Strain the mushrooms and reserve the liquid separately. Coarsely chop the mushrooms and reserve.

While mushrooms are steeping, in a saucepan over medium heat, heat the olive oil until it ripples. Turn heat to low. Add the shallots and cook until translucent (about 4 minutes). Add the garlic and cook for another minute. Turn the heat to high and add the chopped fresh mushrooms. Cook until they release their juices and cook dry, about 5 to 6 minutes.

Add the barley and stir for 1 minute. Pour in ¼ cup of the Marsala wine and enough of the reserved mushroom broth to just cover the barley. Add the reserved dried mushrooms, bring to a gentle simmer, and stir. As the barley absorbs the liquid, add more mushroom broth, a ladleful at a time, stirring before and after each addition. Add the other ¼ cup of Marsala wine with the last ladleful of broth. After about 20 to 25 minutes the barley should be tender. If it is still chewy, add a little more broth and continue to stir until tender.

Stir in the Parmesan, salt, pepper, and thyme. Taste for seasoning. Serve immediately in warm bowls.

Harvest Fruit Crisp

Serves 12   *Harvest fruits are all of the gorgeous fruits the farmers bring to market during the summer and early autumn—apples, pears, apricots, grapes, cranberries, cherries, blueberries—and any combination of them can be baked into a bubbling crisp that will make your mouth water. It can be made in the morning and warmed just before serving. Serve topped with vanilla yogurt or a drizzle of buttermilk if desired.—Kevin*

TOPPING

1 cup firmly packed light brown sugar

1 cup unbleached all purpose or whole wheat pastry flour

1½ cups rolled oats

1 teaspoon ground cinnamon

½ teaspoon ground ginger

¼ teaspoon salt

1 cup coarsely chopped pecans

¼ pound (1 stick) cold unsalted butter, cubed

FILLING

4 large, firm, tart apples, such as Granny
    Smith, McIntosh, or Ida Red, cored and
    sliced

3 ripe pears, such as Bartlett or Bosc, cored
    and sliced

1 cup seedless red grapes, stems removed

1 cup fresh or thawed frozen cranberries

1 cup light-colored honey

3 tablespoons cornstarch

2 teaspoons ground cinnamon

1 teaspoon ground ginger

½ teaspoon ground cloves

Preheat the oven to 350° F. Butter a 9 x 13–inch baking dish.

To make the topping: Combine the brown sugar, flour, oats, cinnamon, ginger, salt, pecans, and butter in the bowl of an electric mixer fitted with the paddle attachment. Blend on low speed until the butter is incorporated and the topping is the consistency of coarse meal (about 2 minutes). Reserve. If you don't have an electric mixer, you can also use two forks or a pastry cutter and cut it together.

To make the filling: Combine the apples, pears, grapes, and cranberries in a large mixing bowl. Combine the honey, cornstarch, cinnamon, ginger, and cloves in a separate bowl and mix well. Add the honey mixture to the fruits and toss to coat evenly. (It may be easier if you use your hands.)

Spread the fruit mixture into the prepared baking dish. Cover with the crumb topping. Place baking dish on a cookie pan in case it boils over. Bake until the juice is thick and the topping is browned (about 50 minutes). If the topping browns before the fruit is cooked, cover with foil and bake until the fruit is tender.

Serve warm, or let cool to room temperature, cover, and refrigerate for up to 2 days. Re-warm before serving.

RESTAURANT NORA

Washington, D.C.

Chef/Owner Nora Pouillon

- *Arugula and Melon Salad with Lime Dressing*
- *Grilled Eggplant Steak with Roasted Red Peppers, Feta Cheese, Black Olives, and Pita Bread*
- *Russian Blueberry and Raspberry Pudding*

Since the 1970s, Nora Pouillon's goal has been to show people that healthful, chemical-free food tastes delicious, and to consistently campaign for organics and a more sustainable lifestyle. Her restaurant was the first certified organic restaurant in the country. Nora believes the food she serves—grown or raised without chemical additives or hormones—is not only healthier for us, but simply tastes better, too. Nora is the author of *Cooking with Nora: Seasonal Menus from Restaurant Nora: Healthy, Light, Balanced, and Simple Food with Organic Ingredients.*

Arugula and Melon Salad with Lime Dressing

Serves 6 to 8

The cool pastel balls of melon contrast with the spicy green of arugula in this eye-and-palate pleaser—the perfect way to start or end a summer meal.—Nora

2 tablespoons lime juice (1 large lime)	½ medium cantaloupe, seeds removed
1 tablespoon water	½ medium honeydew, seeds removed
¼ teaspoon salt	1 medium wedge watermelon, seeds
¼ teaspoon freshly ground black pepper	removed
3 tablespoons olive oil	8 to 10 cups arugula (approximately 10
1 tablespoon fresh mint, minced	ounces)

Mix the lime juice, water, salt, pepper, oil, and mint in a small bowl. Taste for seasoning and adjust.

Use a melon baller to make balls from each kind of melon. Set aside in separate bowls, so that you can divide them easily when composing the salad.

Wash and spin dry the arugula leaves. Toss with the lime dressing and divide among 6 large or 8 smaller salad plates. Garnish each salad plate with an assortment of melon balls.

Grilled Eggplant Steak with Roasted Red Peppers, Feta Cheese, Black Olives, and Pita Bread

Serves 4 *In this colorful Mediterranean taste feast, the potent garlic and salt tastes are balanced by the calm of the grilled eggplant. Add a green vegetable or spinach salad to balance color and flavor. You can serve on warmed dinner plates or at room temperature.—Nora*

TAMARI-BALSAMIC MARINADE

3 tablespoons balsamic vinegar

1 tablespoon tamari

1½ tablespoons garlic (3 cloves), finely minced

salt to taste

¼ teaspoon freshly ground pepper

2 tablespoons olive oil

REMAINING INGREDIENTS

1 large eggplant (about a pound)

1 cup red peppers (2 medium)

¼ pound feta cheese, cubed or crumbled

½ cup black olives (Greek or Moroccan), pitted

2 tablespoons fresh oregano or flat leaf parsley, chopped

4 small pita breads

4 teaspoons balsamic vinegar

sprigs of fresh oregano or parsley for garnish

Preheat grill or broiler. To make the marinade, in a small bowl whisk together the vinegar with the tamari, garlic, salt, and pepper. Slowly add the olive oil, stirring until blended.

To make the eggplant steaks, cut the eggplant lengthwise into 4 ½ inch thick slices to resemble steaks. Place steaks in 9 x 13–inch glass pan. Pour tamari-balsamic marinade over eggplant and marinate for 15 minutes, turning occasionally.

Grill or broil peppers, turning them until skin blisters and chars. Put peppers in a bowl, seal with plastic wrap, and let them steam for 6 to 8 minutes. When peppers are cool enough to touch, peel off charred skin and seed them. Cut peppers into ½-inch cubes.

Put the red peppers, feta, olives, and oregano in a small bowl. Season to taste with salt and pepper. When the eggplant has marinated, pour the marinade from the pan into the bowl. Stir to coat peppers, feta, and olives.

Grill or broil eggplant slices for 2 to 4 minutes on each side, until tender but not too soft. Toast or grill the pita bread and cut it into wedges.

Place an eggplant steak on each of 4 dinner plates. Place spoonfuls of red pepper–olive–feta salad on top of the eggplant, dividing it equally. Sprinkle each steak with a teaspoon of balsamic vinegar. Garnish with pita bread wedges and fresh oregano or parsley.

Russian Blueberry and Raspberry Pudding

Serves 4   *This dessert is quick and easy and delicious when made at the height of berry season.—Nora*

1 pint blueberries, washed and drained

1 pint raspberries, washed and drained

4 tablespoons of brown sugar

1 cup low-fat yogurt

mint for garnish

Preheat the broiler. Divide the berries among 4 individual oven-proof dishes. Top each with ¼ cup of yogurt and sprinkle each with 1 tablespoon of brown sugar. Broil for about 3 minutes or until the sugar melts and caramelizes on the top. Serve with a garnish of mint.

COMING TO OUR SENSES

DESSERTS

FOOD FOR THOUGHT

A SHORT LIST OF RECOMMENDED BOOKS & FILMS

HUMAN NATURE, CULTURE, AND MARKETS

- *The Anatomy of Human Destructiveness*
  Erich Fromm (New York: Holt, Rinehart and Winston, 1973)

- *Bowling for Columbine* (documentary, 2002)
  Directed by Michael Moore, www.michaelmoore.com

- *The Culture of Make Believe*
  Derrick Jensen (New York: Context Books, 2002)

- *The Divine Right of Capital*
  Marjorie Kelly (New York: Berrett-Koehler, 2001)

- *Everything for Sale: The Virtues and Limits of Markets*
  Robert Kuttner (New York: Alfred A. Knopf, 1997)

- *Mindfulness*
  Ellen J. Langer (Boston, Massachusetts: Perseus Publishing, 1990)

FOOD, POLITICS, AND BIOTECHNOLOGY

- *Against the Grain: Biotechnology and the Corporate Takeover of Your Food*
  Marc Lappé and Britt Bailey (Monroe, Maine: Common Courage Press)

- *Fast Food Nation: The Dark Truth Behind the All-American Meal*
  Eric Schlosser (Boston, Massachusetts: Houghton-Mifflin, 2001)

- *Food Politics: How the Food Industry Influences Nutrition and Health*
  Marion Nestle (Berkeley, California: University of California Press, 2002)

- *The Food Revolution: How Your Diet Can Help Save Your Life and the World*
  John Robbins (Berkeley, California: Conari Press, 2001)

- *Trust Us, We're Experts! How Industry Manipulates Science and Gambles with Your Future*
  Sheldon Rampton and John Stauber (New York: Tarcher/Putnam, 2001)

GLOBALIZATION AND DEVELOPMENT

- *Ancient Futures: Learning From Ladakh*
  Helena Norberg-Hodge (San Francisco, California: Sierra Club Books, 1991)

- *Globalization and Its Discontents*
  Joseph E. Stiglitz (New York: W. W. Norton, 2002)

- *Life and Debt* (documentary, 2001)
  Directed by Stephanie Black, www.lifeanddebt.org

ENVIRONMENTAL JUSTICE AND NATURE'S WISDOM

- *Biomimicry: Innovation Inspired by Nature*
  Janine M. Benyus (New York: Morrow, 1997)

- *Blue Vinyl* (documentary, 2002)
  Directed by Judith Helfand and Daniel B. Gold, www.bluevinyl.org

- *Natural Capitalism: Creating the Next Industrial Revolution*
  Paul Hawken, Amory B. Lovins, and L. Hunter Lovins (Boston, Massachusetts: Little, Brown and Co., 1999)

- *The Web of Life: A New Scientific Understanding of Living Systems*
  Fritjof Capra (New York: Anchor Books, 1996)

HOPE'S EDGE
DISCUSSION CIRCLES

SUGGESTED QUESTIONS TO ENLIVEN THE TALK

We've been delighted to learn of groups across the country using *Hope's Edge* to ignite discussion. Below you will find ideas we've gathered. Consider them as starting points and brainstorm triggers—not as hard-and-fast directions. We welcome your ideas and tips based on your own experiences.

—ANNA & FRANKIE

- **Make it a potluck.** Consider inviting participants to make recipes from *Hope's Edge* to share before the discussion begins—or afterward.

- **Preparing people.** Think about asking participants to come with one or two burning questions or topics that they would like to talk about.

- **Opening the session.** Consider beginning with a moment of silence or a reading from the book. You might invite participants to state what they hope to gain from the experience together.

- **Commitments and entry points.** At the end of the discussion, perhaps participants would like to share a personal commitment to change that they'd like to make.

- **Local connection.** Consider inviting local organizations whose energy is devoted to themes in *Hope's Edge* and/or having materials available with ideas for practical action.

- **Closing the session.** Before you begin, think about how long you would like the discussion to last and how it might close. Maybe choose a passage, poem, or thought to end with.

QUESTIONS AND DISCUSSION POINTS

Depending on the time you have, you may want to explore just a few of these topics. Each could spark long conversations!

GENERAL THEMES AND CONCEPTS

- **Hope.** What is your reaction to the word? What does "hope" mean in your life? How do the authors and the people in *Hope's Edge* understand hope? What is meant by "hope's edge"? In talking about this question, you might want to read aloud from pages 136 and 307–308, and from the Epilogue.

- **Thought traps and springing free.** See pages 328–329. Discuss the ideas behind each thought trap. For each trap and liberating idea, you might want to explore how it appears in the book and how it may apply to your life. Looking back, have you felt yourself limited by thought traps at work, at home, in your community? What has released you?

- **Courage.** See page 307. What do the authors mean by "the courage of an expanding heart"? What would such an understanding of courage mean in your own life?

- **Rethinking fear.** What ideas do you have about fear after reading *Hope's Edge*? Consider the stories of people transforming fear into action in the book. Were there individuals with whom you especially identified? For example, Cathrine Sneed of the Garden Project, Vandana Shiva in India, Wangari Maathai and Reverend Njoya in Kenya, members of the MST in Brazil, Muhammad Yunus in Bangladesh, or John Kinsman in Wisconsin.

- **Seeing with new eyes.** At the beginning of Chapter 11, "Traveling the Edge of Possibility," the authors say that their book is really about perception. What does this mean? Has this been true for you? Reflecting on your life, are you aware of ways in which your perception has suddenly shifted, allowing you to see "with new eyes"?

- **Moments of dissonance.** What does this phrase suggest to you? Have you had moments of dissonance while reading this book? What have been the most significant moments of dissonance in your life? Have they propelled you forward? See pages 218, 280–281, and 302–303.

- **Bringing democracy to life.** What do the authors mean by "living democracy"? How would you define "democracy"? See pages 31 and 155–156.

- **Solving for pattern.** What does this phrase mean to you? Have you experienced or witnessed the effects of *not* solving for pattern in your own life or community? How might the outcome have been different, or be different, if you had solved for pattern? Think of a local problem. Imagine how you might resolve it by solving for pattern versus solving by dissection.

- **Creating citizens.** On page 80, reread the last paragraph in the section about the Landless Workers' Movement. What do the authors mean by the "creation of citizens"?

SPECIFIC CONCERNS AND ENTRY POINTS

- **Food.** Reread the paragraph on page 251 that begins "Now I see . . ." What is meant by "knowledge can kill taste"? Do you agree? Have you had a similar experience? What are ways to access healthy food—for your home, for schools, and for elsewhere? How might you help make these connections?

- **Diet.** What lessons did you learn about diet? What's happening to our nation's diet? How has your own diet been shaped by the stories of this book or by the original *Diet for Small Planets*? Did your choice to eat differently have ripples beyond food? What are actions that we can take to make healthy food accessible to all?

- **Genetically modified organisms.** Reread the paragraph on page 17 that begins, "Instead of . . ." What do the authors mean by GMOs being the "ultimate wake-up call"? Do you agree? What is your impression about GMOs after reading *Hope's Edge*?

- **Conscious consuming.** In Chapter 8, what do the authors mean by "stirring the sleeping giant"? Do you agree with Paul Rice when he uses this phrase? If so, what actions could you take, or have you taken, in your own life to manifest this power?

- **Food citizenship.** What does this phrase suggest to you? Think about the stories from Belo Horizonte, Brazil (Chapter 4). What would it look like to make food a human right in your own community?

- **Banking and poverty.** What role do you think microcredit can play in helping people escape from poverty? Why? Do you think that microcredit may just be the "miniaturization of capitalism"? Reread pages 134–136 and explore what Muhammad Yunus means by the distinction between the "grammar" and the "philosophy" of Grameen Bank.

- **Corporate globalization.** Through these stories, how has corporate globalization—the expansion of power and control of corporations—affected the lives and livelihoods of the people in this book? You might want to think about Kenya and the IMF, India and the WTO and patents, or Jean Yves and his realization of the interconnectedness of his farm in France and farmers in Brazil.

- **Global governance.** Reread pages 234–237, the section on the World Trade Organization (WTO) in Chapter 9. What lessons does this case hold about the nature of global corporate capitalism? How does our inherited definition of democracy jibe with new global institutions like the WTO?

- **Re-embedding economic life in community.** What does this phrase suggest to you? What examples best illustrate this idea for you? What possibilities do you see in your community?

- **People-to-people globalization.** How are people in the book participating in a different kind of globalization—people connecting across borders? How is this type of globalization happening in the stories in the book and in your own life?

- **Entry points.** In Chapter 11, "Traveling the Edge of Possibility," the authors talk about "entry points." Discuss the difference between an "issue" and an "entry point." What are some entry points in your own life? Each participant might want to choose one of the groups in the Entry Points section, page 315, to explore and report back on its work.

BIBLIOGRAPHY

Michael Ableman, *On Good Land: The Autobiography of an Urban Farm* (San Francisco, California: Chronicle Books, 1998).

Sarah Anderson, John Cavanagh, Thea Lee, and Institute for Policy Studies, *Field Guide to the Global Economy* (New York: The New Press. Distributed by W. W. Norton, 2000).

Alan AtKisson, *Believing Cassandra: An Optimist Looks at a Pessimist's World* (White River Junction, Vermont: Chelsea Green, 1999).

Robert M. Axelrod, *The Evolution of Cooperation* (New York: Basic Books, 1984).

Ben H. Bagdikian, *The Media Monopoly* (Boston, Massachusetts: Beacon Press, 1997).

Kevin Bales, *Disposable People: New Slavery in the Global Economy* (Berkeley, California: University of California Press, 1999).

Benjamin R. Barber, *Jihad vs. McWorld* (New York: Ballantine Books, 1996).

Neal Barnard, *Eat Right, Live Longer: Using the Natural Power of Food to Age-Proof Your Body* (New York: Crown, 1997).

Richard J. Barnet and John Cavanagh, *Global Dreams: Imperial Corporations and the New World Order* (New York: Simon & Schuster, 1994).

Michael Barratt Brown, *Africa's Choices After Thirty Years of the World Bank* (Boulder, Colorado: Westview Press, 1996).

David Bornstein, *The Price of a Dream: The Story of the Grameen Bank and the Idea that is Helping the Poor to Change their Lives* (New York: Simon & Schuster, 1996).

Douglas H. Boucher, *The Paradox of Plenty: Hunger in a Bountiful World* (Oakland, California: Food First Books, 1999).

John Briggs and F. David Peat, *Seven Life Lessons of Chaos: Timeless Wisdom From the Science of Change* (New York: HarperCollins Publishers, 1999).

Lester Russell Brown and Worldwatch Institute, *State of the World 2000: A Worldwatch Institute Report on Progress Toward a Sustainable Society* (New York: Norton, 2000).

Severyn Bruyn, *A Civil Economy: Transforming the Market in the Twenty-First Century. Evolving Values for a Capitalist World* (Ann Arbor, Michigan: University of Michigan Press, 2000).

Roland Bunch, *Two Ears of Corn* (Oklahoma City, Oklahoma: World Neighbors, 1982).

J. Baird Callicott, *Beyond the Land Ethic: More Essays in Environmental Philosophy* (Albany, New York: State University of New York Press, 1999).

Fritjof Capra, *The Tao of Physics: An Exploration of the Parallels Between Modern Physics and Eastern Mysticism,* 4th ed., updated, 25th anniversary ed. (Boston, Massachusetts: Shambhala. Distributed in the U.S. by Random House, 2000).

Chuck Collins, Felice Yeskel, and United for a Fair Economy, *Economic Apartheid in America: A Primer on Economic Inequality and Insecurity* (New York: The New Press, 2000).

Ann Cooper and Lisa M. Holmes, *Bitter Harvest: A Chef's Perspective on the Hidden Dangers in the Foods We Eat and What You Can Do About It* (New York: Routledge, 2000).

Alex Counts, *Give Us Credit* (New York: Times Books, 1996).

Mihaly Csikszentmihalyi, *The Evolving Self: A Psychology for the Third Millennium* (New York: Harper-Collins Publishers, 1993).

Herman E. Daly, *Beyond Growth: The Economics of Sustainable Development* (Boston, Massachusetts: Beacon Press, 1996).

Jared M. Diamond, *Guns, Germs, and Steel: The Fates of Human Societies* (New York: W. W. Norton, 1997).

Ami Domini, *Socially Responsible Investing: Making a Difference and Making Money* (Chicago, Illinois: Dearborn Trade, 2001).

Mark Dowie, *American Foundations: An Investigative History* (Cambridge, Massachusetts: MIT Press, 2000).

Joel Dyer, *Harvest of Rage: Why Oklahoma City is Only the Beginning* (Boulder, Colorado: Westview Press, 1997).

Paul R. Ehrlich, *Human Natures: Genes, Cultures, and the Human Prospect* (Washington, D.C.: Island Press, 2000).

———, *The Population Bomb* (New York: Ballantine Books, 1968).

Cliff Feigenbaum, Hall Brill, and Jack Brill, *Investing with Your Values: Making Money and Making a Difference* (Princeton: Bloomberg Press, 1999).

Michael W. Fox, *Beyond Evolution: The Genetically Altered Future of Plants, Animals, the Earth—Humans* (New York: Lyons Press, 1999).

Richard W. Franke and Barbara H. Chasin, *Kerala: Radical Reform As Development in an Indian State* (San Francisco, California: The Institute for Food and Development Policy, 1991).

Paulo Freire, *Pedagogy of the Oppressed,* New rev. 20th-Anniversary ed. (New York: Continuum, 1993).

Thomas L. Friedman, *The Lexus and the Olive Tree* (New York: Farrar Straus Giroux, 2000).

Jeffrey R. Gates, *Democracy at Risk: Rescuing Main Street from Wall Street: A Populist Vision for the 21st Century* (New York: Perseus Books, 2000).

Susan George, *The Lugano Report: On Preserving Capitalism in the Twenty-First Century* (Sterling, Virginia: Pluto Press, 1999).

Malcolm Gladwell, *The Tipping Point: How Little Things Can Make a Big Difference* (Boston, Massachusetts: Little, Brown and Co., 2000).

Trauger Groh and Steven McFadden, *Farms of Tomorrow Revisited: Community Supported Farms, Farm Supported Communities* (Kimberton, Pennsylvania: Biodynamic Farming and Gardening Association, 1997).

Joan Dye Gussow, *Chicken Little, Tomato Sauce, and Agriculture: Who Will Produce Tomorrow's Food?* (New York: Bootstrap Press, 1991).

Betsy Hartmann and James K. Boyce, *A Quiet Violence: View From a Bangladesh Village, Third World Studies* (San Francisco, California: Zed Press. Institute for Food and Development Policy, 1983).

Paul Hawken, *The Ecology of Commerce: A Declaration of Sustainability* (New York: HarperBusiness, 1993).

Dee Hock and VISA International, *Birth of the Chaordic Age* (San Francisco, California: Berrett-Koehler Publishers, 1999).

Jane Jacobs, *The Nature of Economies* (New York: Modern Library, 2000).

Derrick Jensen, *Listening to the Land: Conversations About Nature, Culture, and Eros* (San Francisco, California: Sierra Club Books, 1995).

Kevin Kelly, *New Rules for the New Economy: 10 Radical Strategies for a Connected World* (New York: Viking, 1998).

Brewster Kneen, *Farmageddon: Food and the Culture of Biotechnology* (Gabriola Island, British Columbia, Canada: New Society Publishers, 1999).

Frances Moore Lappé, *Diet for a Small Planet,* 20th anniversary ed. (New York: Ballantine Books, 1991).

———, *Rediscovering America's Values* (New York: Ballantine Books, 1989).

Frances Moore Lappé and Joseph Collins, with Cary Fowler, *Food First: Beyond the Myth of Scarcity* (Boston, Massachusetts: Houghton-Mifflin, 1977).

Frances Moore Lappé, Joseph Collins, and David Kinley, *Aid as Obstacle: Twenty Questions about our Foreign Aid and the Hungry* (San Francisco, California: Institute for Food and Development Policy, 1980).

Frances Moore Lappé and Rachel Shurman, *Taking Population Seriously* (London: Earthscan, 1989).

Frances Moore Lappé and Paul Martin Du Bois, *The Quickening of America: Rebuilding Our Nation, Remaking Our Lives* (San Francisco, California: Jossey-Bass Publishers, 1994).

Frances Moore Lappé, Joe Collins, and Peter Rosset, *World Hunger: Twelve Myths,* Second Edition (New York: Grove Press, 1998).

Marc Lappé, *Breakout: The Evolving Threat of Drug-Resistant Disease* (San Francisco, California: Sierra Club Books, 1995).

———, *Germs that Won't Die: Medical Consequences of the Misuse of Antibiotics* (Garden City, New Jersey: Anchor Press/Doubleday, 1982).

Marc Lappé and Britt Bailey, *Against the Grain: The Genetic Transformation of Global Agriculture* (London: Earthscan, 1999).

James B. Lieber, *Rats in the Grain: The Dirty Tricks and Trials of Archer Daniels Midland* (New York: Four Walls Eight Windows, 2000).

Steve Lerner, *Eco-Pioneers: Practical Visionaries Solving Today's Environmental Problems* (Cambridge, Massachusetts: MIT Press, 1997).

Howard Lyman and Glen Merzer, *Mad Cowboy: Plain Truth From the Cattle Rancher Who Won't Eat Meat* (New York: Scribner, 1998).

Jerry Mander and Edward Goldsmith, *The Case Against the Global Economy and for a Turn Toward the Local* (San Francisco, California: Sierra Club Books, 1996).

Bill McKibben, *Hope, Human and Wild True Stories of Living Lightly on the Earth* (Boston, Massachusetts: Little, Brown and Co., 1995).

Anuradha Mittal and Peter Rosset, *America Needs Human Rights* (Oakland, California: Food First Books, 1999).

John Nichols and Robert Waterman McChesney, *It's the Media, Stupid,* Open Media Pamphlet Series, 17 (New York: Seven Stories Press, 2000).

Karl Polanyi, *The Great Transformation* (Boston, Massachusetts: Beacon Press, 1971).

Sheldon Rampton and John C. Stauber, *Mad Cow U.S.A. Could the Nightmare Happen Here?* (Monroe, Maine: Common Courage Press, 1997).

David Richard and Dorie Byers, *Taste Life! The Organic Choice* (Bloomingdale: Vital Health Publishing, 1998).

Matt Ridley, *The Origins of Virtue: Human Instincts and the Evolution of Cooperation,* 1st American ed. (New York: Viking, 1997).

Jeremy Rifkin, *Beyond Beef: The Rise and Fall of the Cattle Culture* (New York: Dutton, 1992).

Jeremy Rifkin, *The End of Work: The Decline of the Global Labor Force and the Dawn of the Post-Market Era* (New York: Tarcher/Putnam, 1995).

Ocean Robbins and Sol Solomon, *Choices for Our Future: A Generation Rising for Life on Earth* (Summertown, Tennessee: Book Pub, 1994).

Dani Rodrik, *Has Globalization Gone Too Far?* (Washington, D.C.: Institute for International Economics, 1997).

E. F. Schumacher, *Small Is Beautiful: Economics As If People Mattered* (New York: Harper & Row, 1973).

Barry Schwartz, *The Battle for Human Nature: Science, Morality, and Modern Life* (New York: Norton, 1986).

Amartya Kumar Sen, *Development As Freedom* (New York: Knopf, 1999).

Vandana Shiva, *Biopiracy: The Plunder of Nature and Knowledge* (Boston, Massachusetts: South End Press, 1997).

————, *Monocultures of the Mind: Perspectives on Biodiversity and Biotechnology* (Atlantic Highlands, New Jersey: Third World Network, 1993).

————, *Staying Alive: Women, Ecology, and Development* (London: Zed Books, 1988).

————, *Stolen Harvest: The Hijacking of the Global Food Supply* (Cambridge, Massachusetts: South End Press, 2000).

————, *The Violence of the Green Revolution: Third World Agriculture, Ecology, and Politics* (Atlantic Highlands, New Jersey: Zed Books, 1991).

Vandana Shiva, Afsar H. Jafri, Shalini Bhutani, and Research Foundation for Science, Technology, and Ecology, *Campaign Against Biopiracy* (New Delhi: Research Foundation for Science Technology and Ecology, 1999).

Thomas E. Skidmore, *Brazil: Five Centuries of Change* (New York: Oxford University Press, 1999).

Vaclav Smil, *Enriching the Earth: Fritz Haber, Carl Bosch, and the Transformation of World Food Production* (Cambridge, Massachusetts: MIT Press, 2001).

————, *Feeding the World: A Challenge for the Twenty-First Century* (Cambridge, Massachusetts: MIT Press, 2000).

Adam Smith, *The Theory of Moral Sentiments* (London: A. Millar, 1759).

J. W. Smith, *The World's Wasted Wealth 2: Save Our Wealth, Save Our Environment* (Cambria, California: Institute for Economic Democracy, 1994).

Lori Wallach and Michelle Sforza, *The WTO: Five Years of Reasons to Resist Corporate Globalization* (New York: Seven Stories Press, 2000).

Edward Osborne Wilson, *In Search of Nature* (Washington, D.C.: Island Press, 1996).

James Q. Wilson, *The Moral Sense* (New York: Maxwell Macmillan International, 1993).

Robert Wright, *The Moral Animal: The New Science of Evolutionary Psychology* (New York: Pantheon Books, 1994).

Muhammad Yunus, *Grameen Bank, As I See It* (Dhaka, Bangladesh: The Bank, 1994).

————, *Jorimon of Beltoil Village and Others: Faces of Poverty* (Dhaka, Bangladesh: University Press, 1987).

Muhammad Yunus and Alan Jolis, *Banker to the Poor: Micro-Lending and the Battle Against World Poverty* (New York: PublicAffairs, 1999).

Stone Zander and Benjamin Zander, *The Art of Possibility* (Cambridge, Massachusetts: Harvard Business School Press, 2000).

ENDNOTES

THE BEGINNING

PROLOGUE: PUSHING THE EDGE OF HOPE

1 Gary Gardner and Brian Halweil, "Overfed and Underfed: The Global Epidemic of Malnutrition," WorldWatch Institute, WorldWatch Paper 150, March 2000, 34, 35, 43. See also Ellen Ruppel Shell, "The World Food Syndrome," *The Atlantic Monthly,* June 2001.

2 Data from United for a Fair Economy, see www.ufenet.org. United for a Fair Economy, 37 Temple Place, 2nd Floor, Boston, Massachusetts, 02111, (617) 423-2148. See, in particular, Chuck Collins and Felice Yeskel, *Economic Apartheid in America: A Primer on Economic Inequality and Security* (New York: The New Press, 2000).

3 *The Economist,* June 23, 2001, 13.

CHAPTER I: MAPS OF THE MIND

1 Based on UN Food and Agriculture Organization and UN Development Programme statistics.

2 Estimates of the percent of world grain fed to livestock vary, from a low of one-third. We are relying here on Vaclav Smil, author of *Feeding the World.* After considerable research, he arrives at 45 percent but cautions that it is impossible to know precisely. The amount of grain to livestock could be as low as 40 or as high as 47 percent, he told us. Some other estimates are lower still. When I wrote the original *Diet for a Small Planet,* the estimate was one third.

3 Dr. David Pimentel, Cornell University, author correspondence.

4 Estimates range from 2,000 to 12,000 gallons per pound of beef. See, for example, David Pimentel, Laura Westra, and Reed Noss, editors, *Ecological Integrity: Integrating Environment, Conservation and Health* (Washington, D.C.: Island Press, 2001).

5 David Pimentel, et al., "Will Limits of the Earth's Resources Control Human Numbers?" *Environment, Development and Sustainability,* 1: 19–39, 1999, 23.

6 David Pimentel and Celia Harvey, "Ecological Effects of Erosion," in *Ecosystems of Disturbed Ground,* L. R. Walker, ed. (Amsterdam: Elsevier, 1999), 123, citing M. Simons, "Winds Toss Africa's Soil, Feeding Lands Far Away," *The New York Times,* October 29, 1992, A1, A16.

7 Ibid., 125, citing *World Resources 1994–1995,* World Resource Institute, Washington, D.C., 400.

8 Paul Hawken, Amory and Hunter Lovins, *Natural Capitalism* (Boston, Massachusetts: Little, Brown and Co., 1999), 14. Quoting Robert U. Ayres, "Industrial Metabolism," in Jesse Ausubel and Hedy E. Sladovich, eds., *Technology and Environment,* (Washington, D.C.: National Academy Press, 1989), 25–26.

9 See International Service for the Acquisition of Agri-biotech Applications (ISAAA) for country-by-country listings of transgenic crops planted and an annual report on the planting of genetically modified crops worldwide, www.isaaa.org. See also WorldWatch Institute, *Vital Signs 2001: The Trends That Are Shaping Our Future* (New York: Norton, 2001) 102.

10 Ben Bagdikian, *The Media Monopoly,* Sixth Edition (Boston, Massachusetts: Beacon Press, 2000), xviii.

11 Data from the United Nations Children's Fund, 1999.

12 Carol Kaesuk Yoon, "Study Jolts Views on Recovery from Extinctions," *The New York Times*, March 9, 2000, A20, study by Dr. James W. Kirchner at the University of California–Berkeley and Dr. Anne Weil, a paleontologist at Duke University.

13 Quoted in a report by The Center for a Livable Future, Leo Horrigan, Robert Lawrence, and Polly Walker, "Our Food, Our Health: How Sustainable Agriculture Can Address the Environmental and Human Health Harms of Industrial Agriculture," (Baltimore, Maryland: Johns Hopkins University, December, 2000), 9. To order a copy of the report, contact: The Center for a Livable Future, Johns Hopkins University, 613 North Wolfe Street, #8503, Baltimore, Maryland, 21205, phone: 410-502-7578, or email: clf@jhsph.edu.

14 Chuck Collins and Felice Yeskel, *Economic Apartheid in America: A Primer on Economic Inequality and Security* (Boston, Massachusetts: The New Press, 2000).

15 D. O. Hebb, "Science and the World of Imagination," *Canadian Psychology* 16 (1975), 4–11, quoted by Rosamund Stone Zander and Benjamin Zander, *The Art of Possibility*, (Cambridge, Massachusetts: Harvard Business School Press, 2000), 11.

16 Ibid. *The Art of Possibility*.

17 Erich Fromm, *The Anatomy of Human Destructiveness* (New York: Holt, Rinehart and Winston, 1973), 149.

18 Naylor, R. L., J. Goldberg, J. H. Primavera, N. Kautsky, M. C. M. Beveridge, J.Clay, C. Folke, J. Lubchenco, H. Mooney, and M. Troell, 2000. "Effect of aquaculture on world fish supplies," *Nature* 405:1017–1024. See also: D. Pauly, V. Christensen, J. Dalsgaard, R. Froese, and F. C. Torres, Jr., 1998. "Fishing down marine food webs." *Science* 279: 860–863.

19 U.S. Senate Committee on Agriculture, Nutrition and Forestry, "Animal Waste in America: An Emerging National Problem." Compiled for Senator Tom Harkin, December 1997.

20 WorldWatch Institute, *Vital Signs 2001: The Trends That Are Shaping Our Future*, (New York: Norton, 2001), 101.

21 Pat Roy Mooney, "The ETC Century, Erosion, Technological Transformation and Corporate Concentration in the 21st Century," *Development Dialogue*, Dag Hammarskjold Foundation and the Rural Advancement Foundation International, 1999, published January 2001, 9–10.

22 Howard Lyman, *Mad Cowboy* (New York: Scribner, 1998). See also www.eatwild.com.

23 Union of Concerned Scientists, "70 Percent of All Antibiotics Given to Healthy Livestock," January 8, 2001. To read more from the Union of Concerned Scientists, visit www.ucsusa.org.

24 "Stop Using Antibiotics for Livestock, AMA Says," *USA Today*, June 25, 2001, 9B.

25 Francis Bowen and Phillips Bradley, ed., *Democracy in America* (New York: Alfred A. Knopf, 1960), 1 and 246.

26 Maude Barlow, "Water Privatization and the Threat to the World's Most Precious Resource: Is Water a Commodity or a Human Right?" *IFG (International Forum on Globalization) Bulletin*, Summer 2001, 7.

27 Jane E. Brody, "A World of Food Choices, and a World of Infectious Organisms," *The New York Times*, January 30, 2000.

28 Joby Warrick, "Modern Meat: Buyer Beware, An Outbreak Waiting to Happen, Beef-Inspection Failures Let In a Deadly Microbe," *The Washington Post*, April 9, 2001, A1. Estimate of .01 percent from Felicia Nestor and Menonah Hauter, Government Accountability Project and Public Citizen, Washington, D.C., September 2000. The Government Accountability Project report "Jungle 2000" can be viewed online at www.citizen.org.

29 Sheldon Rampton and John Stauber, *Trust Us, We're Experts!* (New York: Tarcher/Putnam, 2001), 166–169. See also www.foxrBGHsuit.com.

30 Andrew Pollack, "Green Revolution Yields to Bottom Line as Crop Research Goes Private," *The New York Times*, May 15, 2001, D2. The professor cited is Dr. Rod A. Wing of Clemson University.

31 Rampton and Stauber, *Trust Us, We're Experts!*, 165.

32 Ibid., Chapter 7.

33 David Pimentel, T. W. Culliney, and T. Bashore, "Public Health Risks Associated with Pesticides and Natural Toxins in Foods," in E. B. Radcliffe and W. D. Hutchison, eds., *Radcliffe's IPM World Textbook* (St. Paul, Minnesota: University of Minnesota, last revision, September 2000). Available online at http://ipmworld.umn.edu.

34 David Pimentel, Professor of Entomology, Cornell University, author communication.

35 Thomas L. Friedman, *The Lexus and the Olive Tree* (New York: Farrar, Straus, Giroux, 1999), 86.

THE JOURNEY

CHAPTER 2: THE DELICIOUS REVOLUTION

1 "The Delicious Revolution," keynote speech to the Environmental Grantmakers Association 1999, Pacific Grove, California.

2 Gary Gardner and Brian Halweil, "Overfed and Underfed: the Global Epidemic of Malnutrition," WorldWatch Institute, WorldWatch Paper 150, March 2000, 15.

3 Eric Schlosser, "Fast Food Nation: The True Cost of the American Diet," *Rolling Stone,* Issue 794, September 3, 1998. See also Eric Schlosser, *Fast Food Nation: The Dark Truth Behind the All-American Meal* (Boston, Massachusetts: Houghton Mifflin Company, 2001).

4 John Robbins, *The Food Revolution* (Berkeley, California: Conari Press, 2001).

5 Gary Gardner and Brian Halweil, "Escaping Hunger, Escaping Excess," WorldWatch, July–August 2000, 26, 29, 33.

6 Brian Halweil, "The United States Leads World Meat Stampede," WorldWatch Issues Paper, July 2, 1998.

7 Beef exports from U.S. Department of Agriculture. In 1970 the U.S. exported 40 million pounds of carcass-weight beef. Major markets were Canada, Bahamas, Jamaica, and Japan. By 1999 the U.S. export market had expanded to 2.417 billion pounds of beef. Major markets were Japan, Mexico, Korea, and Canada.

8 Brian Halweil, "The United States Leads World Meat Stampede," WorldWatch Issues Paper, July 2, 1998.

9 Judy Putnam, Linda Scott Cantor, Jane Allshouse, "Per Capita Food Supply Trends: Progress Toward Dietary Guidelines," *Food Review,* Vol. 23, No. 3.

10 John Robbins, *The Food Revolution* (Berkeley, California: Conari Press, 2001), see especially Chapter Three: Joyrides on the Great American Diet Roller-Coaster. Robbins notes that Dr. Richard Leakey concluded that our early ancestors, Cro-Magnons, who some have claimed to be big meat eaters, were likely to have only rarely eaten meat, just like our closest genetic relative, the chimpanzee.

11 Centers for Disease Control Behavioral Risk Factor Surveillance System (BRFSS) at www.cdc.gov. See also National Health and Nutrition Examination Survey (most recent 1999–2000), "Overweight Among U.S. Children and Adolescents," from the National Center for Health Statistics, Centers for Disease Control.

12 WorldWatch Institute, *Vital Signs 2001: The Trends That Are Shaping Our Future* (New York: Norton, 2001). See "Being Overweight Now Epidemic," 136–137.

13 J. E. Manson, M. J. Stampfer, C. H. Hennekens, and W. C. Willet, "Body weight and longevity. A reassessment," *JAMA,* 1987, 257:353–58. N. D. Barnard, A. Nicholson, J. L. Howard "The medical costs attributable to meat consumption." *Preventive Medicine,* 1995, 24:646–55.

14 David B. Allison, Kevin R. Fontaine, JoAnn E. Manson, June Stevens, and Theodore B. VanItallie, "Annual Deaths Attributable to Obesity in the United States," *JAMA,* 1999, 282:1530–1538. See also other articles in the same *Journal of the American Medical Association* (*JAMA*) October 17, 1999 issue: "The Spread of the Obesity Epidemic in the United States, 1991–1998" Ali H. Mokdad, Mary K. Serdula, William H. Dietz, Barbara A. Bowman, James S. Marks, and Jeffrey P. Koplan, 282:1519–1522; and "The Disease Burden Associated With Overweight and Obesity,"

Aviva Must, Jennifer Spadano, Eugenie H. Coakley, Alison E. Field, Graham Colditz, William H. Dietz, *JAMA*, 1999, 282:1523–1529;

15 Data from the International Diabetes Foundation.

16 American Diabetes Association, "Economic Consequences of Diabetes Mellitus in the U.S. in 1997," *Diabetes Care*, Vol. 21, No. 2, 296.

17 WorldWatch Institute, *Vital Signs 2001: The Trends That Are Shaping Our Future* (New York: Norton, 2001). See "Being Overweight Now Epidemic," 137, quoting Graham Colditz, "The Economic Costs of Obesity and Inactivity," Harvard School of Public Health, Cambridge, Massachusetts, unpublished manuscript, undated.

18 Virginia Messina and Mark Messina, *The Dietician's Guide to Vegetarian Diets: Issues and Applications* (Gaithersburg, Maryland: Aspen Publishers, 1996), 58, cited in John Robbins, *The Food Revolution*.

19 Ibid., 20, cited in John Robbins, *The Food Revolution*.

20 National Research Council. *Diet, Nutrition, and Cancer* (Washington, D.C.: National Research Council, 1982).

21 See, for example, Walter C. Willett, MD, DrPH, "Goals for Nutrition in the Year 2000," *CA Journal: A Cancer Journal for Clinicians.* 1999, 49:331–352. In the abstract, Dr. Willett states: "Quantitative estimates of the proportion of preventable cancers in Western countries remain at approximately 30 to 40 percent." See also Willett, P. J. Skerett, and Edward L. Giovannucci, *Eat, Drink, and Be Healthy: The Harvard Medical School Guide to Healthy Eating* (New York: Simon and Schuster, 2001). See also the international report on diet and cancer prevention, commissioned by the American Institute for Cancer Research and the World Cancer Research Fund: *Food, Nutrition and the Prevention of Cancer: A Global Perspective* (Washington, D.C.: American Institute for Cancer Research, 2000). The American Institute for Cancer Research's toll-free hotline (U.S. and Canada only) is (800) 843 8114.

22 Dr. Anne E. Becker, Assistant Professor of Medical Anthropology, Department of Social Medicine, Harvard Medical School, author communication. For further background on body image and eating-disorder trends internationally, see Dr. Becker's book, *Body, Self, and Society: The View from Fiji* (Philadelphia: University of Pennsylvania Press, 1995).

23 From Deborah Tamannie, A Garden in Every School Project Director, California State Department of Education. To find out more about school gardens, or to find a school garden project near you, visit the A Garden in Every School registry online at www.kidsgardening.com/School/register.asp.

24 Public Health Institute, "2000 California High School Fast Food Survey," from the Public Health Institute, Sacramento, California, p. ii. http://www.phi.org.

25 Marion Nestle, "Soft Drink 'Pouring Rights': Marketing Empty Calories," *Public Health Reports 2000*; 115:308–319.

26 WorldWatch Institute, *Vital Signs 2001: The Trends That Are Shaping Our Future* (New York: Norton, 2001), 19.

27 Eric Schlosser, *Fast Food Nation: The Dark Truth Behind the All-American Meal* (Boston, Massachusetts: Houghton Mifflin Company, 2001), 243.

28 California Endowment, "A Special Report on Policy Implications from the 1999 California Children's Healthy Eating and Exercise Practices Survey." To see a copy of the report visit www.calendow.org.

29 For a complete account of commercialism in schools, see Alex Molnar, "What's in a Name? The Corporate Branding of America's Schools," *The Fifth Annual Report on Trends in Schoolhouse Commercialism Year 2001–2002*, Commercialism in Education Research Unit (CERU), College of Education, Arizona State University, September 2002. http://edpolicylab.org.

30 Vincent Schiraldi, Jason Ziedenberg, and John Irwin, "America's One Million Nonviolent Prisoners," (Washington, D.C.: The Center for Juvenile and Criminal Justice, 1996).

31 Margaret Andrews, Mark Nord, Gary Bickel, and Steven Carlson, "Household Food Security in the United States 1999," Food and Rural Economics Division, Economic Research Service, U.S. Department of Agriculture, *Food Assistance and Nutrition Research Report*, No. 8, Fall 2000.

32 From the California Department of Corrections, quoted by Fox Butterfield, "Often, Parole Is One Stop on the Way Back to Prison," *The New York Times*, November 22, 2000, A1.

33 Jason Ziedenburg and Vincent Shiraldi, "The Punishing Decade: Prison and Jail Estimates at the Millennium," Justice Policy Institute Report, (Washington, D.C.: The Center for Criminal and Juvenile Justice, May 2000).

34 Robert B. Gunnison, "1998 Prison Guards Win 12% Pay Increase," *San Francisco Chronicle*, August 26, 1998.

35 The State of America's Children Yearbook 2000, Children's Defense Fund, for information see www.childrensdefensefund.org.

36 Greg Critser, "Let Them Eat Fat," *Harper's Magazine*, March 2000, 42.

37 David S. Ludwig et al. "High Glycemic Index Foods, Overeating, and Obesity," *Pediatrics*, Vol. 103, No. 3, March 1999. The authors note possible advantages for treating obesity with a diet with abundant quantities of vegetables, legumes, and fruits. See also David S. Ludwig, Karen E. Peterson, and Steven L. Gortmaker, "Relationship Between Consumption of Sugar-sweetened Drinks and Childhood Obesity: a Prospective, Observational Analysis." *The Lancet*, February 17, 2001. See also Michael F. Jacobson, "Liquid Candy: How Soft Drinks are Harming Americans' Health," Center for Science in the Public Interest, October 21, 1998.

38 N. D. Barnard, A. R. Scialli, P. Bertron, D. Hurlock, K. Edmonds, L. Talev, "Effectiveness of a low-fat, vegetarian diet in altering serum lipids in healthy premenopausal women." *American Journal of Cardiology*, 2000; 85:969–72.

39 See, for example, Marion Nestle et al., "Behavioral and Social Influences on Food Choice," *Nutrition Reviews*, May 1998; B. J. Rolls and E. A. Bell, "Intake of Fat and Carbohydrate: Role of Energy Density," *European Journal of Clinical Nutrition*, April 1999; J. E. Blundell and J. I. MacDiarmid, "Fat as a Risk Factor for Overconsumption: Satiation, Satiety, and Patterns of Eating," *Journal of American Dietetic Association*, July 1997, cited in "Overfed and Underfed," 22. See also, Paul Ehrlich, *Human Natures: Genes, Cultures, and the Human Prospect* (Washington, D.C.: Island Press, 2000).

40 Alice Waters, 16th Annual Ecological Farming Conference, Asilomar, California, 1996.

CHAPTER 3: THE BATTLE FOR HUMAN NATURE

1 Global Justice Center, the Pastoral Land Commission, and the Landless Workers' Movement, "Agrarian Reform and Rural Violence," *Annual Report, Human Rights in Brazil 2000*. See also, National Report on the Situation of Human Rights and Agrarian Reform in Brazil, United Nations High Commissioner for Human Rights, May 17, 2000. For more information visit SEJUP (Servico Brasilero de Justica e Paz) online at www.oneworld.org/sejup.

2 Michael A. Serrill, "Of Land and Death: A shocking encounter between police and squatters forces the pace of land reform in Brazil," *Time International*, Volume 147, No. 19, May 6, 1996.

3 Official estimates from Instituto Nacional de Colonizaçãoe Reforma Agrária, the government land-reform agency based on data from the 1995 Brazilian Census.

4 Thomas E. Skidmore, *Brazil: Five Centuries of Change* (New York: Oxford University Press, 1999), 155–157.

5 MST, Summary of Current Projects, www.mstbrazil.org, viewed on October 11, 2000.

6 Lonely Planet, *Brazil* (Oakland, California: Lonely Planet Publications, 1998), 51.

7 Michael A. Serrill, "Of Land and Death: A shocking encounter between police and squatters forces the pace of land reform in Brazil," *Time International*, Volume 147, No. 19, May 6, 1996.

8 Freedom House, *Freedom in the World 1999–2000 Country Reports: Brazil*. For more information see www.freedomhouse.org.

9 Jack Epstein, "For Brazil's Glamour Set, It's the Crusade of Choice," *Time Magazine: Latin America*, January 18, 1998, Vol. 151, No. 2. See also: Wendy Wolford, "Grassroots-Initiated Land Reform in Brazil: The Rural Landless Workers' Movement," in *The Changing Role of the State in*

Latin American Land Reform, paper presented at WIDER-FAO workshop, Santiago, Chile, April 27–29, 1998.)

10 Quoted by Alma Guillermoprieto in *The Heart that Bleeds: Latin America Now* (New York: Vintage, 1995), 293.

11 Based on the 1996 Brazilian Land Atlas, 62 percent of Brazilian land is unproductive. In 1985, 44 percent of total arable land in Brazil was unproductive; among the 46 largest land holdings, only 17 percent of land was being used. From Wendy Wolford, "Grassroots-Initiated Land Reform in Brazil: The Rural Landless Workers' Movement," in *The Changing Role of the State in Latin American Land Reform,* paper presented at WIDER-FAO workshop, Santiago, Chile, April 27–29, 1998.

12 From *Jornal da Manhã,* from Ponta Grossa, *News From Brazil,* April, 19, 1999, supplied by SEJUP (Servico Brasileiro de Justica e Paz).

13 From MST, "Slaughter of Landless Workers in Curitiba-Paraná," May 2, 2000. See, for example, www.mstbrazil.org.

14 From reports by the Pastoral Land Commission, an organization created by the Catholic Church in the late 1980s to monitor land questions.

15 Bill McKibben, *Hope, Human and Wild* (New York: Little, Brown and Co., 1995).

16 See for example, Peter Rosset, "On the Benefits of Small Farms," Food First Backgrounder, Vol. 6, No. 4, Winter 1999, quoting FAO report on MST settlements. The national average income for formerly landless settled is about 3.7 times the Brazilian minimum wage. The average for a landless person is seven-tenths the minimum wage.

17 "Harvesting farming's potential," *The Economist* (September 9, 2000), 36.

18 James B. Twitchell, "In Praise of Consumerism: When the going gets tough, the tough go shopping. And sometimes even get happy," *Reason Magazine,* August-September, 2000.

CHAPTER 4: BEAUTIFUL HORIZON

1 Between 1994 and 1998 the average income of farmers in Brazil fell by 49 percent. See the National Report on the Situation of Human Rights and Agrarian Reform in Brazil, United Nations High Commissioner for Human Rights, May 17, 2000.

2 Cecilia Rocha, "An Integrated Program for Urban Food Security: The Case of Belo Horizonte, Brazil," Unpublished Paper, Department of Economics, Ryerson Polytechnic University, Toronto, Ontario, April 2000, 9.

CHAPTER 5: THE HYACINTH PRINCIPLE

1 See Garrett Hardin, "Lifeboat Ethics: The Case Against Helping the Poor," *Psychology Today,* September 1974.

2 Data from the United Nations Children's Fund.

3 Muhammad Yunus, *Banker to the Poor* (New York: PublicAffairs, 1999). See also David Bornstein, *The Price of a Dream* (New York: Simon & Schuster, 1996), 106.

4 Barry Bearak, "Women Are Defaced by Acid and Bengali Society Is Torn," *The New York Times,* June 24, 2000, A1.

5 Steve Minkin, M. Mokhlesur Rahman, and Mahmudur Rahman, Chapter 5, "Fish Biodiversity, Human Nutrition and Environmental Restoration in Bangladesh," *Openwater Fisheries of Bangladesh,* Chu-Fa Tsai and M. Youssouf Ali, eds., Bangladesh Center for Advanced Studies (India: Vedams Books, 1997).

6 Seventy-five percent of microcredit borrowers are women and 14 million of these borrowers live on less than a dollar a day. Alex Counts author correspondence. See also www.microcredit summit.org.

7 Chuck Collins and Felice Yeskel, *Economic Apartheid in America: A Primer on Economic Inequality and Security* (New York: The New Press, 2000).

CHAPTER 6: SEEKING ANNAPOORNA

1 Frances Moore Lappé, Joseph Collins, and Peter Rossett, with Luis Esparza, *World Hunger: Twelve Myths,* second edition, (Grove Press: New York, 1998). See, in particular, Chapter 5: The Green Revolution Is the Answer.

2 Vandana Shiva, *Stolen Harvest,* (Cambridge, Massachusetts: South End Press, 2000), 11–12.

3 Dr. Charles Benbrook, "Troubled Times Amid Commercial Success for Roundup Ready Soybeans: Glyphosate Efficacy is Slipping and Unstable Transgene Expression Erodes Plant Defenses and Yields," AgBio Tech InfoNet Technical Paper Number 4, May 3, 2001, (Sandpoint, Idaho: Northwest Science and Environmental Policy Center). Dr. Benbrook is a former executive director of the Board on Agriculture, National Academy of Sciences.

4 *Human Development Report 2000,* United Nations Development Program, (New York: UNDP, 2000), 84.

5 See, for example, Vandana Shiva, *The Violence of the Green Revolution: Third World Agriculture, Ecology and Politics* (New York: Zed Books, 1991).

6 See, for example, Brewster Kneen, *Farmageddon: Food and the Culture of Biotechnology* (Gabriola Island, Canada: New Society Publishers, 1999).

7 See World Food Prize, www.worldfoodprize.org.

8 W. R. Grace was ranked as the 26th largest chemical corporation in the world by Fortune 1,000 in the year 2000. For more about W. R. Grace, visit their website at www.grace.com.

9 For more information about neem and its uses, see the website of the Research Foundation for Science, Technology, and Ecology at www.vshiva.net.

10 Neem tree oil case: European Patent No. 0436257 revoked, Munich, May 10, 2000. For more information, see www.european-patent-office.org.

11 Initiators in the U.S. include the Foundation on Economic Trends and the National Family Farm Coalition, both in Washington, D.C. For more information, contact the Foundation on Economic Trends, 1660 L Street, NW, Suite 216, Washington, D.C. 20036, phone (202) 466-2823.

12 Research Foundation for Science, Technology, and Ecology, "Neem Patent (No. 0436257) Revoked by EPO: A Report," (New Delhi: Research Foundation for Science, Technology, and Ecology, 2000). Also see Michela Wrong, "Challenge to patent over neem tree oil fungicide," *Financial Times,* May 10, 2000, 13.

13 Hope Shand, "Legal and Technological Measures to Prevent Farmers from Saving Seed and Breeding Their Own Plant Varieties," in J. Janick ed., *Perspectives on New Crops and New Uses* (Alexandria, Virginia: ASHS Press, 1999). See especially pages 124–126. For more information on corporate concentration in the seed industry, see Action Group on Erosion, Technology and Concentration, www.ETCgroup.org.

14 WorldWatch Institute, *Vital Signs 2001: The Trends That Are Shaping Our Future* (New York: Norton, 2001). See especially, "Growth in Transgenic Area Slows," 103.

15 See the ETC Group at www.etcgroup.org.

16 Vandana Shiva, *Biopiracy: The Plunder of Nature and Knowledge* (Boston, Massachusetts: South End Press, 1997). See also ETC Group at www.etcgroup.org.

17 *Business Line,* "RiceTec withdraws crucial claims on basmati patent," September 27, 2000.

18 Erin Moriarty, "Coca-Cola: Growing sales mean India is it," *American City Business Journals Inc.,* March 13, 2000.

19 Gary Gardner and Brian Halweil, "Overfed and Underfed: The Global Epidemic of Malnutrition," WorldWatch Institute, WorldWatch Paper 150, March 2000, 42.

20 Professor M. S. Swaminathan, UNESCO-Cousteau Chair in Ecotechnology and Chairman of the M. S. Swaminathan Research Foundation, India, author correspondence.

21 *Species Extinctions: Causes and Consequences,* 1992. World Resources Institute, 10 G Street, NE (Suite 800), Washington, D.C. 20002 (202/729-7600; fax: 202/729-7610). For more information, contact lauralee@wri.org

22 Roland Bunch, "An Odyssey of discovery: principles of agriculture for the humid tropics," *ILEIA Newsletter* Vol. 11, No. 3, October 1995.

23 U.S. Patent No. 5,723,765, awarded March 3, 1998, "Control of Gene Expression." For more information see U.S. Department of Agriculture Research Service, "The Control of Plant Gene Function," visit, www.ars.usda.gov/misc/fact.htm.

24 *The Statesman,* "Excessive Fear of Genetics Hurts Indian Farmers," January 11, 1999, published on Monsanto Indian website, www.monsantoindia.com. See also Jennifer Thomson, "Poor Nations Can't Afford Debate on Gene-Altered Crops," *Christian Science Monitor,* November 13, 2000.

25 Mark Dowie quoting Lowell Hardin, Ford Foundation agriculture program director, at a speech in 1971 to American farmers and agronomists. Hardin told his audience: "A truly widespread green revolution [was] a promise, not a reality . . . The green revolution is exerting a destabilizing influence on traditional social and political institutions . . . Increased output is not necessarily associated with positive social change." See Mark Dowie, *American Foundations: An Investigative History* (Cambridge, Massachusetts: MIT Press, 2000), 114.

26 Vandana Shiva, *The Violence of the Green Revolution: Third World Agriculture, Ecology and Politics* (New York: Zed Books, 1991).

27 Afsar H. Jafri, "Navdanya's Seeds of Hope Programme in Bhatinda Punjab," Research Foundation for Science, Technology, and Ecology, New Delhi, 2000.

28 Madhu Gurung, *Female Foeticide,* 1999. c/o Colonel (Retired) R. B. Gurung, P. Ranjhawala, O. Raipur, Dehra Dun. U.P., India. Report can be viewed at Harvard University's Global Reproductive Health Forum South Asia Site: www.hsph.harvard.edu/grhf/SAsia/forums/foeticide/articles/foeticide.html.

29 Lester Brown, WorldWatch Institute, *State of the World 2000,* (New York: Norton, 2000).

30 Gary Gardner and Brian Halweil, "Overfed and Underfed: The Global Epidemic of Malnutrition," WorldWatch Institute, WorldWatch Paper 150, March 2000, 12. "FAO estimates that 21 percent of India's population is chronically hungry . . . but on-the-ground surveys suggest that 49 percent of adults and 53 percent of children in India are underweight." See also "The Crisis of Malnutrition in India," World Bank Reports, November 18, 1999.

CHAPTER 7: WALKING TO NAIROBI

1 World Bank, *World Development Report 2000–2001.* Survey year 1994.

2 Freedom House, *Freedom in the World 1999–2000 Country Reports: Kenya.* For more information about human rights in Kenya, see www.freedomhouse.org.

3 National Research Council, Board on Science and Technology and International Development, *Lost Crops of Africa Volume 1: Grains* (Washington, D.C.: National Academy Press, 1996).

4 Frances Moore Lappé, Joe Collins, and Peter Rosset, *World Hunger: Twelve Myths,* Second Edition (New York: Grove Press, 1998), 12, quoting Gunilla Andrae and Bjorn Beckman, *The Wheat Trap: Bread and Underdevelopment in Nigeria* (London: Zed Books, 1985).

5 Bane Onimode quoted in Michael Barratt Brown, *Africa's Choices After Thirty Years of the World Bank* (Boulder, Colorado: Westview Press, 1996), 139.

6 Frances Moore Lappé and Joe Collins with Cary Fowler, *Food First: Beyond the Myth of Scarcity* (New York: Ballantine Books, 1979).

7 From Paul Rice, Executive Director, TransFair USA, author correspondence.

8 G. van Roozendaal, "Kenyan Cut Flower Export Blooming," *Biotechnology and Development Monitor,* No. 20, 1994, 6–7.

9 National Research Council, *Lost Crops of Africa Volume 1: Grains,* Board on Science and Technology and International Development (Washington, D.C.: National Academy Press, 1996), xiii.

10 Data from the World Health Organization.

11 Sarah Anderson and John Cavanagh with Thea Lee, *Field Guide to the Global Economy* (New York: The New Press, 2000). According to Jubilee 2000, $2.5 trillion is owed in aid if developing countries are included, based on World Bank definition, which would include countries such as Pakistan, China, India, and Brazil.

12 Data from Jubilee 2000. In 1998, the latest figures posted, sub-Saharan Africa paid $1.41 to creditors for every $1.00 received in grants, up from $1.36 in 1997 and $1.38 in 1996.

13 *World Development Report 2000–2001,* World Bank.

14 For more information about structural adjustment and the poor, see Giovanni Andrea Cornia, Richard Jolly, and Frances Stewart, eds., *Adjustment with a Human Face* (Oxford: Clarendon Press, 1988); Lance Taylor and Ute Pieper, *Reconciling Economic Reform and Sustainable Human Development: Social Consequences of Neo-Liberalism,* Office of Development Studies, Discussion Paper Series (New York: U.N. Development Programme, 1996). See also, Michael Barratt Brown, *Africa's Choices After Thirty Years of the World Bank* (Boulder, Colorado: Westview Press, 1996) especially p. 98.

15 Frances Moore Lappé, Joe Collins, and Peter Rosset, *World Hunger: Twelve Myths,* Second Edition (New York: Grove Press, 1998). See especially, Chapter 1: There's Simply Not Enough Food.

CHAPTER 8: STIRRING THE SLEEPING GIANT

1 For more information contact FLO International, Kaiser-Friedrich-Strasse 13, 53113 Bonn, Germany, or visit their site online at www.fairtrade.net.

2 Geert De Lombaerde, "Starbucks aims to grind up P&G's market share," *BizJournals,* June 13, 1997. Also, Max Havelaar Foundation, www.maxhavelaar.nl/english.

3 Research from Robert A. Rice and Justin R. Ward, "Coffee, Conservation, and Commerce in the Western Hemisphere," Smithsonian Migratory Bird Center and the Natural Resources Defense Council, June 1996.

4 WorldWatch Institute, *Vital Signs 2001: The Trends That Are Shaping Our Future* (New York: Norton, 2001). See "Global Coffee Production Hits New High," 36–38.

5 Ibid.

6 From Committee of the North American Bird Conservation Initiative. For more information online go to www.bsc-eoc.org/nabci.html. See also the Northwest Shade Coffee Campaign, www.seattleaudobon.org.

7 The U.S. Department of Agriculture estimates, on average, 889,000 farmworkers are working any given week based on 1995–1997 studies. Others, such as the Migrant Health Program Atlas, estimate 4.1 million farmworkers.

8 For more information, see U.S. General Accounting Office, "Hired Farmworkers: Health and Well-Being at Risk," Washington, D.C.: U.S. General Accounting Office, 1992; GAO/HRD-092-46, 3. See also Lee Tucker, "Fingers to the Bone: United States Failure to Protect Child Farmworkers" (New York: Human Rights Watch, June 2000); online at www.hrw.org.

9 From Patricia Reagan and Jodi Brookins-Fisher (Eds.), *Community Health in the 21st Century* (San Francisco: Benjamin Cummings, 2002), 313. Other life expectancy figures from the World Development Indicators 2000–2001.

10 United Farmworkers White Paper, "Five Cents for Fairness: The Case for Change in the Strawberry Fields," The Strawberry Workers Campaign, November 1996. See also Tracy L. Barnett, "Fresh Campaign," *Santa Cruz Sentinel,* May 19, 1996.

11 Edward Alden, "America Wakes up to the Smell of Fair Trade Coffee," *Financial Times,* October 4, 2000.

CHAPTER 9: THE LAST TASTE OF PARIS

1 To learn more about Pellworm, visit www.pellworm.de.

2 For more information about alternatives to national accounting measures like the Gross National Product, contact Redefining Progress, www.redefiningprogress.org. See also *Calvert-Henderson Quality of Life Indicators,* The Calvert Group, Washington, D.C., 1999.

3 Frances Moore Lappé and Joseph Collins with Cary Fowler, *Food First: Beyond the Myth of Scarcity* (Boston: Houghton-Mifflin, 1977). See also Frances Moore Lappé, Joseph Collins, and David

Kinley, *Aid as Obstacle: Twenty Questions About our Foreign Aid and the Hungry* (San Francisco: Institute for Food and Development Policy, 1980).

4 Rik Langendoen, "Milk Imports Threaten Indian Diary Farmers," *Yes!*, Winter, 2001.

5 Otto Doering, "The Impact of Modern Agricultural Technologies: Economies Usefulness in the Debate about Future Directions for Agriculture," *Globalization and the Rural Environment*, in Otto T. Solbrig et al., eds., *Globalization and the Rural Environment* (Cambridge: Harvard University Press, 2001), 305–307. For more information on nitrates, see Vaclav Smil, *Enriching the Earth: Fritz Haber, Carl Bosch, and the Transformation of World Food Production* (Cambridge, Massachusetts: MIT Press, 2001). Additional research from Dr. David Keeney, researcher with the Institute of Agriculture and Trade Policy, www.iatp.org.

6 Vaclav Smil, *Enriching the Earth* (Cambridge, Massachusetts: MIT Press, 2001), 186.

7 A recent report from the Leopold Center for Sustainable Agriculture analyzed USDA produce-arrival data in Chicago and found that the average food had traveled 1,245 miles in 1981; by 1998 that distance had climbed to 1,518 miles. For more information, see Rich Pirog, Timothy Van Pelt, Kamyar Enshayan, and Ellen Cook, "Food, Fuel, and Freeways: An Iowa Perspective on How Far Food Travels, Fuel Usage, and Greenhouse Gas Emissions," Ames, Iowa: Iowa State University. See also Brian Halweil, "Homegrown: The Case for Local Food in the Global Market," Worldwatch 2002.

8 Based on totals of all advertising for food and beverages in the U.S. From *Advertising Age*, 1999.

9 U.S. Department of Agriculture, Economic Research Service.

10 David C. Korten, *The Post-Corporate World: Life After Capitalism* (San Francisco: Kumarian Press, 1999), 165.

11 Mary Hendrickson, William Heffernan, Philip Howard, and Judith Heffernan, "Consolidation in Food Retailing and Dairy: Implications for Farmers and Consumers in a Global Food System," Department of Rural Sociology, University of Missouri, January 8, 2001, for a report commissioned by the National Farmers Union, 3.

12 John Robbins, *The Food Revolution* (Berkeley, California: Conari Press, 2001).

13 Francesco di Castri, "Rural Values and the European View of Agriculture," in *Globalization and the Rural Environment*, in Otto T. Solbrig et al., eds., *Globalization and the Rural Environment* (Cambridge: Harvard University Press, 2001), 502.

14 Max J. Pfeffer, et al., "Forging New Connections between Agriculture and the City," in *Globalization and the Rural Environment*, in Otto T. Solbrig et al., eds., *Globalization and the Rural Environment* (Cambridge: Harvard University Press, 2001), 435.

15 European figures from article by Pierre-Yves Guiheneuf with the Forum-Synergies network. Subsidy levels in the U.S. from Clark Williams-Derry and Ken Cook, "Green Acres: How Taxpayers are Subsidizing the Demise of the Family Farm," April 2000, Environmental Working Group. To see this report and other EWG publications visit www.ewg.org.

16 Leo Horrigan, Robert S. Lawrence, and Polly Walker, "Our Food: Our Health: How Sustainable Agriculture Can Address the Environmental and Human Health Harms of Industrial Agriculture," Center for a Livable Future, Johns Hopkins University, submitted for publication, 2001. For more information see the Humane Society of the United States, www.hsus.org.

17 See International Service for the Acquisition of Agri-biotech Applications (ISAAA) for country-by-country listings of transgenic crops planted and an annual analysis of genetically modified crops worldwide, www.isaaa.org.

18 For more on this approach, see, for example, Joel Tickner and Lee Ketelsen, "Precaution: Who Decides? Why Democratic Methods of Decision-Making are Critical to Implementing the Precautionary Principle," *Loka Alert* 8:3, April 20, 2001. For more information, contact the Loka Institute, P.O. Box 355, Amherst, Massachusetts 01004-0355, phone (413) 559 5860 or online at www.loka.org.

19 Miguel A. Altieri and Clara Ines Nicholls, "Ecological Impacts of Modern Agriculture in the United States and Latin America," in Otto T. Solbrig et. al., eds. *Globalization and the Rural Environment* (Cambridge, Massachusetts: Harvard University Press, 2001), 134.

20 Ibid., 131–132.

21 To learn more about the campaign to label GMOs in the U.S., visit: www.truefoodnow.org. See also TomPaine.com report on the labeling decisions.

22 From "The Revolving Door," a report from the Edmonds Institute, a non-profit, public interest organization dedicated to education about environment, technology, and intellectual property rights, 20319 92nd Avenue West, Edmonds, Washington 98020, phone (425) 775 5383. Report is available online at www.edmonds-institute.org/olddoor.html. See also Jennifer Ferrar, "Revolving Doors: Monsanto and the Regulators," *The Ecologist,* September/October 1998.

23 Kristine Kieswer, "PCRM Wins USDA Lawsuit," *Physicians Committee for Responsible Medicine Magazine,* Winter 2001, Volume X, Number 1, www.pcrm.org.

24 *United Nations Development Report 1998,* United Nations Development Program, overview.

25 Sarah Anderson and John Cavanagh with Thea Lee, *Field Guide to the Global Economy* (New York: The New Press, 2000), 67.

26 United Nations, 1997, speech by John Langmore, Department of Economic and Social Affairs.

27 Alexander Stille, "Thinkers on the Left Get a Hearing Everywhere but at Home; Europeans, Wary of Globalization, Embrace American Economists Who Heed Social Needs," *The New York Times,* November 11, 2000, B7.

28 U.S. Department of Agriculture, Economic Research Service, Ronald A. Gustafson, author correspondence.

29 For more information on the debate about the WTO, see Public Citizen Global Trade Watch, www.citizen.org/trade. See also World Trade Organization Agreement on Agriculture, especially Article 4 and Article 5, see also Annex 5. The Agreement on Agriculture is available online at www.wto.org.

30 Opinion of the Scientific Committee on Veterinary Measures Relating to Public Health, "Assessment of Potential Risks to Human Health from Hormone Residues in Bovine Meat and Meat Products," European Commission, Directorate General, April 30, 1999. To view the full report, visit europa.eu.int/comm/food/fs/sc/scv/out21_en.pdf (viewed January 2001).

31 Export figures from the U.S. Department of Agriculture, Economic Research Service, Ronald A. Gustafson, author correspondence.

32 Lori Wallach and Michelle Sforza, *The WTO: Five Years of Reasons to Resist Corporate Globalization* (New York: Seven Stories Press, 1999). For more information, see Public Citizen's Global Trade Watch, www.tradewatch.org.

33 Graham Dunkley, *The Free Trade Adventure: The WTO, the Uruguay Round and Globalism, a Critique* (New York: Zed Books, 2000), 217.

34 Sandra Blakeslee, "Stringent Steps Taken by U.S. on Cow Illness," *The New York Times,* January 14, 2001.

35 *The New York Times,* "Fear of Diseased Beef Deepens in France's Supermarket Aisles," November 15, 2000, A1. For more about mad cow disease in the U.S. see Sheldon Rampton and John Stauber, *Mad Cow USA: Could the Nightmare Happen Here?* (Monroe, Maine: Common Courage Press, 1997).

36 For more information about organics in Europe and France, visit www.organic-europe.net.

37 Timothy Egan, "'Perfect' Apple Pushed Growers into Debt," *The New York Times,* November 4, 2000, A1 and A8.

38 To read more about France's Week of the Taste, visit www.legout.com.

CHAPTER 10: TAKING OFF THE COWBOY HAT

1 Eric Schlosser, *Fast Food Nation: The Dark Truth Behind the All-American Meal* (Boston, Massachusetts: Houghton Mifflin Company, 2001), 5.

2 To learn more about antibiotics resistance see for example, Marc Lappé, *Breakout: The Evolving Threat of Drug-Resistant Disease,* (Sierra Club Books: San Francisco, 1995). See also, MT Osterhol, "Emerging Infections—another warning," *New England Journal of Medicine* 2000: 342: 1290–1281.

3 See for example, "Time to Act," report from the National Commission on Small Farms (Washington, D.C., 1998). See also, Willis L. Peterson, "Are Large Farms More Efficient?" Staff Paper Series, Department of Applied Economics, College of Agricultural, Food and Environmental Sciences, University of Minnesota, St. Paul, Minnesota, January 1997. The report can be viewed online at www.reeusda.gov/agsys/smallfarm/report.htm.

4 Clark Williams-Derry and Ken Cook, "Green Acres: How Taxpayers are Subsidizing the Demise of the Family Farm," April 2000, Environmental Working Group. To see this report and other EWG publications visit www.ewg.org.

5 Elizabeth Henderson with Robyn Van En, *Sharing the Harvest: A Guide to Community-Support Agriculture* (Chelsea Green Publishing Company: April 2000), xvi. This book is an excellent resource for farmers interested in starting a CSA and for consumers interested in supporting one.

6 CSA estimate based on most recent figures available from U.S. Department of Agriculture Alternative Farming Systems Information Center. For more information about CSAs and to see a state-by-state listing, visit www.nal.usda.gov/afsic/csa.

7 Jennifer Bauduy, "The End of Family Farms? Big Farmers Are Getting Fat on Uncle Sam's Dough as Old Family Farms Die Out," May 5, 2001. www.tompaine.com. Average small farm income from U.S. Department of Agriculture.

8 Miguel A. Altieri and Clara Ines Nicholls, "Ecological Impacts of Modern Agriculture in the United States and Latin America," Otto T. Solbrig, Robert Paarlberg, and Francesco di Castri, eds., *Globalization and the Rural Environment,* Harvard University Press, 2001, 128. To find out about New York City–area CSAs, contact Just Foods at Just Food, 307 7th Avenue, Suite 1201, New York, NY, 10001; (212) 645 9880, www.justfood.org; info@justfood.org.

9 See discussion in Ann Cooper and Lisa M. Holmes, *Bitter Harvest: A Chef's Perspective on the Hidden Dangers in the Foods We Eat and What You Can Do About It* (New York: Routledge, 2000), especially Chapter 5: We Are What We Eat. See also U.S. Department of Agriculture food composition tables available online at www.usda.org.

10 For many helpful peer-reviewed citations compiled by Jo Robinson for her book, *Why Grassfed Is Best!* (Vashon, Washington: Vashon Island Press, 2000), see: www.eatwild.com.

11 N. D. Barnard, A. R. Scialli, P. Bertron, D. Hurlock, K. Edmonds, L. Talev. "Effectiveness of a low-fat, vegetarian diet in altering serum lipids in healthy premenopausal women." *American Journal of Cardiology,* 2000; 85:969–72.

12 Brian Halweil, "The United States Leads World Meat Stampede," WorldWatch Issues Paper, July 2, 1998.

13 From the National Beef Cattlemen's Association, www.beef.org.

14 For more information, contact Kim Cates, coordinator of the Great Lakes Grazing Network, www.glgn.org, a project of the Wisconsin Rural Development Center. See also Program on Agricultural Technology Studies, University of Wisconsin, Madison, www.wisc.edu/pats.

15 Charlie LeDuff, "At a Slaughterhouse, Some Things Never Die: Who Kills, Who Cuts, Who Bosses Can Depend on Race," *The New York Times,* June 16, 2000, A1.

16 Joby Warrick, "They Die Piece by Piece: In Overtaxed Plants, Humane Treatment of Cattle Is Often a Battle Lost," *Washington Post,* April 10, 2001, A01.

17 Felicia Nestor and Wenonah Hauter, *The Jungle 2000,* (Washington, D.C.: Global Accountability Project and Public Citizen, 2000).

18 Joseph Weber, "Will Agribusiness Plow Under the Family Farm?" *Business Week,* October 23, 2000.

19 Professor Jim Gerrish, Forage Systems Research Center, University of Missouri, author correspondence.

20 Trauger Groh and Steven McFadden, *Farms of Tomorrow Revisited: Community Supported Farms, Farm Supported Communities* (Kimberton, Pennsylvania: Biodynamic Farming and Gardening Association, 1997), 60.

21 From Farm and Land in Farms final estimates 1993–1997, U.S. Department of Agriculture National Agricultural Statistics Service quoted by Farm Aid from www.farmaid.org.

22 Agriculture Outlook, May 2000, Economic Research Service, U.S. Department of Agriculture.

23   Ted Schettler, Gina Solomon, Maria Valenti, and Annette Huddle, *Generations at Risk: Reproductive Health and the Environment* (Cambridge, Massachusetts: MIT Press, 1999), 107.

24   Dr. David Pimentel, author correspondence. See also David Pimentel et al., "Environmental and Economic Impacts of Reducing U.S. Agricultural Pesticide Use," *Handbook of Pest Management in Agriculture,* Vol. 1, 679–718. (Boca Raton, Florida: CRC Press, 1991), also printed in Pimentel and Lehmen, eds., *The Pesticide Question: Environment, Economics and Ethics* (Chapman Hall, 1993), 223–278.

25   Steve Gorelick, "Facing the Farm Crisis," *The Ecologist,* October 24, 2000. See also Joel Dyer, *Harvest of Rage: Why Oklahoma City is Only the Beginning* (Boulder, Colorado: Westview Press, 1997). Dyer's book is an investigative look at the impact of the loss of family farms on rural communities.

26   Jules Pretty and Rachel Hine "Reducing Food Poverty with Sustainable Agriculture," Centre for Environment and Society, University of Essex, UK, February 2001. See also www.i-sis.org.

27   Todd Hettenbach and Richard Wiles, "A Few Bad Apples . . . Pesticides in Your Produce, Why Supermarkets Should 'Test and Tell'" (Washington, D.C.: Environmental Working Group, April, 2000). For more information, contact EWG, 1718 Connecticut Avenue, N.W., Suite 600, Washington, D.C. 20009, or online at www.ewg.org.

28   John P. Reganold, Jerry D. Glover, Preston K. Andrews, and Herbert R. Hinman, "Sustainability of three apple production systems," *Nature,* 410, 926–930, April 19, 2001.

29   E. Koohan Paik, "Homogenized Planet," WorldWatch, Vol. 14, No. 2, March/April 2001, 25.

30   Richard Burroughs was the FDA veterinarian fired. He filed a lawsuit against the Department of Health and Human Services and won on appeal in February 1990. Court: Washington Regional Office, U.S. Merit Systems Protection Board. See "Hear No Evil," in *Eating Well,* July–August, 1991, 41–47.

31   A good source for information about rBGH, genetically modified foods, and related issues is the Organic Consumers Association, 6101 Cliff Estate Road, Little Marais, Minnesota, 55614. See also www.purefood.org and www.organicconsumers.org. See also, Sheldon Rampton and John Stauber, *Trust Us, We're Experts! How Industry Manipulates Science and Gambles With Your Future* (New York: Tarcher/Putnam, 2001).

32   Rampton and Stauber, Ibid., 168.

33   Ronnie Cummins, author correspondence. See also Ronnie Cummins, *Genetically Engineered Food: A Self-Defense Guide for Consumers* (New York: Marlowe & Co., 2000).

34   See www.foxrBGHsuit.com. Here you can view the original documentary by Jane Akre and Steve Wilson.

35   E. Giovannucci, E. B. Rimm, A. Wolk, A. Ascherio, M. J. Stampfer, G. A. Colditz, W. C. Willett, "Calcium and fructose intake in relation to risk of prostate cancer," *Cancer Research,* 1998a, 58:442–7. This is from the Health Professionals Follow-Up Study, a cohort of U.S. male dentists, optometrists, osteopaths, pharmacists, and veterinarians.   Relative risk of advanced prostate cancer associated with daily consumption of more than two glasses of milk was increased by about 60%, compared to those who drank no milk. Of the milk consumed, 83% was skim or low-fat. See also: J. M. Chan, M. J. Stampfer, U. Ajani, J. M. Gaziano, E. Giovannucci, "Dairy products, calcium, and prostate cancer risk in the Physicians' Health Study." Presentation, American Association for Cancer Research, San Francisco, April 2000. This is the Physicians' Health Study cohort, which found that consumption of two-and-a-half dairy servings daily was associated with increased risk of prostate cancer, compared to having less than one half serving daily, after adjustment for age, smoking, exercise level, and body mass index (BMI).

36   Paul Hawken, Amory and Hunter Lovins, *Natural Capitalism* (Boston, Massachusetts: Little, Brown and Co., 1999), 71.

37   There are fourteen Living Machines® constructed in the United States and a total of twenty-two in the world. For more information about Living Machines®, Inc., www.livingmachines.com.

38   Miguel Altieri, "Multifunctional dimensions of ecologically based agriculture in Latin America," *International Journal of Sustainable Development and World Ecology,* 7 (2000), 62.

39 Edward O. Wilson, *In Search of Nature* (Washington, D.C.: Island Press, 1996).

40 Mary Hendrickson, William Heffernan, Philip Howard, Judith Heffernan, "Consolidation in Food Retailing and Dairy: Implications for Farmers and Consumers in a Global Food System," Department of Rural Sociology, University of Missouri, January 8, 2001, report for National Farmers Union. The report can be viewed online on the National Farmers Union site, www.nfu.org.

41 From U.S. Department of Agriculture Economic Research Service, quoted by Farm Aid, www.farmaid.org.

42 To learn more about Organic Valley, visit www.organicvalley.com.

43 There are 150,000 community gardens across the U.S. and Canada. Although the number of new gardens is increasing, the number of gardens plowed under for development is, too. To learn more about community gardens, visit American Community Garden Association's website: www.communitygarden.org.

44 From the Organic Consumer Association, www.organicconsumers.org.

45 For more information, or listings of farmers' markets near you, see the National Farmers' Market Directory and the U.S. Department of Agriculture website www.ams.usda.gov/farmersmarkets/facts.htm.

46 For more information, contact Just Food in New York City, www.justfood.org.

THE HOMECOMING

CHAPTER II: TRAVELING THE EDGE OF POSSIBILITY

1 Condensed from a letter by William Blake written in verse to the Reverend Dr. Trusler on August 23, 1799, reprinted in *Resurgence Magazine*.

2 Erich Fromm, *The Anatomy of Human Destructiveness* (New York: Holt, Rinehard and Winston, 1973), 260.

3 Jon Christensen, "Golden Rice in a Grenade-Proof Greenhouse," *The New York Times,* November 21, 2000, D1, 5.

4 From the Nutrition Foundation of India, see also www.nutritionfoundationofindia.org.

5 "Demons in Disguise?" *The Telegraph* (Calcutta), November 13, 2000.

6 Vaclav Smil, *Feeding the World: A Challenge for the Twenty-First Century* (Cambridge, Massachusetts: MIT Press, 2000), 237, using U.N. Food and Agriculture Organization 1999 data, 236–237.

7 Ibid., 237.

8 D. Ornish, L. W. Scherwitz, J. H. Billings, S. E. Brown, K. L. Gould, T. A. Merritt, S. Sparler, W. T. Armstrong, T. A. Ports, R. L. Kirkeeide, C. Hogeboom, R. J. Brand. "Intensive Lifestyle Changes for Reversal of Coronary Heart Disease," *JAMA,* 1998; 280:2001–7.

9 Smil, *Feeding the World,* 237.

10 Dr. David Pimentel, Cornell University, author correspondence.

11 Smil, *Feeding the World,* 195.

12 WorldWatch Institute, *Vital Signs 2001: The Trends That Are Shaping Our Future,* (New York: Norton, 2001). See "Commodity Prices Weak," 122.

13 Amartya Sen, *Development as Freedom* (New York: Knopf, 1999), 207–209.

14 Michael Pragnell, CEO Syngenta, interviewed by Clancy Gebler Davies in *The Independent,* UK, April 11, 2001. He added: "If agriculture went organic again, we would suffer a tremendous lack of food."

15 To learn more, write to Ecology Action, 5798 Ridgewood Road, Willits, California 95490-9730, or visit www.growbiointensive.org.

16 Minor Sinclair, "From Big to Small, Toxic to Green, New Strategies to Grow Food in Cuba," *Latin America DRCLAS NEWS,* David Rockefeller Center for Latin American Studies, Harvard University, Spring/Summer 2001.

17 Richard Manning, *Food's Frontier: The Next Green Revolution* (New York: North Point Press, 2000), 16–17.

18 Nicholas Wade, "Tree of Life Turns Out to Have Complex Roots," *The New York Times,* April 14, 1998.

19 Kevin Kelly, *New Rules for the New Economy: 10 Radical Strategies for a Connected World* (New York: Viking, 1998).

20 William Ury, *Getting to Peace* (New York: Viking, 1999), 102–3 (later released as *The Third Side*).

21 Ibid., 106.

22 Ibid., 107.

23 Ibid., 107.

24 *World Bank Development Report,* World Bank, 1999.

25 Paul Ehrlich, *Human Natures: Genes, Cultures and the Human Prospect,* (Washington, D.C.: Island Press, 1999).

26 Erich Fromm, *The Anatomy of Human Destructiveness* (Henry Holt, New York: 1973), 264.

27 Adam Smith, *The Theory of Moral Sentiments,* 1790, D. D. Raphael and A. L. Macfie (Indianapolis: Liberty Classics, 1982. Part 1, section 1, chapter 1, 9.

28 Charles Darwin, *Descent of Man and Selection in Relation to Sex,* Vol. 1, (London: John Murray, 1871), Chapter III, 96–97.

29 William Ury, *Getting to Peace* (New York: Viking, 1999), 40 (later released as *The Third Side)*

30 Frances Moore Lappé and Paul Martin Dubois, *The Quickening of America* (San Francisco: Jossey-Bass Publishers, 1994).

31 Thomas L. Friedman, *The Lexus and the Olive Tree* (New York: Farrar, Straus, Giroux, 1999), 269–273.

32 For an excellent historical overview, see Karl Polanyi, *The Great Transformation* (Boston, Massachusetts: Beacon Press, 1944).

33 Henry Fountain, "Now the Ancient Ways Are Less Mysterious," *The New York Times,* January 20, 1999, Week in Review, 5.

34 See, for example, Fritjof Capra, *The Web of Life: A New Scientific Understanding of Living Systems* (New York: Anchor/Doubleday, 1996).

35 Friedman, *The Lexus and the Olive Tree,* 273.

36 David C. Korten, *The Post-Corporate World: Life After Capitalism* (San Francisco: Kumarian Press, 2000). See especially Chapter 2.

37 Thomas A. Lyson and Annalisa Lewis Raymer, "Stalking the Wily Multinational: Power and Control in the U.S. Food System," *Agriculture and Human Values,* 17:199–209.

38 Gary Gardner and Brian Halweil, "Overfed and Underfed: the Global Epidemic of Malnutrition," WorldWatch Institute, WorldWatch Paper 150, March 2000, 29, quoting Advertising Age website, www.adage.com/dataplace, October 1999.

39 Kurt Eichenwald, "Archer Daniel Midland, Fine-Payer to the U.S.," *The New York Times,* October 20, 1996, Section 4, Page 2. To read more about the ADM case see James Lieber, *Rats in the Grain: The Dirty Tricks and Trials of Archer Daniels Midland* (New York: Four Walls Eight Windows, 2000). See also, James Bovard, "Archer Daniels Midland: A Case Study In Corporate Welfare," Cato Policy Analysis, No. 241, September 26, 1995. Department of Justice Press Release, "Archer Daniels Midland Co. To Plead Guilty And Pay $100 Million For Role In Two International Price-Fixing Conspiracies," October 15, 1996.

40 Dwayne Andreas quoted by Dan Carney in "Dwayne's World," *Mother Jones,* January 1995.

41 Peter Rosset, Institute for Food and Development Policy, quoting Food and Agriculture Organization study. Peter Rosset, "On the Benefits of Small Farms," *Food First Backgrounder,* Vol. 6 No. 4, Winter 1999.

42 Robert A. G. Monks, *The New Global Investors* (London: Capstone Publishing, 2001), 93, 134.

43 Cory Rosen, Center for Employee Ownership, for more information, see www.nceo.org.

44 See Cliff Feigenbaum, Hall Brill and Jack Brill, *Investing with Your Values: Making Money and Making a Difference* (New York: Bloomberg Press, 1999) and their website: www.naturalinvesting.com. See also, *Socially Responsible Investing: Making a Difference and Making Money,* Ami Domini and see also www.socialinvest.org.

45 "GM Firms Top of Ethical Investors' Blacklist," *The Scotsman,* August 31, 1999. Citing study by the Ethical Investment Trust.

46 Shorebank, 7054 S. Jeffery, Chicago, IL 60649, phone (773) 288 1000, www.shorebankcorp.com, info@shorebankcorp.com.

47 The Natural Step US, P.O. Box 29372, San Francisco, California 94129-0372, phone: (415) 561 3344, tns@naturalstep.org.

48 Initiators in the U.S. include the Foundation on Economic Trends and the National Family Farm Coalition, both in Washington, D.C.

49 Thomas Friedman, *The Lexus and the Olive Tree* (New York: Farrar, Straus, Giroux, 1999), 273.

50 Abraham H. Maslow, *The Farther Reaches of Human Nature* (New York: The Viking Press, 1971), 199–212. See especially "Synergy in the Society and the Individual."

EPILOGUE

1 Mirian Vilela, Executive Director, Earth Charter Secretariat, Earth Council, P.O. Box 319-6100, San Jose, Costa Rica, www.earthcharter.org.

ACKNOWLEDGMENTS

From Frankie . . . How grateful I am for my dear friends far and wide who gave me the strength for this journey: Hathaway Barry, Sue Bumagin, Derrick Jensen, Bruce Kaiper, Susan Kanaan, Paul Korn, Paul Lacey, Judy and Howard Luttrell, Nancy Moorehead, Jeff Perkins, Linda Pritzker, Dick Rowe, Anna Whyatt, and Mary Walsh. And to my Vermont "family" whose unconditional support buoyed me at every step: Anne Black, Carol and Monroe Whitaker, Sylvie Blanchet, Andrea Diehl, and Mary Ann Carlson.

I'm grateful also to the Department of Urban Studies and Planning and its Center for Reflective Community Practice at the Massachusetts Institute of Technology, especially professors Ceasar Mc-Dowell, Bishwapriya Sanyal, and Larry Suskind, for providing just the environment I needed for this undertaking.

From Anna . . . A tremendous number of people have been supportive and patient throughout this entire process; to each of them my deep gratitude. I want to thank especially my friends and family who put up with my stress and urgency as I said, "No really, these are the final, final edits!" A special thanks to Lisa Jobson, Christina Kappaz, and Adam Lubinsky who gave their early and smart-as-ever feedback. And a toast to Chris Allieri, Andrea Calise, Jeana Frost, Kate Hallward, Noah Leff, Jake Sherman, Cassandra Stubbs, and Shawna Wakefield for letting me crash on their couches at various points in the journey (in some cases many, many times). Thanks to my dad whose poetry and courage have inspired me to tap my own. And my thanks to Eric for being my biggest fan, for helping me trust myself, *et bien sur,* for breaking the stereo at just the right moment.

From us both . . . First to Anthony Lappé without whom this book would not have been born—for your loving support from its conception to lengthy birth.

Our deepest gratitude goes to all of our translators, both literal and figurative. Traveling to four continents in seven months, we could never have learned what we did without the organizing help and generous time given to us everywhere. This book is filled with the voices of dozens of people who opened their homes and their lives to us. To each of them we're grateful. To the many whose names and stories do not appear directly in this book we are also deeply indebted—and we hope this book pays honor to their lives as well.

A special thanks to Marilyn Borchardt, Peter Rosset, and Anuradha Mittal whose energy sustains the important work of the Institute for Food and Development Policy, better known as Food First.

In California, we thank Alice Waters and her helpful staff at Chez Panisse; Cathrine Sneed, Ron Roth, and Anthony Travis at The Garden Project; Ene Osterraas-Constable, Esther Cook, David Hawkins, Mildred Howard, and Neil Smith at Martin Luther King Jr. Middle School and The Edible Schoolyard; Zenobia Barlow, Janet Brown, and Fritjof Capra of the Center for Ecoliteracy; and Tom

Bates and Jered Lawsen at the Food Systems Project. We're also grateful for the help of Ann Evans who works with Delaine Eastin to spread school gardens statewide. Thanks to them, the San Francisco Bay Area is a national leader in bringing communities together through growing and sharing food.

In Brazil, a special thanks to Vilmar and Dirceu Boufleuer, Geraldo Fontes, João Pedro Stédile, and the members, volunteers, and staff of the Landless Workers' Movement (MST) in Curitiba, São Paulo, as well as in the countryside of Paraná, all of whom are taking risks to create communities that value each of their members. Thanks also to Leonardo Laurio and to guidance from Gianpaolo Baiocchi, Judith Tendler, Wendy Wolford, and others here in the U.S.

In Belo Horizonte, our gratitude to Adriana Aranha and her staff in the city government.

In Bangladesh, thanks to Nurjahan Begum, Fazley Rabbi, Jannat-e-Quinine, Professor Muhammad Yunus, and the dozens of other Grameen staff and members whom we met and who shared with us their stories. Thanks also to Shireen and Nasreen Huq in Dhaka and their work with the pro-women organization Naripokkho. In the U.S., Alex Counts at the Grameen Foundation (helping spread Grameen's philosophy, not just its "grammar") also gave astute advice, as did Jim Boyce, Betsy Hartmann, and Steve Minkin.

In India, our thanks to Vinod Kumar Bhatt, Claire Datta, Afsar Jafri, Darban Singh Negi, Dr. Vandana Shiva and Mira Shiva, and the wonderful staff at the Research Foundation on Science, Technology, and Ecology. Thanks also to translation help from Sumel Singh in the Punjab.

In Kenya, our deepest appreciation to Wangari Maathai, Muta Maathai, and Donald Mumbo who helped us learn about the Green Belt Movement. Thanks to our host family and all of the Green Belt members we met in Kyaume; their dedication, vision, and dancing we'll remember for a lifetime. Thanks also to Sarah Ghiorse and Carter Via for helping to bring the Sokoni Project to life, enabling more Americans to learn from the wisdom of the Green Belt, and to all the Sokoni participants whose good cheer and support were much appreciated.

In the fair trade chapter, thanks to Jonathan Rosenthal and Rosario Castellon from Equal Exchange, Thomas Fricke and Sylvie Blanchet of ForesTrade, Deborah James at Global Exchange, Hans Bolscher at The Max Havelaar Foundation in the Netherlands, Paul Rice at TransFair USA, Scott Exo at The Food Alliance, and Erik Nicholson at Northwest Treeplanters and Farmworkers United. And, of course, to the millions of farmers and consumers who are building a fair-trade movement, bringing dignity to the growing and sharing of food.

In Europe, thanks to Hannes Lorenzen in the European Parliament and to Kees Elgerhuizen. We're grateful to José Bové, René Louail and the Confederation Paysanne, Jean-Yves Griot at the Réseau Agricole Durable, Bruno Rebelle at Greenpeace, and for translation help from Eric Reiffsteck. In Poland, Anna's gratitude to Jadwiga Lopata and her dedication to preserving organic, small farms there; thanks also to all the farmers who welcomed her into their homes.

In Wisconsin, a special thank-you to Jack Kloppenburg and Sharon Lezberg at the University of Wisconsin, who generously arranged our interviews there. Our deepest gratitude to the farmers and nonfarmers who told us their stories and shared with us their work—both those whose names appear in this book and those whose don't.

In *Coming to Our Senses,* our big thank-you to the chefs who shared their creations with us and cheered us on. And to Andrea Diehl for helping us select recipes and artfully test each and every one of them. And to Mollie Katzen, whose encouragement vitalized us from the book's inception and who graciously devoted untold hours to help us make it happen.

Many specialists offered us critical information. Two were particularly tireless in responding to our queries—Dr. Vaclav Smil at the University of Manitoba in Canada and Dr. David Pimentel at Cornell University.

An additional thank you to our fearless readers and editors, including Diana Beliard, Joe Collins, Andrea Diehl, Bruce Kaiper, Susan Kanaan, Paul Lacey, Cory Marshak, Dick Rowe, and Billy Wimsatt.

Heartfelt thanks to our indefatigable agent, Tracy Fisher, and her assistants, Shana Kelly and Tanya Warren, at the William Morris Agency. You helped us find the perfect publisher in Joel Fotinos at Tarcher/Putnam and the perfect editor in Stacy Creamer. More thanks at Penguin Putnam to Allison Sobel and publicist Kelly Groves and his team, who deserve kudos for their tireless and creative efforts.

We are grateful as well to our assistants early in the process, including Michelle Graham, Tom Scanlon, and Heather Upton; to our research interns, Kristna Evans, Karoline Gruelke, Pam Rosen, and Alexis Page. Our special thanks to Hannah Burton, whose positive spirit helped make the initial *Hope's Edge* publicity tour a joy and who has superbly abetted all our efforts to spread the word. We're grateful also to Jane Rohman, who provides top-notch publicity savvy, always pushing us to stretch.

Our gratitude also to Marcia Gallo and the Funding Exchange for their encouragement, guidance, and spirit in support of the Small Planet Fund.

Finally, thanks to the oasis where we finished our book, to our fellow "refugees" (especially Andrew Boyd, who kept us laughing and "easing our consciousness" until the very end), and to Peter Barnes for bringing the Mesa Refuge to life.

INDEX

Please note: For an index of recipes from *Coming to Our Senses*, see pages 406–9

ABOUT THE AUTHORS

FRANCES MOORE LAPPÉ wrote the 1971 three-million-copy bestseller *Diet for a Small Planet*—a classic that's still opening readers' eyes to the power of their own choices. While writing *Hope's Edge,* Lappé, author of twelve other books, was a visiting scholar at the Massachusetts Institute of Technology. She is the co-founder of two national organizations—the California-based Institute for Food and Development Policy (known as Food First) and the Center for Living Democracy, a ten-year initiative to accelerate the spread of democratic innovation. Her books have been used in a broad array of university courses in more than fifty countries. Her life and work have been featured in *People Magazine, The Boston Globe Magazine, The Utne Reader, Vegetarian Times,* and many other publications. Lappé's articles have appeared in publications as diverse as *The New York Times, Los Angeles Times, Readers' Digest, Christian Century, Chemistry, Le Monde Diplomatique, National Civic Review, Tikkun,* and *Harper's.* Lappé has received sixteen honorary doctorates and in 1987 became the fourth American to receive the Right Livelihood Award, sometimes called the Alternative Nobel.

ANNA LAPPÉ is a writer, nonprofit consultant, and public speaker. Anna has guest lectured at Allegheny College, Boston University, Brown University, New York University, University of Connecticut, and many other institutions. Her writing has appeared in *The Washington Post, San Francisco Chronicle, Globe and Mail,* and *Los Angeles Times,* and she is a regular contributor to Guerrilla News Network (www.GNN.tv). She holds a Master's degree from Columbia University's School of International and Public Affairs. In 2002 she was named the first recipient of the Bioneers Youth Award, given annually to honor effective and innovative social and environmental activists. At 29, she has traveled to more than twenty countries and has lived and worked in South Africa, England, and France. She lives in Brooklyn, New York, where she belongs to her local community-supported agriculture farm and has finally learned what to do with kohlrabi.

FRANCES MOORE LAPPÉ & ANNA LAPPÉ co-founded the Small Planet Fund. Separately and together, they lecture widely on food, globalization, and the media. They have appeared on dozens of radio programs across the country, including National Public Radio's nationally syndicated *Weekend Edition* and *The Diane Rehm Show.* Their joint writing has been published in many national and international periodicals.

THE SMALL PLANET FUND

a project of the Funding Exchange

We, Anna and Frances, founded *The Small Planet Fund* (www.smallplanet fund.org) in 2002 to support key movements in *Hope's Edge*. We believe that all of us gain energy and hope by linking with those who are addressing the root causes of hunger. They are showing us—through food, farming, and economic innovations—the possibility of re-embedding economic life in community values so that we can heal our relationship with the earth and ensure that all eat healthfully. In our first year, we raised roughly $50,000, mainly through small donations from readers and through community fundraising events. As The Fund grows, we may expand our giving to similar efforts in the United States and around the world. By contributing, you are connecting directly to the courageous work of trailblazers across our planet who are cutting a path for all of us.

The Fund's Five Principles

❶ Ensure that access to safe, nutritious food is a human right

❷ Evolve capitalism to work for social good as well as private profit

❸ Support growing food in ways that promote a healthy earth and healthy workers and communities

❹ Promote gender equality and the safeguarding of women's rights as essential to ending hunger

❺ Celebrate and protect rural communities, family farmers, and indigenous knowledge

The Funding Exchange (www.fex.org) is the grant-making public foundation that provides the administrative and legal home for the Small Planet Fund. The Funding Exchange is based on a membership of community-based foundations and donor-advised funds across the country dedicated to supporting democratic social change through fundraising for local, national, and international grant making.

To contribute at any level and know you are part of a global upsurge of hope, please return the form on the next page to:

The Small Planet Fund
c/o The Funding Exchange
666 Broadway, Suite 500
New York, NY 10012 USA
Tel: (212) 529-5300 Fax: (212) 982-9272

Name: _____

Address: _____

_____

_____

Country: _____

E-mail: _____

Website (or other information): _____

_____

____ Please send me more information about The Small Planet Fund.

____ Yes, I would like to donate to The Small Planet Fund:

    ____ $5,000 (and up) Founding Member ____$1,000 ____$500

    ____$100 ____$50 ____$35 $_____ (other)

____ I have enclosed a check. Make checks payable to **The Funding Exchange** (with a notation for **The Small Planet Fund**).

____ Please debit my credit card for the amount of $ _____ .

    Credit Card (*Circle one*):   American Express   Visa   MasterCard

    Card #: _____ Exp. Date: _____

    Full name of cardholder: _____

    Signature: _____

Every contribution counts. On behalf of all the groups who benefit from The Small Planet Fund, we thank you for your generosity.

For more information, please visit our website:
www.smallplanetfund.org